CANCER SUPPORTIVE CARE:

A Comprehensive Guide for Patients and Their Families

Ernest H. Rosenbaum, MD
Isadora R. Rosenbaum, MA

Preface by Susan Molloy Hubbard, BS, RN, MPA
Director, International Cancer Information Center
National Cancer Institute, National Institutes of Health

Completely Revised and Updated

A Somerville House Book
Toronto

© 1998 Somerville House Books Limited

Text © Ernest H. Rosenbaum MD, and Isadora R. Rosenbaum, MA

Managing Editor: Ruth Chernia
Interior Design: Falcom Design and Communications Inc./
Sona Communication Services

Artwork: Pp 144 and 153 - Images courtesy of Art for Recovery Breast Cancer Quilt Project, University of California/San Francisco, Mount Zion Medical Center.

Back Cover: Quilt image courtesy of Art for Recovery, University of California/San Francisco, Mount Zion Medical Center. Size: 8' x 8'. Media: pencil, fabric, bead work, appliqué, collage, watercolor, marking pen, buttons, dye, pen, ink and gesso. Created in 1996 by the Art for Recovery Breast Cancer Quilt Project.

Canadian Cataloguing in Publication Data

Rosenbaum, Ernest H.
    Cancer supportive care: a comprehensive guide for patients and their families

Includes index
ISBN 1-894042-11-5

1. Cancer – Popular works.   2. Cancer – Psychological aspects.
I. Rosenbaum, Isadora R.   II. Title.

RC263.R645 1998   616.99'4   C98-931807-9

Published by Somerville House Publishing
a division of Somerville House Books Limited
3080 Yonge Street, Suite 5000
Toronto, Ontario   M4N 3N1
Website: www.sombooks.com
E-mail: sombooks@goodmedia.com

Somerville House acknowledges the financial assistance of the Canada Council, the Ontario Arts Council and the Department of Canadian Heritage.

A note regarding names of drugs:
Throughout this book the brand name is capitalized and the generic name is lower case.

We would like to acknowledge the support of the following pharmaceutical companies:

Bristol-Myers Squibb Oncology

Pharmacia & Upjohn Company

Schering Oncology Biotech

This book is dedicated to

our mother, Dora Rosenbaum, who in spite of medical disabilities returned

to active living, through her own determination and indomitable spirit.

At age 91 she is a teacher and pianist.

And to

Ida Friend, who because of her unshakable valor in facing her illness, and for

her gift of love and kindness, will long be remembered by all who knew her,

and to the

Susan G. Koman Breast Cancer Foundation

for their support of breast cancer patients, research and quality of life.

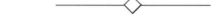

There is destiny that makes us brothers.

None goes his way alone.

All that we send into the lives of others

comes back into our own.

— Edwin Markham

CONTENTS

◇

FOREWORD

Alan Glassberg, MD, Associate Director for Clinical Care,
UCSF/Mount Zion Cancer Center

The Rosenbaums have devoted much of their lives and an enormous amount of their boundless energies to the care, well-being and comfort of cancer patients and their families. Their indefatigable and unending efforts on behalf of their patients are widely recognized and lauded.

This book is a distillation of the Rosenbaums' shared experience gained from years of the constant study, communication and practice of sound and compassionate care for cancer patients. It will give patients and families everywhere an opportunity to benefit from the knowledge and wisdom of these two exceptional caregivers.

This guide will take cancer patients and their families, caregivers and advocates through the myriad of confusing and overlapping paths toward physical and emotional improvement and stability.

Readers will find orderly recommendations based on experience, good sense and science—recommendations designed to help cancer patients to maximize their chances to recover fully, or at least lead lives filled with joy, dignity, serenity and a sense of purpose.

The guide will also be useful to those care providers who have not been exposed to the different and challenging issues involved in helping cancer patients specifically.

A look at the contents reveals the book's comprehensive scope. The authors and contributors understand the heavy emotional toll that cancer has on patients, friends and family, just as they understand the debilitating physical toll it has on patients. They recognize and address the crucial role of a whole array of alternative therapies and complementary social, aesthetic, emotional and physical services in improving a patient's prognosis and quality of life. The authors emphasize the importance of strong personal support from family and friends.

The guide includes medical information about cancer—its causes, diagnosis and standard therapies. There is an exceptionally good chapter describing the elements of an honest and compassionate physician-patient relationship.

Most important, this book acknowledges the huge role that a cancer patient's own determination, positive attitudes and lifestyle and sense of fulfillment can play in his or her rehabilitation, quality of life and, sometimes, full recovery, while acknowledging the extreme anxiety, even terror, that a cancer diagnosis brings to all involved.

Thus the book devotes numerous chapters to topics such as personal coping, nutrition, exercise, sexuality and the concept of one's will to live.

Finally, this book is realistic. It includes a final frank and informative section on life and death issues.

But the bulk of the book is dedicated to living, not dying: to helping cancer patients concentrate on enhancing and cherishing the quality of their lives despite, and sometimes because of, their brush with this frequently life-threatening illness.

To my knowledge, this is the only book that looks so comprehensively at the full spectrum of cancer patients' needs and the medical and other services and supports that are designed to meet those needs.

It has been my personal and professional privilege to be associated with the Rosenbaums and all the other contributors to this guide. They have taught me the expert and compassionate ways to care for patients who encounter challenges every day that most of us fear to ever face.

This book reflects the standards of care that all of us at the UCSF/Mount Zion Cancer Center in San Francisco strive to implement every day with every patient and with their family and friends.

PREFACE

Susan Molloy Hubbard, BS, RN, MPA, Director, International Cancer Information Center, National Cancer Institute, Bethesda, Maryland

When cancer strikes an individual, it strikes the whole family. Fear, turmoil and loss of control are felt by all. The patient and his or her loved ones need a book like this to empower them with information they will need to face the many challenges they may have to deal with during their cancer experience. This book provides a framework for cancer care that focuses on the full spectrum of physical, psychosocial and spiritual needs. Right from the start, it prescribes a team approach of shared decision making. It is chock full of wisdom gleaned from two individuals who have committed their lives to learning about cancer and caring for individuals with a cancer diagnosis. It is an invaluable resource for any family facing the diagnosis of cancer as well as every caregiver trying to provide the best cancer care possible.

Throughout the book there is a series of recurring refrains critical to shared decision making. Work in partnership with your physician and the other members of the health care team that have been assembled to help you. If you do not feel you are being allowed to actively participate in your care, say so. If the situation does not change after you voice your concern, carefully consider other options. Do your own research. Learn how to assess and obtain the care that you need and want—a task that requires articulating your preferences and asking why whenever you don't understand or agree. Share in every medical decision by telling your doctor what you are expecting and asking if your expectations are realistic. Affirm that you want only honest assessments of your options and any side effects that may accompany them—even when this request poses a challenge to your health care team. Discuss the potential adverse effects of any proposed plan of action and inquire about the availability of supportive services that may help you and those you love cope with what you may encounter. While information is not an answer, it is the tool that enables an enlightened patient and family and/or significant other(s) to participate in care in ways that optimize the health care team's ability to prescribe reasonable action.

At issue is responsibility and who has it. The answer is not simple and involves a complex interplay among all members of the health care team if an organized and comprehensive program of care is to be provided for each cancer patient. Again, that is why this book is so valuable. It is a road map that informs cancer patients and their loved ones how to regain an intelligent and measured level of control with active participation of the health care team. Although informed and shared decision making may not always produce a cure, it will ensure that each patient's desires and values are given adequate consideration in the selection of a course of action.

Among the myriad of issues carefully considered by the Rosenbaums are the nature of cancer and its management; the all-important unwritten and contractual relationship between a patient and a physician; and the critical components of a healthy rehabilitation and recovery. Well over half of the book is devoted to mind and body issues that range from the will to live, stress, depression and spirituality to nutrition, therapeutic massage and sexuality. Almost a third of the book is focused on the medical and social support services, the financial aspects of cancer care, dealing with death and bereavement, and coping with a future without a loved one. Having lost my best friend to ovarian cancer last year, I can attest to the importance of these issues and the crying need for greater understanding and emphasis of these critical areas of comprehensive and high-quality cancer care.

However, the beauty of this book is its emphasis on physical, psychological, social and spiritual health in the context of a life-threatening illness that can incapacitate and isolate people who are not taught how to mobilize their own resources. The book is a wellspring of perceptive advice and practical information about personal action, strength, health, hope and recovery—and a font of astute wisdom.

A PATIENT'S POINT OF VIEW

Diane Behar

It has been a great privilege for me to contribute to the second edition of this exceptional book. In addition to my involvement as an editor, I come to this subject from a very personal perspective. Like many of you, I have been diagnosed with cancer. I have been living with this illness—in my case, breast cancer—for close to ten years and am all too familiar with the difficulties and challenges that many of you face each day as you deal with your condition, absorb new information, make decisions about your care and continue to lead productive and meaningful lives. As a long-term survivor, I know that a diagnosis of cancer is not a death sentence. Nor does it have to be a barrier to living a full and active life. Today, half of all cancer patients can be cured, and those of us who cannot be can look forward to leading lives with the same life expectancy as people with other chronic diseases. And besides, tomorrow always brings the hope and promise of a cure.

Learning that I had cancer was an unexpected wake-up call that has changed my world forever. It forced me to take a closer look at my life and to re-evaluate my goals and priorities. It made me aware of the important role of good health care, proper nutrition, exercise and relaxation in strengthening the immune system and prolonging life. Most important, it has taught me to live life to the fullest, with a more positive outlook and a deeper appreciation for every precious moment while we are here.

At the same time, coping with a life-threatening disease is not easy and certainly not something that any of us would have taken on willingly. There are many times when dealing with the demands and dimensions of having cancer can be overwhelming, even with the love and support of family and friends and a dedicated health care team. This is why an overall program that can enable you to take the right steps toward finding suitable treatment, gain greater control over your situation and, it is hoped, achieve full recovery is so essential.

This remarkable book can show you the way. Written by a team of experts who possess a rare combination of knowledge, sensitivity and expertise, it offers you a comprehensive program that focuses on you as the total patient. It will provide you with a full range of tools and strategies to help you manage every aspect of your illness and to make the most of the resources and information available to you. The active participants are you, your family and your friends and your coordinated health care team.

As its name suggests, this book is comprehensive—and best of all, it is highly comprehensible. It is well organized and easy to read. It even has a glossary in the back for looking up scientific and medical terms. And whether you choose to read it from cover to cover (as I recommend you do) or to use it as a reference guide for focusing on those areas of special interest to you, you will find it to be an invaluable resource for making intelligent and informed decisions about your mental and physical well-being.

This book has made a difference in my life. I came away from reading it with more confidence and courage for facing my disease and more determined than ever to forge ahead and not give up. I wish the same for each and every one of you, and hope that it will become a valuable partner in your road to recovery.

I send you my heartfelt wishes for renewed and continued health.

ACKNOWLEDGMENTS

We wish to give special thanks and recognition to our original editor, Mary Anne Stewart, for her dedication and invaluable creative efforts in developing and organizing the first edition of *A Comprehensive Guide for Cancer Patients and Their Families*; to the late David Bull, past president of the Bull Publishing Co. of Palo Alto, California, who published the 1980 edition; to Jane Gaspari-Somerville, who edited the 1980 edition with David Bull, and to James Bull, Bull Publishing Co., for permission to reprint excerpts from *Nutrition for the Cancer Patient* by Janet Ramstack, PhD, and Ernest H. Rosenbaum, MD.

We wish to thank Bernadette Festa Bell for her extensive efforts and editing advice on Chapters 16 to 20 on nutrition for the cancer patient. Chapter 4, Bone Marrow Transplantation by Keren Stronach, is dedicated to Josh, her family and all the people whose love and support carried her through the transplant process.

Keren Stronach would also like to acknowledge the transplant survivors who generously shared their experiences and recommendations. Thanks are also in order to the following list of individuals who took the time to review and edit sections of the chapter: Frederick Appelbaum, MD, Jane Ariel, PhD, Myra Jacobs, MA, CFRE, Nancy Janz, RN, PhD, C. Michele, E. Lloid, RDH, BA, MS, Peggy Maas, PT, Celia Savonen, MSW, Sam Silver, MD, PhD, Saul Silverman, MD, Jean M. Stern, MS, RD, CD.

We also wish to give thanks and recognition to our special editors Tina Anderson, Diane Behar, Mary Heldman; Michael Glover (preliminary editing), Christopher Benz, MD; Gail Gordon; consultants Susan Claman, Francis Perkins and Zoli Zlotogorski, PhD; Whitney Burroughs in the MZH Resource Center and typists Paula Chung and Diane McElhiney. Thanks to Ruth Chernia for project management, Shaun Oakey for skilled copy editing and careful proofreading, Heather Ebbs for creating the index and Sarah Rashid for page layout of a truly complex book.

Thank you to Mary Connell, June Fraps, Jason Gans, Ann Gossman, Brian Greenwald, Noah Kahn, Holly Miller, MD, Fay Volk, Steven Heilig, Stephen Dobbs, Edmund Pellegrino, MD, David Perlman, J. Jerrill Plunkett and Martin Diamond for their editing and general support for the section "Planning for the Future."

We wish to acknowledge Bristol-Myers Squibb Oncology, Schering Oncology Biotech and Pharmacia & Upjohn Company for their generous support of this project.

We wish to thank contributors to the 1980 edition: Stephanie Conger, RN, BA, RA, Diana Denker, RN, MS, Lizabeth Light, BA, RSN, BN, Joanne Meany-Handy, RN, MS, Eileen Shepley, RN, BSN, MSN, Marie Smith, RN, BSN, Carol Stitt, RD, and Julie Williams, RN, BSN.

And, finally, a special thank you to Ann Lazerus, executive director of Mount Zion Health Systems and to the San Francisco chapter of the Susan G. Komen Breast Cancer Foundation.

INTRODUCTION

Ernest H. Rosenbaum, MD, and Isadora R. Rosenbaum, MA

———————◇———————

We are beginning to win the war on cancer declared 25 years ago by President Richard Nixon. But it has taken longer than projected to see the early results. Two recent major studies have confirmed that for the first time there has been a drop in the overall cancer mortality rate. The studies showed a turning point after decades of continuous rise, with a 6.5 percent rise in cancer mortality between 1971 and 1990. The largest mortality reductions have occurred in blacks. From 1990 to 1997, their mortality rate has declined 5.6 percent compared with an 18.3 percent jump from 1971 to 1990. Black men saw a drop of 8.1 percent; the rate declined 2.5 percent in black women. Among whites the decline was 3.6 percent for men and 0.2 percent for women. Breast, colon and prostate cancer mortality are now declining.

Dr. Richard Klausner, director of the National Cancer Institute, said in 1996, "What we report today is not a cause for complacency, but just the opposite. It is a demand for increased commitment. We are on the eve of the twenty-fifth anniversary of the National Cancer Act, the legislation that made cancer research a high national priority. Now our nation's investment is paying off by saving lives."

The evidence shows that lifestyle changes that influence prevention, such as a 50 percent reduction in tobacco use, improved diet, less alcohol consumption and more cancer screening (e.g., mammography and Pap smears), have made a difference. If this trend continues there will be a 20 to 50 percent reduction in the overall cancer mortality rate in the next 20 years.

This book was written especially for you, the patient. It will also be useful to members of your support team—your family, friends, health care providers and other important people in your life. But remember, you are the most important person, and this book can provide you with some valuable tools to help you meet the challenges of living with a serious illness and finding your true path to restored health.

Living with cancer has many different and difficult dimensions, and your needs go well beyond those of receiving basic medical care. Equally important are your psychological, social and spiritual needs, which must also be addressed.

As the healing arts have become more and more specialized, the gap between all these needs has widened to a point where an artificial division now exists between the mind and body. Physicians and other medical practitioners focus primarily on the physical body, while clergy and mental health professionals work to heal the mind and spirit, but in order to heal you—the "whole" patient—an approach is needed that can bring all these important components together for your total care.

This book is designed to provide just that. It will point the way to an organized program of comprehensive rehabilitation to complement the standard forms of cancer therapy (surgery, radiation, chemotherapy and immunotherapy). It specifically examines health, nutrition, exercise, sexuality, and nursing, hospital and community services.

This program also involves the full participation of your physician, who is responsible for its supervision and implementation; your health care team—clergy, educators, nurses, dietitians, social workers and therapists (occupational, physical and recreational)—who assist in their specialized areas; your family and friends, who support and assist in your program, and most important, you, the patient, who is responsible for understanding and using this approach.

We feel that this total team approach offers the best form of therapy. To use less or only part of the team means that you are receiving only partial care. And when you are an active participant in your medical care and rehabilitation, you can maintain a sense of control over your disease and therapy. Only you can take responsibility for your state of mind, nutritional status and physical fitness. The act of taking responsibility is in itself an important factor in promoting self-esteem, independence and faith in your ability to cope. It is a crucial part of getting well.

When you are ill, you have one overriding goal: to get well as quickly as possible to return to an active, fulfilling life. A well-organized, structured program, coordinated by you, your family and your health care team, can facilitate getting well faster and can make the difference between continued good health or illness and chronic disability. Many resources are available, though it can be difficult for you to take advantage of them when you are seriously ill. This book will help make your own healing program—and progress—that much easier and more manageable.

Efforts must be implemented to maintain the body's strength and to encourage endurance, courage and hope. These can greatly enhance the effectiveness of medical therapy or support a comfort care program where efforts are made to relieve pain and suffering.

The goal of cancer treatment is to cure cancer or control and slow the cancer growth so that a person does not need to die of cancer, but can live as long as possible with a full quality of life. And one of the goals of this book is to improve your cancer control no matter how much better or worse your cancer becomes in relation to your therapy. We do know that the better a person's physical status, the stronger the will to live. Thus, a person will have a longer and better quality of life despite the presence, control or growth of disease.

AUTHORS AND CONTRIBUTORS

◇

Ernest H. Rosenbaum, MD
Clinical Professor of Medicine, University of California, San Francisco; Associate Chief of Medicine, University of California, San Francisco/Mount Zion Medical Center; Medical Director, Better Health Foundation, San Francisco

Ernest H. Rosenbaum's career has included a fellowship at the Blood Research Laboratory of Tufts University School of Medicine (New England Center Hospital) and MIT. He teaches at the University of California, San Francisco/Mount Zion Medical Center, and was the cofounder of the Northern California Academy of Clinical Oncology.

His passionate interest in clinical research and good communication with patients and colleagues has resulted in over 50 articles on cancer and hematology in various medical journals. He has participated in many radio and television programs and frequently lectures to medical and public groups.

He has coauthored *Nutrition for the Cancer Patient* and has written numerous books, including *Living with Cancer, A Home Care Training Program for Cancer Patients, Decisions for Life, You Can Live 10 Years Longer with Better Health, A Comprehensive Guide for Cancer Patients and Their Families* and *Everyone's Guide to Cancer Therapy.* For the *Comprehensive Guide* Dr. Rosenbaum et al. received Honorable Mention from the American Medical Writers Association for Excellence in Medical Publications and for *Everyone's Guide* Dr. Malin Dollinger, Dr. Rosenbaum and Greg Cable received the same honor.

Isadora R. Rosenbaum, MA
Isadora Rosenbaum is a medical assistant who has worked in immunology research and an oncology practice offering advice and psychosocial support. She coauthored *The Comprehensive Guide for Cancer Patients and Their Families* and wrote chapters in *Everyone's Guide to Cancer Therapy, Living with Cancer* and *You Can Live 10 Years Longer with Better Health.*

Gary M. Abrams, MD
Assistant Professor of Clinical Neurology, University of California School of Medicine, San Francisco; Interim Chief of Neurology and Director of Rehabilitation, UCSF/MZH

Thomas Addison, MD
Clinical Professor of Medicine, UCSF/MZH

Robert W. Allen, MD
Assistant Clinical Professor, Department of Anesthesia, Division of Pain Management, UCSF/MZH

Joseph S. Bailes, MD
Director, Executive Vice-President and National Medical Director, Physician Reliance Network, Inc., Dallas, TX; President Elect and Member, Board of Directors, American Society of Clinical Oncology (ASCO); American Society of Clinical Oncology; Clinical Assistant Professor of Medicine, University of Texas Health Science Center, San Antonio, TX

Joanna Beam, JD
University Counsel, University of California

Judy Bray, OC
Formerly Chief, Occupational Therapy, UCSF/MZH

Meryl Brod, PhD
Director of the Center for Clinical Aging Services and Research, USCF/MZH Center on Aging

David G. Bullard, PhD
Associate Clinical Professor of Medicine and of Medical Psychology (Psychiatry), University of California School of Medicine, San Francisco

Jean M. Bullard, RN, MS
Utilization Management, Veterans Administration Medical Center, San Francisco; formerly counselor for Patients Sexual Issues, Veterans Administration Medical Center, San Francisco; Lecturer, Department of Nursing, San Francisco State University, CA

Barrie R. Cassileth, PhD
Adjunct Professor of Medicine, University of North Carolina, Chapel Hill; Consulting Professor, Community and Family Medicine, Duke University Medical Center, Durham, NC

Paula Chung
Office Oncology Practice, UCSF/MZH

Catherine Coleman, RN
Consultant, Breast Center Development, Boston, MA

John P. Cooke, MD, PhD
Division of Cardiovascular Medicine, Falk Cardiovascular Research Center, Stanford University School of Medicine

Diane Craig, RN ONC, BSHS
Ida Friend Infusion Center, UCSF/MZH Cancer Center

Janet Amber Damon, MSW
Psychologist, Sausalito, CA

Malin R. Dollinger, MD
Oncology Consultant, John Wayne Cancer Institute, Santa Monica; Clinical Professor of Medicine, University of Southern California School of Medicine, Los Angeles

Mark J. Doolittle, PhD
Professor of Psychology, Sonoma State College, Sonoma, CA

Eric Durak, MSc
Director of Medical Health and Fitness, City of Santa Barbara, CA

Alan B. Glassberg, MD
Clinical Professor of Medicine, UCSF; Director, Hematology and Oncology, UCSF/MZH Cancer Center; Associate Director for Clinical Care, UCSF Cancer Center; Director, General Oncology, UCSF/MZH Cancer Center

Irene Harrison, LCSW
Hospice Care, Kaiser Hospital, Hayward, CA

Anna Hicho
Office Oncology Practice, UCSF/MZH Cancer Center

Susan Molloy Hubbard, BS, RN, MPA
Director, International Cancer Information Center, National Cancer Institute, Bethesda, MD

Robert Ignoffo, PharmD
Professor Oncology Pharmacist, UCSF/MZH

Patricia T. Kelly, PhD
Medical Genetist, Cancer Risk Assessment and Counseling Services, John Muir Medical Center, Walnut Creek, CA; private practice, Berkley, CA

Andrew W. Kneier, PhD
Clinical Psychologist, UCSF/MZH Cancer Center

Jack LaLanne
Physical fitness and nutrition expert

Regina Linetskaya, MA
Oncology Practice, UCSF/MZH Cancer
Center

Nancy Lambert, RN, BSN
Risk Assessment Coordinator, Department of Quality Management,
UCSF/MZH

Betty Lopez, CMA
Office Oncology Practice, UCSF/MZH
Cancer Center

Francine Manuel, RPT
Rehabilitation specialist, private
practice

Eugenie Marek, RN
Inpatient Care Manager, Care
Management Services, Brown & Toland
Physician Services Organization

Lawrence Margolis, MD
Professor of Radiation Oncology,
UCSF/MZH

Julie Matel, MS, RD
Clinical Dietitian, UCSF/MZH

T. Stanley Meyler, MD
Professor of Radiation Oncology,
UCSF/MZH

James Murdock
Art for Recovery, UCSF/MZH, and
the Lorna Barati Music for Recovery
Program, Mount Zion Health Systems, Inc.

Cynthia D. Perlis, BS
Director, Art for Recovery, UCSF/MZH;
Director, the Lorna Barati Music Program,
Mount Zion Health Systems, Inc.

Elmo Petterle
Author, San Rafael, CA

Barbara F. Piper, RN, OCN, DNSc
Associate Professor of Nursing,
University of Nebraska, KS

J. Jerill Plunkett, MD
Private practice

Joel Pollack, CPA
Administrative Director, President's
Office, John Wayne Cancer Institute,
Saint John's Health Center, Santa
Monica, CA

Lee L. Pollak, LCSW
Private practice, Jewish Family and
Children's Services and Coordinator of
the Bereavement Center

Barbara Quinn
Manager, Billing and Collection
Supervisor, UCSF/MZH

Wendy R. Robbins, MD
Assistant Clinical Professor, Department of Anesthesia, Division of
Pain Control, UCSF/MZH

Sabrina Selim, BA
Clinical Research Associate, UCSF/MZH
Cancer Center

Jeffrey Silberman, DMin
Director of Ruach Ami's Jewish
Community Chaplaincy Program,
UCSF/MZH

Stu Silverstein, MD
Attending Pediatrician, St. Vincent's
Medical Center, Bridgeport, CT;
keynote speaker, Medical Humor
Seminars

Patricia Sparacino, RN, MS
Clinical Nurse Specialist, UCSF/MZH

Keren Stronach, MPH
Coordinator, Cancer Resource Center,
UCSF/MZH; Publisher, *Survivors' Guide
to a Bone Marrow Transplant* and *Bone
Marrow Transplant Resource Guide* (coauthor)

Carol S. Viele, RN, MS
Clinical Nurse Specialist, Hematology/Oncology and Bone Marrow
Transplant, UCSF

Kenneth A. Woeber, MD
Chief of Medicine, UCSF/MZH

PART I:
CANCER: DIAGNOSIS AND TREATMENT

1
UNDERSTANDING CANCER: WHAT IT IS AND HOW IT IS TREATED

Ernest H. Rosenbaum, MD, and Isadora R. Rosenbaum, MA

———◇———

Cancer is one of the most feared of diseases, and people wish for a cure. Today we can cure 50 percent of cases. We hope that someday we will have a cure for all cancers, as we do for other diseases.

Cancer is the number-two killer in the United States—heart disease is number one. One out of every three people in the United States will have cardiovascular disease. The lifetime risk of developing cancer in the U.S. is one in two for men and one in three for women. One out of every four will develop cancer. By 2000, cancer is projected to exceed heart disease as the leading cause of death.

In 1998, there were 10 million Americans alive who have had cancer; 7 million have lived five years after treatment and are considered cured. In 1998 there will be 1,228,600 new cases (excluding 800,000 cases of skin cancers), and 564,800 people will die.

Cancer manifests itself by tumor cell growth with invasion.

Not all tumors are malignant. Tumors are of two types: benign and malignant. The benign tumor does not invade or destroy surrounding structures or tissues, but remains local. The malignant, or cancerous, type grows larger by cell division, invades the surrounding tissues (the lymphatic system or the bloodstream) and metastasizes (spreads) to distant areas of the body.

Malignant tumors are invasive and differ from normal cells in their number, structure and chromosomes (composed of deoxyribonucleic acid, DNA). Cancer cells vary from slow-growing, low-grade malignancies to high-grade, more aggressive cancers. The grade of a tumor is classified by tissue examination under a microscope by a pathologist.

Although we speak of cancer as one word, it is not a single disease. There are more than two hundred different cancers, and they can originate in any cell or organ in the body. All cancers have one thing in common: malignant, uncontrolled, invasive growth of cells. When the word *cancer* is used in this book, it means any one of the many forms of cancers.

Sometimes a cancer is reported as in situ. An in situ cancer is a precancerous condition, early and confined to one small area (localized). If it is not treated or controlled, it may never grow, or it may grow and become invasive and malignant. A good example is an abnormal Pap smear with an in situ lesion that, if surgically removed (excised), may never recur.

FORMS OF CANCER

There are three basic forms of cancer, named for the body tissues where they originate:

◆ *Sarcomas* arise from fibrous or soft tissues (muscles, bone or blood vessels).
◆ *Carcinomas* arise from the epithelium—cells that cover the body surface and line body organs (e.g., lung, breast and colon).
◆ *Leukemias* and *lymphomas* arise from the blood cells of the bone marrow or from lymph node cells.

PERIOD OF GROWTH

With both malignant and nonmalignant tumors, there is usually a long latency period of from one to thirty years before a growing tumor can be felt on physical examination or detected by x-ray examination, isotopic scan or chemical or immunology tests. We call this clinically demonstrable. It is believed that a normal cell requires multiple "hits," or injuries, over months or years by a carcinogen before cell mutation can occur, transforming a normal cell into a cancer cell.

Approximately thirty cell divisions must occur for cancer cells to reach a mass that is detectable on physical examination or chest x-ray (usually greater than 1 cubic cm, or 1/3 square inch).

Each form of cancer has its own growth rate and pattern of spread. Some cancers remain localized, some invade adjacent structures, and others metastasize into the blood or lymphatic vessels where they are carried through the body to a distant site.

Cancers in the abdomen or chest cavity are detected late because they have to grow to a size that will cause symptoms. For example, most cases of ovarian cancer remain "silent," or camouflaged, until they have progressed enough to create a distended and painful abdomen due to excessive buildup of abdominal fluid (ascites). Unfortunately, by that time this cancer is usually in an advanced stage.

CAUSES OF CANCER

Because there are so many types of cancer, it is highly improbable that research will unearth a single cause or a single cure. Thus, until we have more specific knowledge, it is open season for speculation about the causes and cures of cancer, and it is impossible to refute some of the wilder speculations that frighten and con-

The malignant transformation of a normal cell and subsequent doublings. After 20 doublings (1 million cancer cells) the cancer is too small to detect.

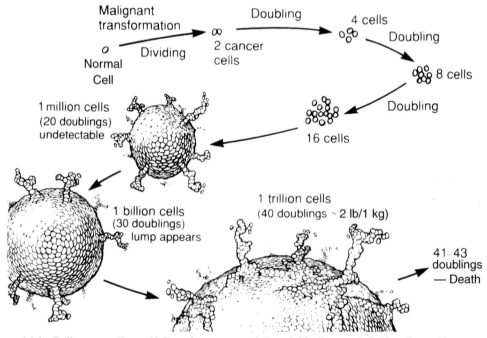

Source: Malin Dollinger, MD, Ernest H. Rosenbaum, MD, and Greg Cable. *Everyone's Guide to Cancer Therapy,* 3rd ed. Kansas City, MO: Andrews McMeel Publishing, 1997.

After two or more "hits" a transformed malignant cell grows into a lump we call cancer. Cells may eventually break off and spread (metastasize) via lymph vessels or blood vessels.

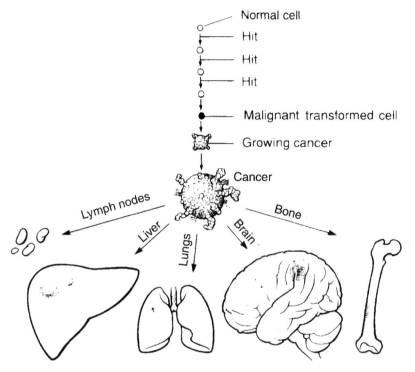

Source: Malin Dollinger, MD, Ernest H. Rosenbaum, MD, and Greg Cable. *Everyone's Guide to Cancer Therapy*, 3rd ed. Kansas City, MO: Andrews McMeel Publishing, 1997.

fuse people, such as the belief that cancer is contagious or that you can get it from using aluminum cookware. Chapter 6, "Alternative and Complementary Therapies," helps to sort out probable from totally speculative ideas.

Our knowledge of cancer is incomplete, but there is common agreement on some points.

External Factors It is widely believed that most cancers develop from normal cells that have been injured by external factors known as carcinogens (e.g., drugs, radiation, smoking and other environmental toxins). For example, smokers have an increased risk (10 times) of developing lung cancer compared to nonsmokers. It

appears that environmental carcinogens initiate over 75 percent of cancers. Occupation, diet and geographic location can also be factors in the development of cancer.

Internal Factors Internal factors that play a role in many cancers include hormones, infection and stress. Animal experiments suggest that viruses may also play a role in causing cancer. So far only a few viruses—the Epstein-Barr virus (Burkitt's, head and neck cancers), HTLV-1 (leukemia and lymphoma) and hepatitis virus (liver cancer)—have been shown to have a causal relationship to cancer in humans. Note that a positive test for the Epstein-Barr virus antibody, confirming past exposure to infectious mononucleosis, can also be found in healthy children and adults. This demonstrates that other factors, such as a specific susceptibility, are required to develop cancer.

Age, sex and race can also be factors in the development of cancer.

In recent years there has been much discussion of the role of the mind and stress in causing cancer. There is no evidence whatsoever that the mind is a major contributing factor in the development of cancer, although it may play a minor role in determining susceptibility or a modest role in accelerating cancer growth. (*See* Chapter 9, "Does Stress Cause Cancer?")

Our bodies have built-in defenses for destroying or containing cancer cells in their earlier stages. These include tumor-suppressor genes, parts of our immune system and gene-repair mechanisms, about which researchers are only beginning to learn. Proper nutrition, exercise and relaxation may also help to keep small, incipient cancers in check. If all these defenses prove inadequate, then the cancerous cells may replicate out of control and eventually spread.

GENETICS AND CANCER

Our knowledge of cancer is incomplete, but there is now common agreement that all cancers arise from abnormalities in a person's genetic material (DNA, or deoxyribonucleic acid)—namely, defective or lost genes. A person who develops cancer has either inherited a genetic defect from his or her parents or has experienced injury to normal genes. It is believed that in some cancers and some persons, both inherited and acquired genetic defects may be necessary before cancer can develop.

It should be emphasized that although all cancers are due to changes in a person's genes, most cancers are not hereditary. That is, most cancers are due to changes in the genes that occur after conception.

Genetic Predisposition A hereditary predisposition (as reflected in a strong family history of cancer) may in part determine one's susceptibility to cancer. The most common forms of inherited cancers occur in the breast, colon and prostate. (However, these cancers also occur in the absence of any genetic predisposition. And not everyone who inherits a predisposition will develop cancer.)

For example, a woman who has a first-degree relative (mother, sister or daughter) who has breast cancer has twice the risk of developing breast cancer (100 percent increased risk) compared to a woman who does not have a family history of breast cancer. As well, women who have two close relatives with breast cancer have a 20 percent chance of developing breast cancer during their lifetimes. Scientists are starting to uncover some of the specific inherited genetic defects that contribute to these and other cancers. At least two "breast cancer" genes have been found in the past few years; together these genes are thought to account for approximately 50 percent of all breast cancers that are inherited.

Genetic mutations can be inherited or can arise after birth from environmental and other causes.

The following special contribution by Patricia T. Kelly explains how genetic damage leads to the unregulated cell division that we call cancer.

GENETIC CHANGES AND CANCER

Patricia T. Kelly, PhD

In the last few years, scientists have learned much about the causes of cancer on the cellular level. It now appears that all cancers originate from changes in a person's genetic material, or DNA. DNA is present in almost every cell of a person's body. It orchestrates the production of the chemicals that cause our bodies to grow and develop.

The genes are composed of DNA and are located on chromosomes, which are long bodies resembling unclasped necklaces. You can think of the genes as multicolored beads on a necklace. Human beings have 23 pairs of these chromosomes. One of each pair is inherited from the father and one from the mother. With the exception of identical twins, triplets, etc., no two individuals' genes are exactly alike.

Throughout life, cells in the body are dividing. When a cell divides, it normally produces two cells, daughter cells, that are just like itself. In many cases, if one member of a gene pair is lost or damaged in the process, the cell can continue to function normally, because of the presence of the second copy. However, if a second event should occur, bringing about the loss of the second member of the gene pair, cancer may occur.

How could a change in only one of 100,000 or more genes result in the formation of a cancer cell? Actually, scientists think that only rare cancers, such as retinoblastoma (an eye cancer found in children) or familial polyposis colon cancer (a form of colon cancer), can be brought about by changes in, or the loss of, a single gene or even a single pair of genes. For most cancers to occur, changes in several genes seem to be required.

Here, however, we will consider the case of cancers that are brought about by a change in, or loss of, a single gene, called a suppressor gene.

Almost all cells in the body are thought to contain the full complement of genetic material—enough to make an entire human being. It has already been possible to grow a whole plant from just a single cell of carrots and other vegetables. Obviously, not all genes in all the cells can be active at all times if the body is to function properly. For example, skin cells, which also contain the genes to make ear cells, eye lenses and so on, must have a way to turn off all genes except those needed to produce and maintain skin. It is as though we have a piano in each cell, with specific keys blocked in different cell types, so that only the appropriate notes are played in any given type of cell.

Clearly, our bodies must have some method of regulating the appropriate expression of genes in the various tissues. Some of this regulatory activity appears to be brought about by genes called tumor-suppressor genes, which help to control cell division. If only one member of a suppressor gene pair is lost or damaged, the cell can rely on the undamaged member of the pair to maintain control. However, if both members of a gene pair are lost or damaged, the cell may lose its growth constraints and begin unregulated cell growth. It is this unregulated cell growth that we call cancer.

What causes suppressor genes to be lost or damaged? Scientists think that some loss or damage may be due to mistakes in cell division. The older a person is, the longer his or her cells have been dividing, and so the more likely it will be that such a mistake or accident in cell division can occur. Environmental carcinogens, such as cigarette smoke, may also play a role in producing changes in the genes or in disrupting regular cell division. Those with an increased hereditary susceptibility to cancer may be born with a change in, or loss of, a suppressor gene. In these people, only one more change in a strong or important gene could lead to the formation of cancer cells.

In the next few years, scientists expect to make great strides in determining which substances in the environment can produce harmful changes to the genes, leading to cancer. The next steps will be to reduce exposure to these substances and to learn how to help the cell repair any damage that occurs.

THE DIAGNOSIS OF CANCER

People hope for a cure for cancer. The best approach is prevention and early diagnosis. Early diagnosis is the prerequisite for cure.

Unfortunately, except for cervical cancer, for which we have the Pap smear; colon sigmoidoscopy examination to detect and remove polyps; mammography for breast cancer, and prostate digital rectal examination and prostate-specific antigen (PSA) for prostate cancer detection, physicians lack routine techniques for diagnosing cancer at its earliest inception, when the likelihood of spread is minimal.

New tests are becoming available, but until they are perfected, most cancers grow for months or years before they cause symptoms that lead to their detection by physical examination, x-ray, chemical or immunological tests, isotope scan or biopsy. In the meantime, the obvious symptoms a person can notice are often ignored, despite the American Cancer Society's public education program and the public statements of many cancer specialists. Any delay allows cancer to spread and often precludes the chance for a cure.

The seven danger signals, as listed in the American Cancer Society brochure "Listen to Your Body," are

C Change in bowel or bladder habits

A sore that does not heal

U Unusual bleeding or discharge

T Thickening or lump in breast or elsewhere

I Indigestion or difficulty in swallowing

O Obvious change in wart or mole

N Nagging cough or hoarseness

Among those diseases for which early detection is important are breast, colon and prostate cancers; melanoma; certain lung cancers, and leukemias.

2

THE PATIENT-PHYSICIAN RELATIONSHIP: THE UNWRITTEN CONTRACT

Ernest H. Rosenbaum, MD, and Isadora R. Rosenbaum, MA

The day I found out I had cancer was the worst day of my life.
— *Senator Hubert H. Humphrey*

———◇———

Not every person who consults with a doctor about a perplexing ailment suspects or assumes that cancer is present; nor does every person who suspects he or she has cancer actually have it. However, because I am a hematologist and an oncologist (a specialist in blood and tumor problems), patients are referred by other doctors and they usually are aware of the reason for the consultation. Some people are referred by their family physicians for a second or third opinion to confirm a diagnosis; others are referred by internists, surgeons or cancer specialists for further evaluation or to reassess a treatment program.

If a doctor is to treat a person for cancer, it is important to have a candid exchange of information during the initial meetings. Because new patients are always apprehensive, oncologists try to give them the basic facts about cancer and its treatment and ask them to describe their symptoms and some of the personal facts that are needed for their physician or consultant to provide the best treatment for each patient.

Information about cancer is readily available and useful to a person who will undergo treatment and live with the disease. Informed patients will be more receptive to treatment and thereby improve their chances of combating the disease. Moreover, the attitudes they acquire in these initial interviews may

well affect the quality of life they are able to maintain for the duration of the illness. The patient is kept informed about why a particular test is being performed and what the results could mean. False hope and subsequent disappointment only lead to distrust of the medical community and wariness of any further treatment.

Patients should be aware that they are entitled to all available information about testing, test results and therapeutic procedures. In the United States, patients now read and sign in the presence of their doctors an "informed consent" form for special diagnostic procedures (such as angiograms) and specific treatments (such as surgery, radiotherapy and experimental chemotherapy and immunotherapy). Each state has its own legal definition of informed consent. For example, in Massachusetts, California and some other states, the law specifies that patients with breast cancer must be fully informed of all alternative forms of treatment.

Knowing that what I say may affect the patient's future, when I meet with a patient, I proceed slowly and carefully, ready to temper my approach as the person reveals how much he or she wants to know at that moment. It is, after all, a patient's prerogative to determine how much he or she wants to hear. I, on the other hand, must be sure to provide an opportunity for someone to find out everything he or she wants to know.

Many patients now bluntly ask, "Do I have cancer?" In such circumstances, I can be frank. But if a patient tells me to take over, that he or she does not wish to know the details of the disease or the treatments, I usually do not press the issue. Each person knows how he or she is best able to function. The only people who I believe must be informed are those who are financially responsible for others.

Whether the meeting takes place in the hospital or in the office, I prefer, whenever possible, to have the closest family members present during the explanation. This eliminates the need for repetition and reduces the possibility of misunderstanding. Sometimes, too, including loved ones lessens a patient's fear of abandonment and provides reassurance that the family is not concealing any facts. Together, the family and the patient can ask questions and consider problems that may arise, for, ideally, the long-term treatment of cancer involves the cooperation of the whole family.

During the initial explanation, patients can be helpful—and ultimately better informed—if they respond to leading questions such as "Do you have any questions about your diagnosis?" A doctor is not helped by a reply of "No," or "You're the doctor. You should know." As I mentioned, the doctor-patient relationship works best when both participants are responsive, as in the following dialogue:

Doctor: "What do you think is wrong?"
Patient: "I'm not sure."
Doctor: "Well, there are several possibilities. Acute infection or arthritic or systemic disease—or some other type, an ulcer or a malignancy. What do you think is causing your problem?"
Patient: "I really don't know. Can you tell me?" or "Do I have cancer?"

When the reply is "Yes, you have cancer," or "Yes, you have a tumor," the doc-tor should give a detailed explanation, repeating much of the basic information the patient may have received during the diagnostic procedures. The doctor should explain the type and extent of malignancy, although not necessarily all at one time, and it is most important to make the patient aware of the treatments that are available to combat the disease. I always explain that we will begin with the mode of therapy prescribed for this particular form and stage of cancer but that there are others that may be equally effective or provide a backup if the first one is not effective.

A lot of misunderstanding can result from the initial discussion of diagnosis and treatment. Patients are usually too stunned to think clearly and need time to assimilate bad news. Often they cannot respond to my final question, "Is there anything you don't understand about your problem?" They may have understood nothing because they heard nothing after the word *cancer* was uttered.

Several years ago, a patient left my office after an extensive 30-minute discussion of her cancer and was met at the office door by her cousin, who asked, "What did the doctor tell you?" Although only 90 seconds had elapsed since our talk, she replied, "I forgot." It was obvious that my explanation had fallen on deaf ears. She was still in a daze from the first few sentences of our conversation.

For this reason, I usually ask my patients if they would like to have a record of our initial conversations concerning diagnosis and treatment on a cassette tape. The patient, and whomever else (family member or friend) the patient wishes to have present for the explanation, can listen to the tape later at home in a less stressful environment. Someone who receives a diagnosis of cancer needs time to absorb the information, to reflect and to plan.

The patient, family members and friends may have misconceptions, fears and anxieties that should be expressed. The tape helps to deal with these and enables those close to the patient to talk with him or her openly.

Also, patients and their families or friends may have left my office with different ideas about what has been said. By listening to the tape, they can clear up misunderstandings or decide on questions for the next visit. The cassette recording can also help maintain vital communication between the cancer patient and those close to him or her when the latter are unable to be present during a consultation. Some patients have sent the recording to concerned relatives in other parts of the country to keep them informed.

The presence of the tape recorder makes me more conscious of the need for clarity, and I therefore tend to present my explanations in a more concise and organized manner. At the same time, the tape recorder tends to make patients more conscious of their right to ask questions and of their responsibility for exercising that right.

Whether or not patients exercise their option to use the tape cassette, I encourage them to write down questions raised during our consultations. In effect, I ask them to make what I call a "shopping list" of all questions that occur to them about their form of cancer, future treatments or anything else that worries them, no matter how unrelated or trivial it may seem to them. Such a list helps them to include worries that they might otherwise suppress or questions they might just forget to ask me during our next talk. (The list of questions also makes the most efficient use of the often limited time of an office visit.)

Questions and concerns run the gamut:
◆ Please explain the whole thing again. What is happening inside my body?
◆ If I lose my hair, will it grow back?
◆ Is there anything I can take if I get nausea from chemotherapy? I have to go to work every day.

◆ I've had no medical insurance since I left my job two months ago. I can't afford to be sick. Are there any sources of financial aid?
◆ Can I play tennis while having chemotherapy?
◆ I know this is going to take a lot out of me. What can I do to make up for the extra nutrition my body will need?
◆ I have to be able to do housework soon after I get home from the hospital. What can I do to keep my muscles strong while I'm hospitalized?
◆ I know cancer isn't catching but I can't quite rid myself of the notion. Is it really all right if I sleep with my partner?

Any facts that I can give patients that will relieve their worries will free them to devote their energies to self-care and living.

THE FAMILY AND THE DIAGNOSIS

Occasionally a family member takes me aside and requests that the patient not be told the diagnosis if it turns out to be cancer. My feeling is that any agreement concerning a patient should be between the patient and the physician. When someone comes to me for medical help, it is with that person that I make the "unwritten contract" for mutual candor and trust, although I welcome the support of family or friends. Supposedly weak patients are usually stronger than anyone thinks and are quite capable of dealing openly with the cancer.

The reverse situation has also arisen. Patients have requested that their disease be kept a secret to protect a spouse or other family member. In these cases, I try to explain to the patient the therapeutic advantages of treating the family as a unit. For instance, a husband who joins his wife during an office visit will share her problems, know her fears and the routine of her therapy and therefore be able to give invaluable backup support. I had one patient who always told me she felt great until her husband interrupted, "That's not true. You felt nauseated last night." I could then prescribe an antinausea medicine.

Everyone has heard of instances when a family member and the patient each thought he or she was alone in knowing the truth. Generally, this protective attitude is self-defeating, not only because precious energy is expended but because the longer the facade is maintained, the greater the fear and anxiety are for both. Therefore, I try to bring the two together.

Sometimes the circumstances are even more difficult. I am occasionally brought in on a case in which the deception of a patient has been going on for some time. The family or the primary physician have decided not to tell the patient the truth, so the question arises of the wisdom of intervening in an established relationship. My policy in such cases is that if patients have no psychiatric problem and are not senile, and they ask me directly, I explain the nature of the disease in as much detail as they wish. If they show no inclination to know about their illness, I tend to comply with the wishes of the family and the primary physician, even though such a policy has often brought unfortunate results.

This situation may occur when a patient and family observe certain cultural customs where in their part of the world a diagnosis of cancer is not given to the patient but is shared with the family. I feel the patient usually knows the diagnosis but takes part in this deception. Sometimes these patients do worse and lose their will to live when informed that they have cancer.

PLANNING TREATMENT

In accordance with the terms of the unwritten contract, I try not to make any medical decisions without taking into consideration the emotional needs of patients. The more we talk about their family, work, religious views, hobbies, moods and gen-

eral lifestyle, the more I learn what those needs are. At the same time, I have to tell them that our choice of therapy, or combination of therapy, will be limited at any given time by their type of cancer and its stage of development. I describe the risks, side effects and anticipated results of the most current therapies, so that there will be no unnecessary shocks in the future.

A therapy that is new to a patient must be given time to work so that the effects can be properly assessed. I try to explain to patients that when they buy a new car, they have no idea how well it is going to function until they have driven it for a few weeks or months. They then will know how it functions in gas mileage and economy, how often it needs repairs and so on. The same analogy applies to cancer therapy. Although the treatment differs for each type and stage of cancer, one must usually wait 6 to 12 weeks after a treatment has begun to assess the early results through laboratory tests, x-rays and scans.

Many people are concerned when changes are made in their therapeutic program, but a change does not always mean that cancer has progressed or that a new problem has appeared. It is not uncommon to change from one mode of therapy to another, to alter the dosage and content of a therapy or even to stop treatment for a short time. Sometimes such a change is made because a therapy is not effective; at other times, a new concept of treatment has proved valid, or a new treatment shows promise. Sometimes an unrelated medical problem or the patient's desire necessitates a change in, or end of, a particular therapy.

Fortunately, there are alternative medical therapies for most forms of cancer. I was told by one of my patients that I sometimes sound like a sorcerer with a magical bag of tricks, an indefinite number of therapies. Yet, it is amazing how often a person who has been successfully treated on a given program and has subsequently relapsed can achieve another remission with a change in therapy. I am not saying that just because a person accepts treatment, success is guaranteed. We all know there are limits to the possibilities of therapy. But a patient will never know what might have happened unless he or she is willing to try another therapy, assume the risks and undergo assessment of the results. This is the commonsense approach to the treatment of cancer.

Oncologists must know what is current and available in cancer therapy, as well as what may be forthcoming from cancer research, so that they can send their patients to specialized centers for treatment unavailable elsewhere. Nevertheless, despite assurances that they are receiving the most up-to-date and effective treatment known, some patients are so terrified that they will not accept standard therapy. This pattern is seen most frequently in patients who have been told that the available therapy for this disease will contain the rate of spread but holds little promise for cure. Unable to accept that fact, they spend much of their remaining lives running in desperation to distant clinics or other countries seeking a miracle cure.

Patients may also choose alternative treatment. (*See* Chapter 6.) One patient who came to me for consultation and therapy had traveled to Germany and Mexico with her husband because they had been unwilling to accept the therapy recommended at a major university cancer center in California. Instead, she took at least 20 types of vitamins, plus carrot juice, various enzymes and Laetrile. I recommended certain alternative medical therapies to this couple, but they were unable to make a choice.

Finally, because valuable time was passing, I said to them, "There is no sense in my discussing this with you any further until you are willing to come to a decision. If you want me to decide for you, I'll be happy to do so. You have two choic-

es at this time: surgery plus medical therapy—hormones and/or chemotherapy—or radiotherapy and chemotherapy. I've explained the pros and cons of both approaches, and although I have a preference, I am not absolutely certain which is the better treatment. That can be assessed only after a therapy has been tried and the results graded. If you don't wish to try either one because of your own fears, that's your business. As far as I'm concerned, I'll wait to hear from you." This may sound like a tough approach after my description of a reciprocal exchange between patient and physician, but a decision had to be made. Subsequently, it was made, and it resulted in a dramatic improvement with radiotherapy and chemotherapy.

Panic and flight are one type of response. There are other reactions—anger, frustration, depression—for which we must be watchful. Obviously some problems are resolvable, whereas others are chronic with no satisfactory solution. In the latter cases, I believe it is good medical practice to consult another physician. Second and third opinions are becoming increasingly acceptable to both patients and physicians because they realize that no one has all the answers and that another point of view can be helpful, both psychologically and therapeutically.

No matter what a patient's anxieties may be, they should be brought to the attention of the doctor during regular office visits. Many of my patients use the shopping list that reminds them of the troubling thoughts and questions that have arisen since the first visit, and discussing them relieves many anxieties.

Anxiety may also be related to the ordinary pressures of life—fear of losing a job or a spouse, or a misunderstanding with a relative or a friend—and be compounded by having to cope with cancer.

One of my patients holds a responsible, demanding job that could be jeopardized by the limitations on her energy resulting from cancer and the therapy required. Her teenage children are always in trouble and her husband is unable to help emotionally or even take care of the children when she is hospitalized. As a result of these worries, she continued to be depressed even after she obtained a remission from anemia and advanced involvement of the liver and bone from breast cancer. However, because she shared her concerns with me, I was able to offer her extra emotional support. The nurses in the office and the nurse and social workers from the hospital are also available to chat or make a referral to such services as group therapy or family counseling or help obtain assistance at home.

I envisage the role of a physician as an adviser and a friend, and in this capacity I try to help patients plan new approaches with the aid of the medical team. This sometimes involves discussions of how a patient's illness or the knowledge of his or her eventual death is affecting each member of the family.

Sometimes, too, when making a will or arranging insurance or other personal affairs becomes an unwelcome acknowledgment that an illness is terminal, I try to encourage a patient to act for the protection of his or her family. I explain that most people spend their entire working lives planning for the protection and support of their family. They buy insurance and make a will years before illness or death to assure that the needed financial support will be available when needed. (*See* Part V, "Planning for the Future.")

Listening and talking, creating an atmosphere of openness and candor, are the means by which an enduring, supportive relationship between the physician and the patient is developed. If a patient will share emotional, financial and other concerns with his or her physician, unexpected and welcome interest and help may be forthcoming. What patients tell me guides me in each decision regarding the treatment of their cancer and their

general well-being; I hope that what I tell them—the knowledge of their disease and its treatment, present and future—reduces their anxiety and frees them to direct their thoughts toward life. But to make such a relationship a reality, patients must have the wisdom to know their needs and be able to discuss them with their doctor.

REMISSIONS AND RELAPSES

A remission is the goal of every cancer patient. As with any other chronic disease, such as heart disease, arthritis or kidney disease, a remission can vary in duration and effect on a person's long-term health. A complete remission can mean a return to good health. A partial remission is a more limited medical response.

A person who gets some good news, such as being told of a partial remission, may feel better and enjoy a complete return to health even though tumor remains. The reason he or she feels well is that the tumor has been significantly reduced. Even a small reduction in size can bring physical relief.

Some patients remain on therapy indefinitely in hope of containing or eradicating their disease. We encourage them not only to remain on therapy but also to resume the activities of daily living— going to work, doing work around the house, participating in social events and taking vacations—even if participation is limited while on therapy.

Completing a course of therapy is similar to graduating from high school or college. But in spite of that first feeling of elation, life is not the same as it was before. No one can go through such an experience without suffering some trauma. Living with cancer affects to a greater or lesser extent one's emotional reactions and intellectual approach to life. Every new ache or pain, which we all experience daily and ignore, raises for the former cancer patient the fear of a recurrence. I have been through this myself. After surgery in 1980 for a chest tumor that proved to be a low-grade malignancy, I experienced new symptoms. Only a chest x-ray examination convinced me that the tumor had not recurred.

A recurrence for a person who has been in remission is devastating. But just as when the cancer was first detected, a therapeutic approach will be planned with the goal of a new remission. Anxiety, fear and depression will again dominate, but they will also be dealt with as they were before.

Most people who achieve a first remission and have a recurrence need only minimal encouragement to sustain their determination for a new round of treatment. Others are reluctant to continue. They may have found the side effects of surgery, radiotherapy or chemotherapy, even when minimal, to be more than they can tolerate. For example, an executive who underwent four intensive courses of chemotherapy combined with immunotherapy was elated during a period of remission. I warned him his case would have to be followed closely. Now another recurrence is suspected, and although an intensive program of chemotherapy might produce another remission, he insists that treatment be kept to a minimum. Of course, this decision is his prerogative.

When patients announce that they no longer wish to be treated, or wish to receive only minimal treatment, I try to be very convincing. A person with a recurrence may have another chance at remission. The potential is there. I believe it is a chance worth taking. The final decision is the patient's. There does come a time when the value of treatment is less than the effort involved, and thus the goal should be to achieve the best possible quality of life.

The condition of all cancer patients, whether cured or in remission, should be closely monitored for years. Patients should also be well informed about the prospects for a recurrence. With this knowledge, they will be more likely to take the preventive measures that may once again save or prolong their lives.

3
CANCER THERAPY

Ernest H. Rosenbaum, MD, *and Isadora R. Rosenbaum,* MA

The desire to take medicine is perhaps the greatest feature
which distinguishes man from animals.
— *Sir William Osler,* MD

───────◇───────

Surgery, radiation therapy and hormone or chemotherapy (drugs) are the three mainstays of cancer treatment.* Using one or a combination of these treatments, physicians are able to effect a definitive cure (5 to 10 years free of cancer) in about 50 percent of all cancers. The cure rate for some types of cancer is much higher and for others much lower than this average. It is important to note, however, that although treatment fails to cure approximately 50 percent of those who have cancer, it is rare that vigorous treatment does not benefit the patient.

Immunotherapy and gene therapy—vaccines and drugs to improve the efficiency of the immune system—is the fourth kind of therapy. Immunotherapy, once considered experimental, has entered some treatment programs as a standard therapy for many cancers.

Even in cases when it is obvious from the onset that a cure is unlikely or impossible, appropriate therapy, including palliative (comfort) therapy, can assure a patient not only freedom from pain but also many months or years of a relatively normal life if the cancer is of the chronic type. A person may even live a normal life span and eventually die of an unrelated cause.

Over the past 75 years many improvements have been made in early detection, diagnosis and treatment of cancer.

Improvement in the five-year survival rate has increased from 20 percent in 1930 to more than 50 percent in 1998. Yet it is surprising how often one encounters a negative attitude toward the treatment of cancer, not only among patients and the public but even within the medical community. This attitude could be summed up as: "If it cannot be cured, why bother treating it?" It seems strange that such thinking persists in a society in which the treatment of other incurable diseases (heart disease, kidney failure and diabetes, to name just three) is readily accepted.

Sometimes people refuse treatment for their disease because they have heard frightening stories about the side effects of treatment and are more afraid of the treatment itself than they are of the cancer. These fears are largely unwarranted, especially today when side effects are better controlled with improved antinausea drugs such as Kytril, Zofran, Compazine and Marinol. Bleeding and infections are also better controlled, and pain and suffering can be reduced, alleviated or even prevented.

There are four types of responses to cancer treatment. They are graded by changes based on physical examination, laboratory tests and x-rays and scans:
1. Complete response (CR): a 95 to 99 percent reduction in cancer as measured by tests or scans.

*This chapter is an overview of standard and experimental and alternative cancer treatments. More detailed and specific information can be found in *Everyone's Guide to Cancer Therapy* by Malin Dollinger, MD, Ernest H. Rosenbaum, MD, and Greg Cable.

2. Partial response (PR): a greater than 50 percent reduction of the cancer as measured by x-rays or scans.
3. Stable response: the tumor, with treatment, remains the same size with no growth or is smaller, but no more than 50 percent smaller.
4. No response: the tumor grows despite various treatments and treatment is considered a failure.

SURGERY

Surgery offers the ideal primary approach to cancer. If you can "cut it out" without major functional impairment, and if there is no residual disease, a person may be considered cured. A surgical excision is appropriate when the cancer is localized and does not involve vital structures. For example, a normal life can be achieved after the removal of a kidney or part of a lung.

In some cases, a biopsy is performed before surgery. The biopsy is a small, surgically removed specimen (part of the tumor). The specimen is sent to a pathologist for a "frozen section" examination. The pathologist immediately reports the findings to the surgeon. If the tumor contains no malignant cells, the surgeon can perform a conservative, or limited, operation to remove the entire suspicious mass. If the tumor does contain malignant cells, the surgeon can immediately perform an operation designed to eliminate all traces of the malignancy.

A surgeon is often able to remove all visible evidence of the cancer in the hope of effecting a cure. However, depending on the type and stage of the tumor, cancer may recur in a percentage of cases either adjacent to its original location or at some distant site (metastasis), such as the liver, lungs, brain or bone. This is one of the hallmarks of cancer—its tendency to metastasize (spread) before the parent tumor is diagnosed and removed. This characteristic constitutes the single most important problem in the management of malignant diseases; it is the reason for the importance of having close medical follow-up after treatment and for the necessity of waiting several months and years after an operation to be certain that a cure has been achieved.

If the tumor cannot be completely removed or if there is a risk of recurrence, adjuvant (simultaneous) therapy may be considered, using radiation, chemotherapy or both.

RADIATION THERAPY

Lawrence Margolis, MD, and T. Stanley Meyler, MD

Radiation therapy can damage or kill cells by injuring the DNA chromosomes of the cancer cell. Normal, healthy cells can recover from the damage. Many types of cancer can be cured by radiation alone or in combination with chemotherapy and/or surgery. Hope for many cancer patients not cured by surgery may lie in this treatment. It is not the last resort, as many people think, but is a practical method of killing cancer cells, restricting cancer growth, controlling pain or reducing a tumor to a size where surgery is more practical.

The most likely candidate for radiation is the patient with localized cancer. But even when the tumor has spread, radiation may still be used because it can reduce a cancer mass that may be causing an organ obstruction, causing pain or presenting a risk for a bone fracture.

By damaging the cells' DNA, radiation therapy usually renders the cells incapable of further growth or cell division. In radiation therapy, a beam of x-rays or gamma rays (from cobalt, linear acceleration or radium) is aimed directly at the tumor from an x-ray machine. Newer, still experimental techniques use heavy particles—pi mesons (pions) and neutrons—to treat cancers that are less sensitive to conventional radiation.

The area to be treated is carefully outlined (simulated) for each patient with a color skin marker. This colored outline remains on the skin throughout the course of therapy. The staff radiotherapist maps out the area of the tumor mass to be treated. The normal tissues surrounding the tumor receive careful consideration to protect them. A lead mold is made, customized for each patient especially to protect the normal organs surrounding the tumor. This work is usually done by the dosimetrist, a specialist who calculates the dose of radiation to be given. During radiotherapy, the mold is placed above the patient on a special tray attached to the radiation machine, so that the beams will strike only the tumor.

Nevertheless, it is impossible to totally avoid some damage to normal cells that lie in the path of the radiation beam. To minimize this problem, as well as to obtain the most efficient results, normal tissues are shielded as much as possible, and the recommended radiation dose is spread out over a period of time.

The complex mathematical calculations for the radiation dose appropriate for each patient (dosimetry) consider the tumor and the tolerance of the surrounding tissues in the area to be treated, as well as the anticipated side effects. These calculations are based on CT (computerized tomography) scans and other sophisticated roentgenographic techniques.

The development of high-energy radiation delivery machines has markedly reduced damage to normal cells. Most major medical centers now have a full range of megavoltage equipment ranging from cobalt to linear accelerators. The radiotherapist will select the most appropriate machine to treat the tumor and spare normal tissues, taking into account the type and location of the tumor.

A patient does not feel any pain or discomfort while receiving radiation therapy. Undergoing treatment is like having a chest x-ray, with the difference being that in radiation therapy the x-ray radiation machine is left on for several minutes to give a higher dose of radiation. In contrast, chest x-rays take only a few seconds and deliver a minute dose of radiation.

Side effects may occur as a result of damage to normal tissues. These side effects are discussed in Chapter 5, "Side Effects: Causes and Treatment." New, more sophisticated equipment and safety techniques have lessened or eliminated some of these side effects (particularly skin irritation, nausea, vomiting and diarrhea) for many patients. Fortunately, radiation therapy is usually limited to one to six weeks and most of the side effects are not permanent.

Sometimes radiation is administered internally, directly into the cancer. IORT (intraoperative radiation therapy) and brachytherapy (implanting radioactive needles or seeds into a tumor or implanting catheters to be loaded with radioactive substances for the delivery of sharply localized doses of radiation) are two forms of internally administering radiotherapy. They can spare surrounding tissues from significantly higher radiation exposure. These procedures are usually carried out in an operating room under anesthesia.

The tubes or needles are allowed to remain in the tumor for a calculated number of hours or days, allowing the tumor to be treated with a high dose of radiation. This radiation treatment can also be used in conjunction with external-beam radiation to concentrate the dose to the local area.

Certain tumors, such as cancer of the cervix, breast and prostate, may be cured by radiation therapy. The hope for many cancers not cured by surgery may lie in treatment with radiation.

Radiation therapy is often given in conjunction with other cancer treatments. For example, a dose of radiation may be given as a preventive measure to sterilize microscopic tumor cells that may have been left behind at surgery when the bulk of the cancer was removed.

Chemotherapy is often used before (neoadjunctive) or during (concurrent) radiation therapy, with drugs such as Adriamycin, 5-fluorouracil (5-FU) and Platinol or Taxol, which are radiosensitizers, to enhance the effects of radiation therapy. The combination of these therapies is often more effective in controlling certain cancers, but may also have more side effects. These side effects can be reduced or minimized by monitoring and adjusting the doses of the chemotherapy and radiation therapy. (*See* Chapter 17, "Nutrition Problems," for hints on reducing drug and radiation side effects.)

CHEMOTHERAPY

Chemotherapy is the treatment for a malignant disease that uses drugs that attack and may destroy cancer cells. Chemotherapy is generally reserved for systemic or invasive cancers that have spread to other parts of the body through the lymphatic system or blood system and for cases where surgery and radiation therapy are no longer effective. More recently, chemotherapy has been used before and as an adjunct to surgical treatment (the primary treatment) to destroy small amounts of undetectable cancer.

Chemotherapy has a bad reputation. Some of this reputation is deserved, but many times it is greatly exaggerated. Not all of the drugs produce serious side effects, and many patients have minimal toxic reactions. There is no publicity about the person who comes to the office or clinic, sticks out an arm, takes chemotherapy shots for breast or ovarian cancer and then goes home or to work and functions fairly well. Often these people don't talk about their disease or therapy, so what is heard is often from the minority of people who suffer severe side effects from chemotherapy.

Most people can tolerate chemotherapy, some patients have moderate to severe reactions, and a few cannot tolerate therapy at all. Fortunately, there are many ways to reduce the side effects, many of which are discussed in Chapter 5.

Chemotherapy is used to treat more advanced or metastatic cancer. It was originally used only in cases where surgery and radiation therapy were no longer effective, but now it is also used as an extra safeguard after surgical removal of a tumor that has a high risk of recurring. For example, chemotherapy may be administered soon after surgery for breast cancer (when cancer cells have been found in adjacent lymph nodes). See "Adjuvant Chemotherapy" below.

In a few diseases, such as Burkitt's lymphoma, choriocarcinoma, acute leukemia, ovarian cancer, testicular cancer and some cases of advanced Hodgkin's disease, the judicious and aggressive use of chemotherapy, with or without radiation therapy, may bring about a remission or cure.

Like healthy cells, cancer cells are involved in a continuous process of alternately resting and dividing (the cell cycle). This is the process of cell division, when a cell makes two daughter cells. Unlike healthy cells, cancer cells divide in an uncontrollable manner. Chemotherapy takes advantage of the way cells multiply by dividing.

Approximately 60 chemotherapeutic drugs are available, although only about 30 of these are used in the majority of cancers. The chemotherapeutic agents are cellular poisons classified as cell-cycle-specific (targeted at dividing cells), non-cell-cycle-specific (aimed at resting or nondividing cells) or miscellaneous. These classifications refer to the stage at which the particular chemotherapeutic agent is effective. There are several classes of drugs that act by various means to injure the cell and prevent growth by inhibiting cell division. Chemotherapeutic agents are frequently used in combination to increase their effectiveness and to prevent drug resistance by cells.

Because many cancer cells are killed more easily during the process of division than when they are resting, the cell-cycle-specific class of drugs (the antimetabolites) are used to attack those cancer cells while they are dividing. The non-cell-cycle-specific class of drugs (the alkylating or mustard group) tend to attack the DNA of all the cells in a tumor, whether they are resting or dividing. These drugs are generally used to reduce the tumor mass. Then the remaining tumor cells (many of which were inactive before the drug was administered) may become active and start dividing, at which time a cell-cycle-specific drug can be given. Non-cell-cycle-specific and cell-cycle-specific drugs are often used in this sequence or

in combination to obtain the maximum effect.

Progress is constantly being made. We know more about the most effective method and frequency of administering drugs, we have devised better combinations of these drugs, and new drugs are always being developed.

Making the Decision to Take Chemotherapy The decision to take chemotherapy is a personal decision based on information, personal philosophy and accurate medical advice. Many who accept therapy despite poor odds are making a decision to choose to live. The benefits can be little, marginal or major. Desperate patients with advanced disease are often willing to accept chemotherapy in hopes of even a small chance to live.

Over 50 percent of cancer patients are eligible for chemotherapy and will receive it. New research has shown that breast cancer patients who are at increased risk for recurrence can increase survival time, achieve cure or delay recurrence by using chemotherapy. This is also true for Hodgkin's disease, lymphoma, testicular cancer, ovarian cancer and leukemias that respond well to treatment.

Despite years of research and increased knowledge on how best to administer chemotherapy and reduce side effects, the cost of therapy continues to escalate and quality of life is often threatened.

Questions to Ask to Help You Make a Decision to Take Chemotherapy
1. Will therapy be effective in controlling and curing my cancer?
2. Will therapy give me a chance to increase my life span?
3. What are the chances disease will recur if I don't accept chemotherapy? What can I expect will happen?
4. Is my cancer early or advanced? Does this make a difference in choosing a chemotherapy program?
5. Should I be enrolled in a research

protocol? What is the advantage?

6. How will success (response) to chemotherapy be measured? (A 70 percent response rate means that 70 percent of treated persons will have a reduction in tumor size or bulk, reflecting a significant improvement for a certain time.)

7. What are the side effects of therapy? How will side effects be modified or controlled? Are there long-term side effects? How will the side effects be modified or controlled?

8. Is my chemotherapy program palliative? (For incurable and advanced cancer, palliation can relieve pain, pressure or other symptoms of cancer without prolonging life.)

9. Can I talk to a patient who has been treated with this chemotherapy program?

10. Where will chemotherapy be given and who will give it?

Hormonal Therapy Hormonal therapy attempts to reduce or control a tumor by the administration of hormones (either orally or by injection) or by the removal of organs that produce hormones (ovaries, testicles, adrenal glands or the pituitary gland). The goal is to reduce the body's production of, or to block the action of, hormones that promote the growth of certain types of tumors. Cancers of the prostate, breast and kidney have been controlled or significantly reduced by hormonal therapy. The mechanisms are still only partly understood, but the role of hormonal-receptor proteins is a key element.

Hormone receptors are special proteins on the surface of both normal and cancer cells that "lock on" to particular hormones manufactured by the body and transport them into the cell. The prevalence and types of hormonal receptors on the cancer cells removed in surgery are impor-

tant in predicting whether a cancer will respond to hormonal therapy. Tests for hormone receptors are a part of the pathologist's examination of the surgically removed tissue. When a specific receptor is absent, it is considered "negative." Negative receptors are associated with an increased risk of a recurrence.

As an example, breast cancers are generally tested for both estrogen and progesterone receptors. A sufficient presence of one or both of these receptors indicates that these hormones stimulate the growth of the tumor cells. If a breast tumor is estrogen- and/or progesterone-negative (as opposed to positive), there is an increased risk of recurrence; when the tumor is receptor-positive, there is a higher likelihood that treatment with a hormone such as tamoxifen, which counteracts the effects of those hormones, will reduce the rate of recurrence.

ADMINISTERING AND MONITORING CHEMOTHERAPY

Chemotherapeutic drugs are given in pill or liquid form, or by injection in either a vein (IV) or an artery. Single or multiple drugs may also be injected (infused) into organs such as the liver, using a small pump that delivers a constant flow of drugs. The method of administration depends on the drugs and on the protocol or program therapy designed for each type and stage of cancer. For example, certain drugs are given only intravenously because, when taken orally, they are not readily absorbed in the gastrointestinal tract or produce gastrointestinal side effects such as nausea or diarrhea.

The number of office visits can be reduced when chemotherapy is given orally, though many drugs must be given by injection or infusion. With oral administration, periodic office visits are still necessary for blood tests to check the amount of oral chemotherapy needed. A more complex chemotherapeutic program may require more frequent office visits, often three to five days in a row, or alternating periods of therapy and rest. Your physician will determine the method by which therapy is given in consultation with you.

It is crucial to monitor and evaluate the body's response to therapy. The chief procedures include blood counts, x-ray tests, CT scans, MRI scans, special isotope scans, blood chemistry panels of liver or kidney function, serum cancer markers (CEA, CA 15-3, CA-125, CA 19-9), physical examinations and assessments of the patient's general body function and physical status.

In addition to their usefulness in evaluating the effectiveness of treatment, these procedures provide a means of detecting toxicity and reducing side effects. They also serve as safeguards before a decision is made to continue with current therapy or to proceed with a new form of therapy.

Adjuvant Chemotherapy Adjuvant chemotherapy is chemotherapy administered to patients who have a high risk of recurrence of their cancer. It is given after the primary treatment; the primary treatment could be surgery or radiation therapy. The goal of adjuvant chemotherapy is to eliminate undetectable microscopic cells that may have traveled to other parts of the body. If this treatment does not lead to a cure, it usually will prolong the interval before a recurrence.

The most widely used adjuvant chemotherapeutic program is for breast cancer, when one of the following three conditions exists: cancer cells have been found in the lymph nodes during surgery; the tumor is large, indicating a possibility of metastasis, or the tumor has negative hormone receptors (*see* "Hormonal Therapy" in this chapter).

Adjuvant therapy for breast cancer is usually administered for 4 to 9 months.

Neoadjuvant Chemotherapy Neoadjuvant chemotherapy refers to the use of drugs as the primary therapy before surgery or radiotherapy. Its goal is to reduce the size of a large tumor. With initially large tumors, such as large breast or head and neck cancers, surgery and radiotherapy can be more successful after the tumors have been shrunk by neoadjuvant chemotherapy treatments. The use of chemotherapy before other treatments may also help to reduce the incidence of metastatic disease.

CANCER TREATMENTS UNDER INVESTIGATION

Bone Marrow Transplantation A bone marrow transplant is a supportive therapy that allows the use of very-high-dose chemotherapy as a means of curing cancer or delaying its growth in patients with metastatic disease. High-dose chemotherapy can be toxic enough to deplete the bone marrow (where white blood cells, red blood cells and platelets are made). To help the bone marrow to recover, healthy bone marrow—from a relative or other person who is a blood (HLA) match (allogeneic donor), or from the patient's own previously donated bone marrow or peripheral venous blood (autologous stem cell donation)—is transplanted into the patient after the high-dose chemotherapy has been administered.

Additional support is needed with this procedure. This consists of regular blood and platelet transfusions, antibiotics for infections and nutritional support. Results are still too preliminary to predict how successful the procedure will become; more time is needed to determine whether the positive results signify a cure or a delay in disease recurrence. Bone marrow transplantation is discussed in detail in Chapter 4.

Hyperthermia Hyperthermia, the use of heat in the treatment of cancer, has been practiced periodically for 4,000 years. Since 1900, there has been mounting evidence that tumor cells can be killed by heating tumors to 108°F (42° to 43°C) for a short time.

Hyperthermia works because cancer cells are more sensitive to heat than normal cells. Additionally, most tumors have poor circulation (blood supply), which means that they tend to retain heat and cannot eliminate it as well as normal cells.

The heat is often delivered by a radio frequency that can heat internally without damaging the skin. Local tumors and many metastatic tumors can be treated in this way. After treatment, the dead tumor cells (known as tumor necrosis) are replaced by scar tissue. The use of radiation therapy or chemotherapy concurrently with hyperthermia may enhance the anticancer therapeutic effect.

Although still considered experimental, hyperthermia may well become a fifth modality of cancer treatment when further improvements in methods of application are combined with appropriate combinations of chemotherapy and/or radiation therapy.

Immunotherapy The concept of immunotherapy is based on the body's natural defense system, which protects us against a variety of diseases. Although we are less aware of it, the immune system also works to aid our recovery from many illnesses.

For many years, physicians believed that the immune system was effective only in combating infectious diseases caused by such invading agents as bacteria and viruses. More recently, we have learned that the immune system may play a central role in protecting the body against cancer and in combating cancer that has already developed. This latter role is not well understood, but there is evidence that in many cancer patients the immune system does slow down the growth and spread of tumors and can be further stimulated to treat and cure cancer. Perhaps equally important is the body's ability to develop an immune reaction to tumors that may help determine which patients are cured of cancer using conventional therapies including surgery, radiation and drugs.

One immediate goal of research in cancer immunology is the development of methods to harness and enhance the body's natural tendency to defend itself against malignant tumors. If this can be accomplished, medicine will have a new and powerful weapon to add to its arsenal of anticancer treatments.

Of all the experimental possibilities on the horizon, immunotherapy seems to offer the greatest promise of a new dimension in cancer treatment. But it is still very much in its infancy. Although some clinical trials of immunotherapy in humans are in progress, an enormous amount of research remains to be done before their findings can be widely applied.

Immunotherapy began about 100 years ago when Dr. William Coley at the Sloan-Kettering Institute showed that he could control the growth of some cancers and cure a few advanced cancers with injections of a mixed vaccine of streptococcal and staphylococcal bacteria known as Coley's toxin. The French tuberculosis vaccine Bacillus Calmette-Guérin (BCG), developed in 1922, is known to stimulate the immune system and is now used to treat bladder, melanoma and other cancers.

Research efforts are now leading to several promising possibilities of treatment with a form of immunotherapy known as biological modifiers Two biological modifiers are cytokines and monoclonal antibodies.

Interferons and Other Cytokines Interferons are proteins that belong to a group of proteins known as cytokines. They are produced naturally by white blood cells in the body (or in the laboratory) in response to a viral infection or similar stimulation. They have been used as a treatment for certain viral diseases such as herpes zoster or "adult chicken pox."

Interferons are being tested as treatment against various cancers including melanomas, breast cancer, lymphomas and bladder cancer. Tumor shrinkage after treatment with interferons has also been reported in non-Hodgkin's lymphoma, renal carcinoma, hairy cell leukemia and chronic myelogenous leukemia. The preliminary results of these interferon studies are promising. Interferon-alpha was one of the first cytokines to show an antitumor effect (both directly and indirectly) through activating the immune system. Interferon-beta and interferon-gamma are newer cytokines that are being investigated.

Cytokines with antitumor activity that are not interferons include the interleukins (e.g., IL-2) and tumor necrosis factor. Some of the problems with all cytokines, interferons, interleukins and tumor necrosis factor are their side effects, such as malaise and flu-like syndromes.

Monoclonal Antibodies Another important biological-modifier technique involves synthesizing new antibodies using hybridoma cells. (A hybridoma is a cell cloned by fusing two different types of cells.) The antibodies produced are called monoclonal antibodies. To produce them, scientists combine single cells from mice and humans, programming them to produce a single specific antibody that is designed to seek out and destroy cancer cells without affecting the body's normal cells. Monoclonal antibodies made from hybridomas also have the potential for diagnosing as well as treating cancer.

By techniques of genetic engineering, the hybridoma cells that are used to produce the antitumor antibodies are mediated and can be maintained indefinitely as microscopic tissue-culture factories. The monoclonal antibody product from these cells is injected into a patient, where it seeks out the patient's cancer cells.

Researchers are studying ways of binding cytotoxic chemicals and radioisotopes to monoclonal antibodies to enhance the former's effectiveness against cancer cells; in this case the antibodies would function as a targeted delivery mechanism as well as a therapy. The result would be like a "guided missile" capable of seeking out a specific target—a cancer cell. From early clinical studies, it appears that the new monoclonal antibody treatment technique will increase our ability to eradicate human cancer.

Immunotherapy with biological modifiers is still an experimental form of treatment. Many scientists and clinicians believe that its greatest utility will be in the treatment of patients with a small but otherwise incurable tumor burden (e.g., a small number of cancer cells scattered throughout the body). Therefore, many of the current clinical studies are set up to prevent recurrence in patients whose cancer has been removed or reduced by conventional therapy such as surgery, chemotherapy or radiotherapy. Helping the body in its attempt to develop an immune reaction to tumors may prove to be a decisive factor in assuming that patients are cured of their cancer after they have received conventional therapy.

Vaccine Therapies Vaccine therapies are being developed and tested in clinical trials as another form of immunotherapy. Preliminary results in the treatment of melanoma and other cancers indicate that vaccine programs show promise and are becoming more available to treat a wider variety of human cancers.

EXPERIMENTAL THERAPEUTIC APPROACHES

Physicians and other scientists are constantly developing new and experimental therapeutic approaches to cancer.* Unique combinations of the three standard anticancer therapies of surgery, radiation and chemotherapy (known as multimodality therapy) and experimental immunotherapy are examples of recent innovations.

Experimental approaches to cancer treatment undergo lengthy testing in the laboratory and in animals before being introduced into human medicine. But we cannot draw conclusions from evidence from animal experiments, and there comes a moment of truth when an experimental treatment is justified for trial with cancer patients (called a clinical trial). Patients participating in experimental treatments are always given a detailed explanation of the reasons why their doctor feels that an experimental treatment is justified in their case. There is an unwritten law that an unproven experimental therapy is never used on any patient for whom there remains a tried and effective nonexperimental treatment. Experimental therapy is used only when there is a reasonable basis for believing it will be superior to conventional therapy.

Clinical Trials Depending on the type and stage of your cancer, your doctor might recommend a new treatment that has not yet been proved effective. The word *investigational* might come up. Or *experimental* might be the term used. If the standard treatment options available to you aren't likely to be effective, your doctor might suggest that you take part in a clinical trial.

All these terms might make you feel more than a little anxious. They shouldn't. Investigational treatments that are being given a clinical trial are used only under very stringent conditions. They wouldn't be used at all if there wasn't some hope they would be more effective than other treatments.

What a Clinical Trial Is Advances in cancer treatment usually come about because of some clever idea or concept for a new therapy proposed by a cancer research physician. After a new anticancer drug has been found to be effective against one or more experimental tumor systems in the lab, it is tested in rats or other small animals to find out which dosage might be both effective and reasonably safe for humans. The treatment is eventually tested in a large number of patients (clinical trial) to find out two things: Is it effective? And is it as good as or better than unconventional treatments? The treatment's safety is also investigated through testing for adverse effects.

It takes several hundred and sometimes several thousand patients to prove quickly and reliably whether a new treatment will work and is worthwhile. It is almost impossible to conduct a trial in any single

*From *Everyone's Guide to Cancer Therapy*, 3rd ed., by Malin Dolllinger, MD, Ernest H. Rosenbaum, MD, and Greg Cable.

hospital or cancer center. The concept of cooperative clinical trials, involving several clinical settings and doctors, was developed for just this reason. The rules and procedures for clinical trials are standardized and quite specific.

The Clinical Protocol A clinical trial consists of an exact written description of a treatment program that is called the clinical protocol. This is formulated and written with great care. Not only do the researchers need to be sure that the trial will answer the two main questions about effectiveness, but they must also safeguard the rights of the patients being treated. The risks involved have to be minimized and disclosed to all participants. The clinical protocol outlines the criteria for patients who might participate in the trial. It also describes what tests will be done and how the researchers will determine whether a tumor is responding. Systems for monitoring the patient and checking for any adverse effects will be detailed. And there will be provisions for "informed consent" and for the patient's right to drop out of the trial at any time.

Who Approves the Trial The entire project has to be approved by a human use committee made up of physicians and nonphysicians who have no relationship with the study. The members of this committee certify that the patients' rights are protected, that the trial is reasonable and logical and that the study will answer the questions it is supposed to answer. The same committee reviews the progress of the trial and its results. The Cancer Therapy Branch of the National Cancer Institute also keeps watch on these investigational studies.

The Importance of Clinical Trials Almost every advance in cancer treatment over the past 20 years has come about because of clinical trials. In fact, just about every

chemotherapy drug and radiation treatment now considered standard therapy was first given in a clinical Phase I trial. These treatments were given to patients who were willing to be in the forefront of advances in medical knowledge.

For example, the willingness of thousands of women to participate in clinical trials by the National Surgical Adjuvant Breast Project (NSABP) has resulted in answers to extremely important treatment questions. These trials have formed the basis for adjuvant chemotherapy in breast cancer patients with a high risk for recurrence even though no apparent tumor is left after surgery. This treatment has saved many lives.

The Three Phases of Clinical Trials Whether for surgery, chemotherapy, radiotherapy or biological therapy, clinical trials are always conducted in three phases.

Phase I About 20 human patients are treated with the same drug. There is no assurance or certainty that a significant tumor response will occur, although, again, every single anticancer drug now useful in therapy was initially a Phase I agent. During this phase, various dosage levels are tried.

Patients selected for these trials are almost always in cancer research centers and have already received all known effective anticancer therapy. After the proposed treatment is explained to them, they must volunteer to receive the new treatment. There is, therefore, no moral objection to giving this new treatment. Since there is "nothing to lose," it is hoped that a specific new agent may in fact prove effective.

This phase is completed when no unusual problems or toxic effects have been found and the dose necessary to produce a biologic effect has been determined. The study can then move to the next phase.

Phase II In this phase, 10 to 20 patients are treated, each having one of the various types of tumors known to be responsive to chemotherapy. These might include lymphomas, breast cancer or colon cancer. Since these tumor types are known to be responsive, the patients will be those who have already received all standard forms of chemotherapy that seem reasonable; therefore, participation in a Phase II trial does not deprive anyone of any therapy already proven to be effective. If a significant number of patients with each type of tumor respond to the therapy, the trial moves to the next phase.

Phase III In this phase, the number of participants is increased greatly, and the new drug therapy is compared with standard treatment to see if there is an improvement in the response or if the same response rate is achieved but with fewer toxic side effects. Usually there is a control group that receives the chemotherapy already proven to be effective.

A therapy tested in a drug-related clinical trial does not necessarily involve a drug not already in clinical use. A new treatment or therapy often consists of standard drugs used in a new combination or a new sequence, in new dosages or even administered in a new way. If a new drug is involved, and the Phase III trial is successful, the National Cancer Institute will approve the drug for general use. Eventually, the new therapy might become the standard treatment.

Clinical Trials and the "Approved" Uses of Drugs When using anticancer chemicals, it is important for both you and your doctor to be aware of how the pharmaceutical industry works. Once drug companies have fulfilled the lengthy and complex testing and the drawn-out legal procedures required to market a new drug, they tend not to devote a lot of effort to discovering new uses for that drug. They more or less delegate this responsibility to the cancer physicians conducting clinical trials.

Every drug comes with an official package insert detailing what dosage to use for what illness. This information is also listed in the *Physician's Desk Reference*. These summaries usually contain only the information "passed" by the government's approval agencies. Why this is important is that many drug programs in standard use for cancer are not listed as "approved." Such drugs are used because experience with patients has shown them to be effective. About half of the current uses of anticancer drugs in the United States and Canada are for indications and schedules that are not given in the official inserts.

Since the inserts do not necessarily reflect the most up-to-date cancer research, the current standard use of these drugs, or even their optimum use, your doctor should not be restricted to printed drug-listing materials. In fact, the appropriate use of anticancer drugs may be for indications not listed in such official sources.

This is another reason why an oncologist can be a useful member of your health care team. Cancer physicians are up-to-date on the most recent research findings and important advances in treatment even though that information may not appear in the drug-related literature.

UNPROVEN AND QUACK TREATMENTS

Living with cancer creates a state of uncertainty, insecurity and fear that at times is unendurable. It is understandable that anxiety can reach so high a level that a person will be willing to try an unproven method of treatment that has been publicized in the press as a "miracle cure." Among those who resort to these therapies are people who are receiving good medical support as well as those who are not. Neither a high level of education nor the ability to reason will deter the desperate patient.

A person who has cancer wants a cure. When standard therapy cannot guarantee a cure, that person may go to any length to obtain a treatment that has not been sanctioned by any reputable doctor, researcher or government agency. No one wants to die without exhausting every possible means of a cure, and a patient is often encouraged by well-meaning friends and family members who have no knowledge of cancer treatment.

Depression and panic alone can make a patient prey to any speculator who claims to have a cure. So can being told that there is no further conventional therapy that offers a reasonable chance of improving one's health.

Some quack practitioners may sincerely believe their methods are effective; others are just capitalizing on other people's misfortune. In any event, quacks with their false cancer cures cost American patients $2 to $3 billion a year. Furthermore, some quack cures can be extremely dangerous.

The clinical course of cancer is highly variable. A remission or a cure can occur without a patient's having received conventional medical treatment, although this is very rare. (Medical literature documents these cases.) However, if this happy event should coincide with or follow treatment by an unproven therapy, the patient will invariably credit that treatment with the improvement.

Whenever newspaper and magazine articles on miracle cures appear, physicians are bombarded with questions about these unorthodox methods of treatment. "What about diet?" "What about megavitamin therapy?" "What about that new drug that is only available abroad?"

Physicians can only reply that in their experience and the experience of other practitioners, these methods have not proved to be of any benefit to cancer patients.

Unfortunately, the press and the public have given enormous attention to the rare success of unproven treatments, without mentioning the thousands of failures of these unproven treatments reported by physicians in medical journals—those tragic cases of failure are due not only to worthless therapies but often to the general poor medical management that accompanies these treatments.

Some of my patients supplement conventional treatment with megadoses of vitamins, Laetrile (a drug derived from apricot pits), coffee enemas and other unorthodox methods. Although I neither approve nor condone the use of these methods, I do not reject such patients for medical therapy, and, if required, I provide them with medical literature on the useless treatment. I also tell them about cases of poisoning and even of death from taking Laetrile. But I do not try to argue with them. It is their choice, and I accept the compromise as long as they also take conventional medical therapy.

In over 35 years of practice, I have yet to see a single positive result from unorthodox treatment, but my colleagues and I have seen hundreds of patients with progressive advancing cancers who first tried a quack therapy. Sometimes, we were able to reverse the process after beginning traditional therapy, but many of these patients lost their chance for a cure by initially opting for a quack therapy.

Some of these treatments and drugs are available in many parts of the United States in spite of federal and state laws forbidding their use. Laetrile is legal in some states under special circumstances (such as when administered at a university research hospital); it is also administered in an unlicensed clinic in Tijuana, Mexico, and in other countries.

In May 1981 researchers from four cancer centers reported the results of the first government-sponsored tests on Laetrile carried out by the National Cancer Institute. The researchers found the drug to be useless. Patients participating in the test showed no improvement or slowing of growth of their advanced cancer, and no easing of the symptoms of the disease.

The federal Pure Food, Drug and Cosmetic Act stipulates that a producer of a new drug (or treatment method) must prove that it is not only safe but also effective if it is to be licensed for public use. The act also provides for strict controls over investigational and experimental drugs and the sale of prescription drugs.

Unless drugs are approved by the FDA, they cannot legally be distributed through interstate commerce. It is a federal crime, reinforced by our postal laws, to advertise or ship such products. Nine states prohibit the distribution and sale of unlicensed drugs and methods within the state, but until more states reinforce the federal legislation, unproved treat-ments will continue to be promoted and sold. In the states that have not passed their own laws, ways have been found to circumvent the federal ban against false claims in advertising.

The FDA has published booklets, such as "The Big Quack Attack: Medical Devices," that describe various methods of quackery and tell consumers how to register complaints about practitioners of these methods.

The Office of Alternative Medicine was established in 1992 as a part of the National Institutes of Health. Its mission is to evaluate the merits of complementary and alternative methods to cure or relieve symptoms of cancer and other illness. This is an important step in the effort to clarify the role of complementary and alternative treatments for cancer.

Considering the fear, insecurity, frustration and ignorance of the average patient or family in despair, the readiness to believe in promised cures is understandable. The best solution is knowledge, understanding and communication.

4
BONE MARROW TRANSPLANTATION

Keren Stronach, MPH

A bone marrow transplant (BMT) is similar to a blood transfusion. In a bone marrow transplant, high-dose chemotherapy, and in some cases radiation, is used to destroy cancerous or diseased cells in the body. The treatment also destroys a person's bone marrow, the site where blood cells are produced. To restore the ability to make blood cells, a person must be given healthy marrow to replace the marrow that was destroyed.

The bone marrow transplant was developed in the late 1960s to treat cancers and diseases of the bone marrow. Since then the procedure has been refined and expanded to treat many other conditions, including cancers and diseases that do not involve the bone marrow. In the last few years, for example, it has become increasingly common to treat breast cancer, ovarian cancer and testicular cancer with a BMT. In these cases, when the bone marrow is healthy, a person's own marrow can be used. There are three types of transplant: autologous, allogeneic and syngeneic. The type you will have depends on whether you use your own bone marrow or the marrow of a donor.

AUTOLOGOUS TRANSPLANT

In an autologous transplant, a person's own healthy bone marrow cells are removed and stored until the time of the transplant. Chemotherapy, and in some cases radiation, is then administered to destroy diseased cells. This treatment also destroys the remaining bone marrow. The marrow cells that were removed before the treatment are then returned to the patient.

Usually, autologous transplants are done when the bone marrow is healthy and the disease lies elsewhere in the body. In some instances, however, autologous transplants are done even when the bone marrow is diseased. When this is the case, the bone marrow that is removed may be purged, or treated to clear out cancer cells. BMT centers across the country use different methods to purge marrow. It will be up to you and your physician to decide how your marrow will be treated if it needs to be purged.

ALLOGENEIC TRANSPLANT

When a person cannot be his or her own donor and the marrow needs to be taken from someone else, the transplant is called an allogeneic transplant. If the donor is a relative, the transplant is called a related allogeneic transplant. If it is from an unrelated donor, it is an unrelated allogeneic transplant. To find a donor, you will need to have your blood tested and typed so that it can be matched to blood samples of potential donors. This is done through a test called the human leukocyte antigen (HLA) test that examines certain antigens, or proteins, on the surface of your white blood cells. These antigens serve as a kind of "fingerprint" and play an important role in the body's ability to distinguish between "self" and "other." Three pairs of antigens, known as HLA-A, HLA-B and HLA-DR, are considered most important in determining the degree of fit between you and your donor. If you match your donor on these important sites, there is a good chance that your new marrow will recognize you as self and will function effectively in your body. If you do not match your donor on these sites, the donor's marrow may recognize certain organs or tissues in your body as foreign and may attack them. This is called graft-versus-host disease (GVHD). The more closely matched you are to your donor, the less likely you are to get GVHD. (*See* "Graft-Versus-Host Disease" later in this chapter.)

SYNGENEIC TRANSPLANT

In a syngeneic transplant, the donor is an identical twin and the new marrow will be genetically identical to the destroyed bone marrow.

WHAT IS BONE MARROW?

Bone marrow is the spongy center of your bones where blood is produced. It is also the home of your immune system. Bone marrow contains the parent cells, called stem cells, that later mature into white blood cells, red blood cells and platelets. The numbers of your blood cells will be closely monitored throughout the transplant process. As your transplanted marrow begins to produce blood cells, your blood counts will begin to rise and you will begin to regain your immunity, strength and energy.

◆ *White blood cells*, or leukocytes, are cells that fight infection and are an important part of your immune system. When your white count is low, you are at greatest risk for infection. During the transplant, your white count will be carefully monitored. Neutrophils are a common type of white cell that play an important role in fighting infection by bacteria and yeast. During the transplant, your medical team will be closely monitoring your neutrophil count, which is also referred to as your ANC (absolute neutrophil count).

◆ *Red blood cells*, or erythrocytes, are cells that carry oxygen from the lungs to the rest of the body. The oxygen is carried in the red blood cell on a molecule called hemoglobin. During the transplant, your hemoglobin levels will be monitored to determine when you will need a red blood cell transfusion.

◆ *Platelets* are essential in the process of clotting, thus preventing excess bleeding and bruising. When your platelet count is low, your risk of bleeding is high. Your platelets will therefore also be monitored to assess your risk of bleeding and to determine when a platelet transfusion is needed.

◆ Once the *stem cells* in the bone marrow are destroyed by chemotherapy or radiation treatment, you will no longer be able to produce life-sustaining blood cells unless you receive new stem cells to replace those that were destroyed. The stem cells will be taken either from you or from your donor and will be given to you during the transplant.

PREPARING FOR THE TRANSPLANT

Once the difficult decision to undergo a transplant has been made, several important steps can be taken to prepare for the experience. On an emotional level, preparing for a transplant may entail spending time with friends and family or taking time out to be alone to experience one's feelings about the transplant. On a physical level, this may include eating a healthful diet, getting good dental care and maintaining an exercise routine. On a practical level, it may mean choosing a transplant center, organizing caregiving arrangements and obtaining items for the hospital stay.

EMOTIONAL PREPARATION

Facing the prospect of a transplant can be devastating, evoking feelings of dread, panic and helplessness. Coming to grips with the idea that you may have a life-threatening disease while simultaneously dealing with a tremendous volume of information and new medical jargon can be mind numbing. As you face the transplant and the most serious questions of life, it is common to feel overwhelmed by emotions. During this time, you are likely to experience feelings of anxiety, self-pity and self-blame. It is also normal to feel betrayed by your body, and feel anger and jealousy toward others who do not have to face the same ordeals that you face. At times, you may find that your feelings undergo intense fluctuations, alternating between hope, anticipation and fear.

Another reaction you may have is denial. You may find yourself responding to the situation by becoming emotionally numb and very task oriented. As you go through various emotional responses, be understanding and gentle with yourself. After all, you are facing some of the most difficult choices and most stressful conditions you will ever face.

The transplant may also be seen as a new lease on life and, as such, a source of great solace and hope as well as a great challenge to be overcome. Radical alterations in emotions and moods, as well as periods of relative calm, are all part of the common ways of reacting to the transplant.

How you choose to cope with the prospective transplant depends on how you perceive it, your feelings, your personality and your own individual way of coping. You may wish to take a highly active stance in the process and research all medical and alternative options, or hand over control to others, or do some combination of the two. Do whatever works for you. In the following sections you will find suggestions and strategies that others have found useful. I hope that you will find some suggestions that will be of benefit to you.

Express Your Emotions If you are experiencing great anxiety or fear, give yourself permission to express these emotions so that you can process them. Choose to express your emotions to people who are personally meaningful to you and who can be supportive. If certain people are unhelpful, don't feel guilty about avoiding them and focusing on your own needs. Seeing a professional therapist, particularly one who has had experience counseling people with life-threatening diseases, can be very helpful.

Contact a BMT Survivor Contacting someone who has undergone a transplant can be very helpful and calming. This can be done through the National Bone Marrow Transplant Link, where you can leave a message requesting to speak to a BMT survivor who has been in a situation similar to your own. A peer volunteer who has undergone a transplant will usually return your call within a few days. Another possibility is to ask a member of your medical team or your social worker to put you in touch with someone who has undergone a transplant. If you are on the Internet, one way to get in touch with many transplant survivors is to sign on to a computer mailing list that specializes in bone marrow transplants or certain kinds of cancer.

Explore Books and Tapes Books describing the experiences of others with cancer can be particularly helpful, as can many of the self-help books about coping and relaxation. Some survivors have found that certain self-help books make them feel responsible for causing their disease. In reading these books, remember that you are not in any way to blame for your condition. Cancer is caused by complex reasons having to do with environmental, genetic, social and individual factors. Cancer can strike anyone. If a book you are reading makes you feel upset, put it down. You are not obligated to read a book just because a well-meaning friend has recommended it to you. You may even consider asking a friend to read and summarize the main points of a book or article for you.

Reduce Stress During this stressful and anxiety-producing time, it might be helpful to think of ways that you can reduce superfluous stress in your life. Although you may not be able to avoid some of the factors that are producing stress, such as the cancer, there may be ways to cope with your stress. Establishing a clear set of priorities and letting go of less important obligations can reduce the amount of pressure that you feel. Some people find it useful to make a list of the factors contributing to stress and examining ways to reduce the pressures. One suggestion is to allocate tasks to family and friends who want to help. Some friends may be willing, for example, to help you gather information about different transplant centers or to help you find books and tapes about visualization or some other topic of interest.

Many of those who feel close to you are likely to feel helpless in the face of your diagnosis and impending transplant. By giving them concrete suggestions, you may be not only helping yourself but helping them as well. For some, continuing with their normal routine is the most effective way of reducing stress.

Practice Relaxation Techniques Practicing stress-reduction techniques that feel nurturing, such as muscle relaxation, meditation, hypnosis or imagery, may be helpful to you. Some people find that meditation reduces their level of anxiety and is helpful in combating depression as well as lowering their level of discomfort and pain.

Get in Touch with Your Spirituality Spirituality can be an important source of comfort during this period. Many patients report that prayer or meditation can be a source of support and psychological well-being.

Participate in Activities You Enjoy You can reduce stress by incorporating activities that you find most relaxing, healing and fun. Finding creative outlets for your feelings or creative ways to feed feelings of hope can also be an effective way of coping with emotions and reducing stress. Some people find that it is helpful to write in a journal, for example, or to express themselves through painting or dance.

Take Care of Loose Ends Taking care of loose ends and putting your affairs in order does not necessarily mean you are expecting a negative outcome. Sometimes, by dealing with difficult issues that may come up in the event of one's death, it is possible to put these issues aside and focus on more positive things. Some people have found that they need to put their financial affairs in order and take care of lingering interpersonal issues before fully focusing on the issues of treatment and recovery. This may also be a time to pay off outstanding loans or to arrange for Social Security Disability so as to reduce financial pressures post-transplant. At this time, you may also wish to keep a notebook handy to record important information and phone numbers, particularly since during times of upheaval, it may be more difficult to remember everything.

Don't Take People's Reactions Personally
People who are close to you may be undergoing a lot of emotional turmoil themselves as a result of your diagnosis. They may feel helpless and panicked and may not know how to reach out and communicate. You may feel abandoned at times, or feel angry with loved ones for not comprehending your needs. These emotions are understandable and normal. However, remember that everyone involved may need some extra understanding and compassion during this difficult period. In some cases, friends or family members may withdraw, not because they don't care but because they are too overwhelmed by their own feelings of fear, helplessness and uncertainty about how to treat you. If you do get some unexpected reactions from loved ones, remember that their reactions probably have a lot to do with their own internal turmoil.

Seek Medical Information Seeking medical information can sometimes reduce fear and help people regain a sense of control. This can be done through library research, by talking to doctors or former transplant patients, by visiting transplant centers and by contacting cancer organizations that have knowledgeable people who can respond to your questions and concerns.

In seeking information, remember that it is always appropriate to seek a second or even third opinion. When, where and how you will be transplanted may prove to be the most important decision of your life, and you should feel free, if not obligated, to seek a number of medical opinions.

When consulting a physician, don't hesitate to ask for information a second or third time. Having a close friend or family member attend doctor's meetings with you can be useful, as it will allow you to review the information with someone else and to confirm that you understood the information. Taping the medical sessions can be helpful.

Take Time for Yourself Often, in times of stress, people become forgetful or experience mood swings. In this difficult period, take time to extend understanding and compassion to yourself. Give yourself permission to change your mind, to take things one day at a time, to pamper yourself and to be sad. By taking the time to re-evaluate and to make changes in your life, you may find that some of the best parts of your life may be expanding during the time when you are facing the worst trauma of your life. Allow yourself to think deeply about who you are and what matters to you so that you can prioritize your life and expand those areas that are most meaningful to you. Try, as much as possible, not to give up hope. Michael Lerner writes in *Choices in Healing*, page 7, "Give yourself permission to hope, even in the face of all the statistics that physicians may present to you. Statistics are only statistics. They are not you. There is no such thing as false hope." This does not mean that you need to be positive all the time. You are still entitled to "bad" days.

PHYSICAL PREPARATION

Exercise Many people undertake a regular exercise routine to improve their physical conditioning in preparation for the transplant. The extent and the rigor of the exercise you choose will depend in part on your general activity level and physical condition at the time. Some people will be able to exercise vigorously, whereas others may take on moderate routines involving just short walks or stretches in bed. Ideally, you should find some kind of exercise you enjoy. Joining a gym or finding friends who enjoy similar physical activities may be helpful. In addition to conferring physical benefits, exercise may be a helpful way to channel stress and promote general well-being.

If your medical condition does not allow you to undertake a rigorous exercise routine, be aware that many people enter the transplant in poor physical shape and do extremely well. To the extent that exercise is an option for you, consider doing some mode of exercise suited to your medical condition. Chapter 21 offers many suggestions for activities that you can do at various levels of fitness.

Nutrition Eating a healthful diet and meeting your basic nutritional needs is important before a transplant. We all know that a well-nourished body fights infection, aids healing and deals with the demands of very aggressive treatment protocols better than a poorly nourished one. It is beyond the scope of this chapter to discuss in detail the different alternative nutritional therapies. If you are considering an alternative diet, ensure that it provides all the necessary nutrients. Unless you are severely obese, it is not advisable to undergo rapid weight loss immediately before cancer therapy.

The guidelines for maintaining good health, as recommended by the National Academy of Sciences and the American Cancer Society, are covered in detail in Chapter 16.

Dental Care Good dental care before your transplant is an essential part of your overall preparation for transplant. Healthy gums and teeth can prevent infections and some of the painful mouth sores that may develop during transplant. Meticulous mouth care before and during transplant can also protect against infections by limiting the number of open sores in the mouth. Taking care of lingering gum and tooth problems is also important because it is strongly advised that you refrain from any routine dental care for some time after your transplant,

until your immune system is strong and fully functional again.

To have your mouth in the best shape possible before the transplant, you will need to adopt good personal oral hygiene. This may entail regular flossing and brushing as well as using antiseptic mouth rinses. Before taking on a rigorous dental regimen, however, consult your dentist to review the correct way to floss and brush your teeth and to request a recommendation for a good toothbrush and mouth rinse.

Fertility People undergoing treatment with total-body irradiation and some forms of chemotherapy have a high risk of becoming infertile. If you are considering having children after the transplant, you may consider undergoing fertility treatment before the transplant. For males, sperm banking is a possibility. This entails contacting a sperm bank in your area and freezing and storing sperm for use post-transplant.

For women, the situation is more complicated, as they cannot simply freeze their eggs. Women can, however, freeze fertilized eggs. In this process, women undergo hormonal treatment to induce ovulation. Once the eggs mature, they are surgically removed, fertilized in a test tube with sperm, and then frozen for later implantation. Since the procedure is time consuming, it should be undertaken well before the transplant date. Before undertaking this procedure, women should make sure that their medical condition allows for the procedures involved.

A new and still experimental option for women is to freeze an ovary or a portion of it before transplant and to have it reimplanted post-transplant. The advantage to this procedure is that women may be able to regain ovarian function post-transplant and thus avoid the risks associated with early menopause. Another advantage to this procedure is that there is no need for fertilization of the eggs and the procedure is cheaper than embryo storage. There is also a small possibility that women undergoing this procedure may regain their fertility. At the time of this writing, only a handful of women have had their ovaries stored, and none have had them reimplanted. In animal studies, mice and sheep that had their ovaries reimplanted regained not only ovarian function but also, in some cases, fertility and gave birth to healthy offspring. For more information about fertility treatments, see Resources at the end of this book.

Although the majority of people undergoing a transplant will lose their fertility, some patients may in rare instances regain fertility.

PRACTICAL PREPARATIONS

Choosing a Center There are distinct advantages to having the transplant at a large experienced center with an excellent track record. If you have such a center close to home, the choice of where to do the transplant will be easy. If, however, there is no center near your home or it has a poor track record or has performed fewer than five transplants of the kind you need, the choice may be more difficult.

Undergoing a transplant at a large BMT center with a good track record and a great deal of experience provides you with a sense of security that the physicians and staff will be able to handle unexpected complications should they arise. Bigger centers may, in some cases, also have the advantage of having access to large blood banks that can cater to the needs of transplant patients. Large blood banks, for example, are more likely to set aside CMV-negative blood products, which will reduce the risk of CMV (cytomegalovirus) infection. However, large research centers may have the dis-

advantage of being more impersonal than small centers.

Having the transplant in a BMT center close to home allows you to be close to family and friends and to have a strong support system on hand. You will also save on travel expenses and will not have to deal with the hassle of moving to an unfamiliar place. Your life and the life of your caregiver will be less likely to be disrupted, and you may have the advantage of already being familiar with some of the doctors and staff.

Calling the National Marrow Donor Program (NMDP) to get a listing of BMT centers is an excellent way to get initial information about various BMT centers. The NMDP guide contains phone numbers and addresses of most transplant centers with information about the number and type of transplants performed at each center as well as some statistics about survival rates at each center.

In looking at these statistics, you should be aware that the general statistics often include all categories of age groups and illnesses and thus may be inapplicable to you. In order to really compare survival rates at several BMT units, ask directly about the survival rate for your age group, your illness and the type of transplant you will undergo. Getting this information may be difficult and frustrating, as some centers are reluctant to disclose this information. Since gathering this information can be stressful, you may consider recruiting friends or your doctor to help you with this task.

Signing on to bone marrow transplant information bulletin boards or newsgroups on the Internet can be another useful way to get information. Many transplant survivors read these boards daily, answer questions and share information about their experience. See the section on BMT in Resources at the end of the book.

Calling up centers to ask questions can provide useful information and give you a better sense of the transplant center and its atmosphere. Things you may wish to inquire about include:

1. How many transplants has the center done for people with your specific condition? (Ideally, you should undergo a transplant at a center that has done at least five transplants of the type that you need.)
2. Are you going to have the same staff treating you throughout the transplant? (At many BMT centers the doctors and the physician assistants rotate monthly.)
3. Will you be allowed to walk in the halls or will you be confined to your room? (Some centers allow patients to walk around the unit, whereas others do not.)
4. Will you have access to an exercise machine? Will you be visited by a physical therapist?
5. Will you have access to a social worker or counselor during the transplant?
6. Can the hospital accommodate your dietary needs? Can you ask for food at any time of the day or do you have to order it a day in advance? Are you allowed to eat raw fruits and vegetables? (Having a flexible eating schedule can be helpful as you may be nauseated and may not want to eat during conventional mealtimes.)
7. What is the average time that the nurses have worked in the BMT unit?
8. How experienced are the physicians at the center and are specialists available to handle complications should they arise?
9. Is there a support group for patients or their families?
10. What is the survival rate for patients with your condition in your age group undergoing your type of transplant?
11. How does the staff feel about patients putting up "Do Not Disturb" or "Please Knock" signs on the door?
12. Could someone who has undergone a transplant at the center contact you to tell you about his or her experience?
13. What is the visitor policy? How flexible is it? (Having your caregiver stay at the hospital overnight can be very comforting.)
14. What living arrangements can be made for you and your family if you need to move away from your home to the transplant center? What will living expenses cost?
15. Can the center provide any assistance to defray some of the family's expenses?
16. Does the center have a long-term follow-up department that is easily accessible and will respond to questions once you leave the transplant center? (This is particularly important if your oncologist has little experience with BMTs.)
17. If you are undergoing an allogeneic transplant, does the center have a donor search coordinator and a quality tissue typing facility?

Visiting the transplant center before the transplant to familiarize yourself with the transplant setting and some of the staff is often comforting. While you are there, you might inquire if you can speak to patients undergoing transplants at the center to get their impressions, feedback and tips.

If you need to travel to your transplant center, you may save money by contacting companies that provide discounts for medically necessary travel. Most of the major national cancer organizations will have information about these companies. Often airlines provide discounted fares for patients and their caregivers. Organizations such as the

Leukemia Society of America and Cancer Care often reimburse travel expenses to and from medical centers.

Caregiving Arrangements During the transplant, you will need at least one family member or a friend who can provide you with emotional and physical support. This person is often referred to as a caregiver. In many cases, it will be possible for you to have only one caregiver with you. If this is the case, you may consider arranging occasional visits by other family members or friends who can provide additional support during weekends so that the caregiving task does not fall on just one person.

Even though many people successfully make it through the transplant with only one caregiver, and in some cases alone, having two or more caregivers is a real plus. Then, each one can have time to rest and can return to the hospital more refreshed. Having more than one caregiver also allows you to share your feelings and experiences with more than one person. Since caregivers often experience a high degree of anxiety, sharing the responsibility of caring for you can serve to alleviate some of the tension. Finally, having more than one caregiver provides a safeguard in the event that a caregiver gets sick and is unable to be on the ward.

THE TRANSPLANT PROCESS

Moving to the Transplant Center Leaving your home to go to the transplant center may bring up many strong emotions.

The length of time you will spend in the hospital will depend in part on the type of transplant that you have. Autologous transplants generally require two to three weeks in the hospital or, in some cases, are done on an outpatient basis. Allogeneic transplants often require a hospital stay of four to five weeks or longer, depending on your condition and the pro-

cedures followed at your transplant center.

The Hospital Environment What follows is a description of a typical day at one of the larger transplant centers. It is very likely that the specific times and the details of the routine at your hospital may vary from the one described. The main point to note is that the days at the hospital are often full of activity. People will be coming in and out of your room throughout the day to check on you, to check medical equipment and to clean the room. When your energy level is low, interacting with these various members of the hospital staff and keeping up with the requirements for personal hygiene and exercise can take up a lot of your time and energy. Nevertheless, it is a good idea to have enjoyable things to do for the periods that you are alone and have free time and energy to spare.

A Typical Hospital Day (schedules will vary depending on your condition and medical regimen)

4–6 AM	A nurse draws daily routine blood tests.
7 AM	A nurse's aide checks daily weight.
8 AM	A nurse takes vital signs—temperature, blood pressure and pulse (every four hours).
8:30 AM	Doctors with residents and medical students visit on their daily rounds.
9 AM	Breakfast.

11 AM–3 PM
◆ A person from housekeeping staff cleans the room.
◆ A nurse's aide or nurse changes the bed.
◆ A physician assistant comes by to review general medical condition.
◆ Various people from the hospital staff replenish medical supplies in the room and check the equipment.
◆ A nurse comes in at intervals to administer medication or blood products and

check vital signs.

◆ Once a week, patients are required to have a routine chest x-ray.

◆ Lunch.

4 PM	Vital signs are taken and medications replenished.
6 PM	Dinner.
8–8:30 PM	Bedtime preparations.
12 midnight	Vital signs are taken.

Various medications may be administered throughout the night.

Tip: Organizing a daily schedule of activities can be helpful. In addition to keeping you occupied, a daily schedule can motivate you to keep up important daily activities such as exercising and showering. During the day, you will also have the opportunity to watch movies, walk around the halls, have guests and rest. If the hospital schedule clashes with your desired schedule, discuss your preferences with a nurse to see if you can be accommodated.

STEPS THROUGH THE TRANSPLANT

The Medical Evaluation Upon your arrival to the transplant center, you will often undergo a general medical evaluation involving a physical exam and some lab and diagnostic tests to make sure it is safe to go ahead with the transplant and to provide a baseline for future comparison. These tests may include an eye and dental exam, heart and lung studies, a bone marrow aspiration, a spinal tap and a chest x-ray. These tests may sometimes reveal underlying problems that need to be taken care of before the transplant.

Signing Consent Forms During this period you will be required to sign one or more consent forms for the bone marrow transplant and research procedures if you are doing your transplant at a research center. The consent form is a legal document that protects the hospital from medical liability in case of complications.

Therefore, be forewarned, the consent form often lists some of the most frightening and unsavory complications that may arise from the transplant, including those that may be quite rare.

Central Line Before your transplant, you will have a small flexible plastic tube inserted into the large vein above the heart. This is called a central line, central venous catheter or Hickman catheter. The central line is a useful device that allows blood samples to be withdrawn and drugs and blood products to be given painlessly. The procedure for installing the central line generally requires local anesthesia. For many patients this is a simple and painless procedure.

Bone Marrow or Stem Cell Collection— Autologous Transplant Patients If you are having an autologous transplant, you will be your own donor and your own stem cells or bone marrow will be collected. If you are getting marrow from a donor, your donor will undergo the stem cell or bone marrow collection.

Your bone marrow contains a high concentration of stem cells—the cells that give rise to all the cells that make up your blood. A small number of these stem cells are also released into the bloodstream. Stem cells can, therefore, be collected either directly from the bone marrow or they can be obtained from the bloodstream.

Bone Marrow Harvest If stem cells are collected from your bone marrow, you will have to undergo a surgical procedure in which a needle is inserted into the hip bone several times. Marrow rich in stem cells will be withdrawn and stored until the time of the transplant. During the surgery, you will be anesthetized and will not feel any pain, although the area of the surgery may be sore for a few days afterward.

Peripheral Stem Cell Collection Stem cells can also be collected from the bloodstream. The stem cells in your blood are called peripheral blood stem cells. Since your bloodstream has only a small number of stem cells, you will need to take a drug such as G-CSF to increase the number of stem cells in your blood. Once there are enough of them, they are collected in a procedure called apheresis. In this process, blood is withdrawn from your central line and circulated through a cell separator. The stem cells are removed and stored until the transplant, and the remaining blood is returned to you. This process takes between three to four hours a day. Generally, one to three days of apheresis are required to obtain an adequate number of stem cells for transplant.

Patients generally experience little, if any, discomfort during the apheresis procedure. Others experience numbness or tingling in their fingertips or toes, hand or leg cramps, lightheadedness, dizziness or chills. All of these are easily corrected.

Conditioning (Radiation and/or Chemotherapy Treatment) The next stage of the transplant is conditioning treatment (also called preparative regimen), which involves several days of chemotherapy with or without total-body irradiation (TBI). The type and amount of chemotherapy and/or radiation you receive depend upon your particular disease and the type of transplant you are having. Regardless of your exact treatment, the goal of the conditioning treatment is to destroy all the cancerous or diseased cells in your body.

The chemotherapy is often given through your central line and, in some cases, orally. Generally, you will not feel anything during the administration of chemotherapy, but will experience the side effects later. The same is true for radiation treatment, which is painless.

The effects of the conditioning treatment range from mild to severe. Common side effects of chemotherapy and radiation include nausea, vomiting, diarrhea, hair loss, fatigue, loss of appetite and mouth sores. Some people develop all of these conditions, whereas others develop only a few of them. The side effects of treatment are discussed in detail in Chapter 5.

The conditioning treatment may also irritate the bladder and cause bleeding. Bladder irritation can be prevented by inserting a Foley catheter though your urinary tract into your bladder and flushing out the bladder. Some people do not like the Foley catheter, and should know that bladder irritation can also be prevented with medication such as mesna.

THE TRANSPLANT

The day of the transplant is an exciting day that offers a chance at new life. The procedure itself is surprisingly simple. A bag of bone marrow or peripheral stem cells is infused over the course of several hours through your central line just like any other blood product or medication. Once the new marrow enters your bloodstream, the stem cells migrate into your bones, where they begin to reproduce, giving rise to all the cells that make up your blood. This process is called engraftment.

Engraftment Engraftment occurs when the newly infused cells begin to reproduce within your body. Often the first sign of engraftment is a rising white blood cell count. If you have had a peripheral stem cell transplant, engraftment will usually occur within the first two weeks posttransplant. If you have had a transplant with stem cells taken directly from the bone marrow, engraftment will usually take between two to four weeks. If you are someone who engrafts late, you may feel very anxious during the waiting period.

Throughout this period, your white count will be monitored carefully to check for signs of engraftment. Particular attention will be paid to your neutrophil count, also referred to as ANC.

Many patients like to keep close track of their blood counts and keep a calendar in their room to mark off the days until engraftment. Celebrating the day of your engraftment with loved ones can be a good way to break the monotony of the hospital routine. Once your white count is above a certain level and you are free of infection and other complications, you can leave the hospital.

Physical Effects of the Transplant The transplant process is characterized by tremendous change. In response to the chemotherapy, radiation and medications, your body will undergo many transformations. The changes will affect how you look, your energy level and strength as well as the functioning of organs in your body.

Throughout the process, your blood counts and health status will be monitored carefully. Your weight will be checked daily and your vital signs—temperature, blood pressure and pulse—will be checked every few hours. Often you will be given a diary to record the fluids and food you drink and eat and your output in the form of urine, stool and vomit. This close monitoring of your condition ensures that any change in your health is detected and treated as early as possible.

Nausea Nausea is a very common side effect that can range from moderate nausea for several days to severe nausea over the course of several weeks or even months. Fortunately, there are some effective medications for nausea. Some nausea medications may make you sleepy or cause hallucinations. If this is the case, or your medications are not reducing the nausea, explore other medication options

with your medical staff. You may also try relaxation or meditation to decrease nausea. Other tips for dealing with nausea are detailed in Chapter 5.

Mouth Sores Chemotherapy and radiation often cause the tissues inside your mouth to become thinner and more delicate, leading to irritation and ulceration (mucositis). In some cases, the whole digestive tract may become irritated and painful. The extent of irritation will depend in large part on the type of treatment you receive and on your unique reaction to the treatment. Physicians who specialize in pain management, psychologists and psychiatrists may be available to help you cope with pain and stress. As always, make sure to make your needs known. It is also helpful to keep in mind that the pain is transient and will subside once you engraft and have a better-functioning immune system.

Energy Depletion The transplant will tend to make you feel weak. Don't be surprised if you can accomplish only a limited number of activities during the day. Simple tasks like writing a letter or reading may seem very taxing at times. Be patient with yourself. You will regain your energy, but it will take time.

Body Image Coping with a changing body is an integral part of the bone marrow transplant. You may begin the transplant with lots of hair on your head and will then lose most or all of it. Some people lose their eyebrows and eyelashes. If you take certain immunosuppressive drugs, your face, abdomen, hands and feet may become swollen for some time. Weight can fluctuate during the transplant. Although many people experience weight loss during the transplant, others gain weight because of water retention and bloating.

As you go through the transplant process other changes may take place. Once your hair starts coming back in, it may be a different texture or color than it was before. Medications such as cyclosporine, which is commonly used to treat graft-versus-host disease, may cause additional hair growth. After your initial bald state, you may find that your hair, eyebrows and eyelashes are thicker than ever. Some patients may grow additional body and facial hair.

As you go through these transformations, remember to have a sense of humor. Suggestions by other patients include getting a funny haircut before your hair falls out, buying hats or wigs you like, marveling at the changes, remembering to laugh at yourself and keeping in mind that the changes are almost always temporary. Adjusting to a new and perpetually changing self may be difficult, but remember that it is part of the necessary process you must undergo in order to recover and regain your health.

Other Changes Other changes people experience include restlessness and difficulty sleeping, drowsiness, lack of ability to concentrate, trembling hands, loss of memory, hemorrhoids, diarrhea and difficulty eating. Keep in mind that not everyone goes through these changes. However, it is useful to hear what others have been through and to know that despite the most difficult circumstances, people make it through, recover and return to normal active lives post-transplant.

Graft-Versus-Host Disease—Allogeneic Transplant Patients As your white count rises, you may experience graft-versus-host disease (GVHD). Graft-versus-host disease occurs when the white cells produced by your donor's transplanted marrow do not recognize your organs and tissues as "self." This happens because there are some genetic differences between you and your donor. Because of these differences, your new immune system may identify your own cells as for-

eign and will attack them. Patients getting an autologous transplant or getting a transplant from an identical twin do not get graft-versus-host disease. About half of the patients receiving a transplant from a related donor will develop some form of GVHD. Your chances of getting GVHD are higher if your donor is unrelated.

GVHD manifests itself in two forms. Acute GVHD develops in the first three months post-transplant. Chronic GVHD develops any time after that. Acute GVHD primarily affects the skin, the digestive tract and the liver and can cause symptoms ranging from mild skin rashes that come and go to stomach pains, nausea, cramping of the intestines and diarrhea. In more serious cases, GVHD can affect major body organs and can be life threatening. Acute GVHD may resolve itself with treatment or, in some cases, it merges with the onset of chronic GVHD.

The effects of chronic GVHD include dry eyes, dry mouth, skin and joint problems or problems with organs such as the liver or lungs. The severity of GVHD varies dramatically from patient to patient, as does its time of onset and its duration.

A variety of methods are used to reduce the incidence of GVHD. Many patients receive immunosuppressive drugs such as methotrexate, cyclosporine or prednisone. These drugs weaken your immune system, thus reducing the severity of the attack on your organs. Unfortunately, however, they also increase your susceptibility to infections and prolong the period of immunosuppression. These drugs may also affect your emotional and mental state. While on these drugs, some patients experience drug-induced depression, confusion, anxiety, mood swings and exaggerated feelings of anger or excitement. It is helpful to keep in mind that these effects are temporary and that many people do not experience these side effects.

Some BMT centers reduce the incidence of GVHD through the use of T-cell depletion. In this procedure some or all of the T-cells of the donor's marrow are removed, thus limiting the ability of the new immune system to orchestrate an attack on the host (the patient).

COPING EMOTIONALLY

For some people, going through the transplant is extremely difficult emotionally, whereas others find it easier than they expected. Some people are alert and active during the transplant, whereas others suffer greatly. Losing one's independence and privacy, experiencing physical discomfort and adapting to physical and emotional changes can be extremely taxing. In some cases, the medications you will take affect your mood. Some patients find that while going through the transplant they lash out at the people who are closest and dearest to them. Dealing with a changed status and new role in the family may be difficult. You may find that other people are suddenly too protective or not as understanding as you wish.

Taking it one day at a time and remembering to be gentle with yourself and others is helpful. As always, doing things you enjoy can be an effective way of reducing stress during this period. Suggestions for activities include: listening to relaxation and visualization tapes; talking to other patients; getting gentle massages, or sharing feelings with friends, family or a counselor.

Make Your Needs Known—Be Assertive
Generally, the medical staff and your loved ones will want you to feel as comfortable as possible and will try to accommodate your needs and preferences. Make sure to articulate your preferences and needs to those around you. Things that may seem obvious to you may not be obvious to others. Let people know what you would like—what kind of food, what kind of schedule, what kind of care.

Ask what your options are and find out what services are available to you. It is not uncommon for your medical team and other staff members to neglect to tell you about various services and options that are available to you. If you are interested in a certain service that was not mentioned, ask if it can be made available. Remember, it never hurts to ask.

If you like your privacy respected, put a sign on your door requesting that medical personnel knock before entering. Or if there are certain hours when you would prefer not to be disturbed, let the staff know. If there are certain times of the day that you would like to be disconnected from your medication pump, discuss this with your nurse and organize a medication schedule that will allow you to be free of the pump at that time. If you are a vegetarian and the hospital menu is geared to meat eaters, see what can be done to accommodate you.

If you would like to have your spouse or parent stay the night in your hospital room, request a bed for them or buy a small folding camping bed and bring it to the hospital room. If having an overnight guest in the room is not allowed, see whether an exception can be made in your case.

The key is to communicate with your doctors and nurses! If there is some aspect of your care that you are not satisfied with, make this known, either by speaking directly to a member of your medical team or to a person in charge, or by asking your caregiver to express your concerns. It is only by expressing your dissatisfaction with some aspect of your care that the situation will change.

Maintain a Sense of Humor Laughter and a good attitude can be powerful sources of support and healing. Clearly, if you are not feeling well, this can be quite a challenge. To the extent possible, try to incorporate some fun into your days. Rent some funny movies or ask friends and family to send you videos of themselves. If you like to dance, turn up the music in your room and dance a jig or two. Try to incorporate a few things you enjoy into your day. Remember, every day on this earth is incredibly precious, and we all owe it to ourselves to make the most of this gift of life.

CARING FOR YOURSELF DURING THE HOSPITAL STAY

After the conditioning treatment and the transplant, your immune system will be compromised, or weakened, and thus you will be at risk for infections. To minimize risk of infection, good hygiene, mouth care and exercise are all recommended.

Good Hygiene One of the common routines hospitals use to minimize infections is to require that all visitors and staff entering your room wash their hands. As a patient, you should also wash your hands regularly throughout the day, before meals, before taking your pills and after using the bathroom. Daily bathing is highly recommended as it will help to reduce skin bacteria.

Dental Care One of the best things you can do for yourself during the transplant to reduce discomfort and prevent infections is to take meticulous care of your mouth. By maintaining good oral hygiene during the transplant, you can often prevent or reduce oral infections and bleeding gums.

Remember, optimal mouth care entails frequent mouth rinses throughout the day. You should also brush your teeth regularly with a soft nylon-bristle toothbrush or a sponge toothbrush if the regular toothbrush hurts. While brushing, thoroughly rinse your mouth several times to remove bacteria and debris. Brush or rinse your mouth after taking any food, as this will help minimize infection and pain. If you are good at flossing and are able to do so without injuring your gums, continue to do so.

Exercise During days that you feel weak and sick, it is particularly tempting to curl up in bed and not move. However, exercising and moving is going to be your ticket to doing many of the things you will want to do when you are discharged. Exercising will mean more energy to carry out daily activities and is also likely to lower your risk of injury from falling or twisting an ankle. You do not need to be in top condition to exercise. Many exercises and stretches can even be done in bed.

The benefits of exercise are manifold.
◆ Exercise promotes good circulation and encourages the continued normal functioning of your body.
◆ Exercise prevents or minimizes muscle atrophy from prolonged bedrest and steroid treatment.
◆ Exercise is associated with improved nutritional status as it promotes protein assimilation and decreases body fat.
◆ Exercise and deep breathing help prevent the accumulation of fluids in the lungs that can often lead to pneumonia.
◆ Exercise is known to combat depression and promote feelings of well-being as well as to enhance physical comfort.
◆ Exercise improves cardiac function and circulation.

During your time at the hospital and also as an outpatient, you may have visits from a physical therapist who will work with you in maintaining your strength and endurance and working on particularly important things like ankle strength and chest expansion. If you feel you need more information on exercises and stretches, make your needs known and have a physical therapist visit you more often. (*See also* Chapter 21.)

Nutrition Often your treatment will affect

your appetite and ability to eat and digest food. Eating may be difficult for some people because of changes in taste and smell, nausea, general dryness of the mouth or difficulty swallowing. If you are having difficulty eating, you will be fed intravenously through your central line so that your basic caloric and nutritional needs will be met. Good nutrition is particularly important post-transplant as your body will require additional calories, protein, vitamins and minerals to heal and recover.

Eating Tips Although your nutritional requirements will be met through intravenous feeding, it is highly recommended that you try to continue eating, at least small amounts, throughout the period of the transplant. By eating and keeping your digestive tract active, the muscle tone and function of your digestive tract will be better maintained, thus making it easier for you to eat post-transplant. Your dietitian can help you find ways to meet your nutritional needs.

A helpful suggestion is to begin increasing your oral intake with small meals and snacks every few hours. Nutritious beverages are often well tolerated and can be an excellent source of vitamins, minerals and calories.

To aid digestion and prevent heartburn, eat and drink slowly. Sitting up rather than lying down after meals can also help. If you are not experiencing much nausea, light exercise such as walking can promote digestion and may help you feel more comfortable.

Although there are no hard and fast rules about which foods to eat, many people find that moist, bland, low-fat soups, casseroles or noodle dishes are relatively easy to digest compared to fried foods, meats and some raw fruits and vegetables. The best rule of thumb is to eat the foods that are most appealing to you. If the foods you crave are not on the hospi-

tal menu, see if they can be made available for you. Chapter 17, "Nutrition Problems," and Chapters 19 and 20 on special diets and recipes offer suggestions for dealing with many side effects and boosting your appetite.

Finally, to reduce the probability of food-borne illness, wash your hands before eating meals and follow the food safety guidelines that are recommended by your dietitian.

AFTER THE TRANSPLANT

Planning to Go Home It is a good idea to prepare for your return home before leaving the hospital. This may entail arranging to have someone take care of your pet for the first 100 days post-transplant during the time you are immunocompromised, organizing to have your house well cleaned before you return, and arranging for a housecleaner to come in at regular intervals until you can resume such activities. Getting family and friends to help with your return home can make the transition easier for you.

The Transition to Home We all look forward with great anticipation to the day when we can leave the hospital. Despite the joy that often accompanies leaving the hospital, coming home also brings up a lot of fears and anxiety. Many people find the transition from the hospital to the home is one of the more difficult phases of the transplant. In the hospital everything is taken care of for you—if an unexpected glitch happens, care is right there. Once you return to your home environment, dealing with your new limitations and trying to reacclimatize to a world that does not know your condition can be difficult.

Outpatient Care Post-Transplant In the first few months after the transplant, you are likely to visit the outpatient clinic several times a week, or in some cases every day, for blood tests, physical exams, intermittent blood or platelet transfusions, as well as other tests such as throat, urine and stool cultures to screen for infections. Depending on your protocol, you may also undergo periodic x-rays, bone marrow aspirations, lumbar punctures or other procedures. This intensive follow-up care is necessary to monitor your progress and to treat complications should they arise. As the weeks and months progress and your condition stabilizes, your visits will become more infrequent.

Readmission and Setbacks Returning to the inpatient department of the hospital for treatment post-transplant is very common and is part of the recovery process. Although returning to the hospital or contracting an infection is discouraging, it is important to recognize that recovery is a bumpy road and that many patients experience small complications and may need to be readmitted for short periods to manage symptoms that cannot be safely taken care of in the outpatient department. Returning to the hospital for short stays is often just one of the many steps in the recovery process.

CARING FOR YOURSELF POST-TRANSPLANT

During the period immediately following hospitalization, you will be vulnerable to infections and will need to take extra precautions. The time of immunosuppression varies from person to person and depends upon the type of transplant and the amount of immunosuppressants being taken.

People who have had autologous transplants do not need to take immunosuppressants to combat GVHD. As a result, they are less vulnerable to infections than recipients of transplants from donors. Because of this, autologous transplant recipients have to follow the guidelines only for the first one or two months post-transplant. People who have undergone a transplant from a donor, however, should follow the guidelines more strictly and for a longer period. Since every patient's condition is different, the best way to determine how long to follow these guidelines is to consult directly with your physician. In general, the time will range from a few months to a year or more, depending on the type of transplant and your condition.

Coping with all the restrictions post-transplant requires a lot of energy and effort. Although living with these recommended precautions can be challenging, maintaining good hygiene is a very important part of regaining your health and avoiding infection during the period of immunosuppression.

In the months after the transplant, it is helpful to remember that these restrictions are temporary. In the scheme of a lifetime, six months or a year of avoiding certain foods or certain places is a minor sacrifice. Keep in mind that you will have the rest of your life to pursue these activities.

Hand Washing After the transplant, wash your hands frequently during the day, as hand contact is by far the most common way of contracting infections. Many bacteria and viruses are transmitted by touching doorknobs or other objects and then touching one's mouth, nose or eyes. Frequent hand washing is the best protection against infection and should be done regularly before eating meals, taking medications and after using the toilet or any public restroom. Ideally, everyone who comes into contact with you should wash their hands frequently to minimize transmission of microorganisms that can cause infections. Some patients recommend instituting a "hand-washing policy" in the house, requiring that everyone wash their hands upon entering to minimize the risk of transmitting infection.

Personal Hygiene After the transplant, personal hygiene is of paramount importance. Make sure to bathe daily, using soap and shampoo. Often, your skin post-transplant will be dry and sensitive. If this is the case, frequent applications of body lotion can be helpful. Using a milder soap can also reduce dryness and irritation. As part of general hygiene, towels and clothing should be changed daily.

Contact with People To restrict exposure to bacteria and other infection-causing agents, it is generally recommended that you restrict touching or hugging to a few special people with whom you have frequent contact. It is also important to avoid settings in which you are likely to come into contact with sick people. Although this does not mean that you have to avoid public spaces altogether, it is probably wise to limit your exposure to large numbers of people. This will mean avoiding crowded spaces such as movie theaters and restaurants during peak hours, crowded elevators and auditoriums. In particular, you should avoid day-care and school settings, since children are more likely to be sick than adults. Since the transplant can destroy previous immunity to disease, it is also important to avoid contact with babies or adults who have been vaccinated with live viruses such as polio within the last 30 days.

If someone living with you gets sick, check with your medical provider to determine how much risk the infectious person poses to you and what the best course of action is. It is likely that the sick person will be advised to move temporarily until he or she is no longer infectious. If that is not possible, arrange to have the person stay away from you as much as possible.

If you choose to eat at restaurants, make sure they are ones that have a reputation for cleanliness and serve fresh foods. In the period that you are immuno-compromised, don't hesitate to ask when foods were prepared and to ask that foods be prepared fresh especially for you. Many restaurants will accommodate you.

Hygiene in Your Home Your living quarters post-transplant should be kept clean. Again, there are no hard and fast rules about the degree of cleanliness you should maintain. The recommendations vary according to the type of transplant you have had and your degree of immuno-suppression. In any case, the amount of dust, mold and fungus in your home should be kept to an absolute minimum as these have the potential to transmit infection and disease. Depending on the amount of dust and soil in your home, the home should be cleaned once a week or every few days. The bathroom and eating area should be cleaned most often, and used sponges should be replaced weekly. You may also consider having the refrigerator cleaned before stocking it so that it is free of mold spores that can get into your food. Using a cleaner with antibacterial disinfectant properties such as Lysol or bleach is recommended. Using a damp cloth to dust is more effective than a feather duster, which stirs up dust and disperses it in the air. If you can, hire a housekeeper to do housework. Allocating tasks to family members can be extremely helpful.

Plants and Pets As part of the general cleanliness and hygiene requirements, it is recommended that you avoid keeping fresh plants and flowers in your home, since organisms that grow in dirt, water and on plants can cause infections. In general, you should avoid handling plants in the first few months after the transplant. For the same reason, you should avoid contact with soil, lawn waste and compost. Thus, refrain from gardening or sitting on grass, logs or dirt. This restriction should not prevent you, however, from enjoying the outdoors. If you wish to sit outside, take a clean cover to sit on.

In general, it is recommended that you limit your contact with animals and household pets during the first 100 days post-transplant. During this time, you should not clean up after your pets or touch any human or animal excrement. It is particularly important to avoid cat litter boxes and bird cages. Check with your physician to determine the extent of contact you may have with your pets.

Construction Sites It is recommended that you avoid construction sites, as they often have upturned earth, old wooden beams or other materials that may expose you to dust or fungus. If there is a construction site in your neighborhood, walk upwind from it or go around the block to avoid it. If you are driving by, roll up your windows.

Exposure to the Sun The effects of radiation, chemotherapy and some immunosuppressive drugs may increase your skin's sensitivity to sunlight. During the first year post-transplant, stay out of the sun as much as possible and apply a sunscreen with a sun protection factor (SPF) of 25 or higher before going outdoors, even on overcast days. For at least a year post-transplant, on sunny days wear protective coverings such as hats, sunglasses and long-sleeved shirts.

Swimming Avoid swimming in lakes or untreated water until your immune system has reconstituted itself. If you have had an autologous transplant, the restriction applies for several months. Check with your physician before resuming swimming activities.

Food Safety Until your immune system rebuilds itself, you will be at a greater risk for developing food-related infections. Thus, in the period after your transplant, it is extremely important to follow food safety guidelines. Although the guide-

lines may vary slightly from center to center, a good rule of thumb to follow is to eat only those foods that have been freshly prepared in a clean environment and that have not been sitting out for any length of time.

The following recommendations have been adapted from patient guidelines at the Fred Hutchinson Cancer Research Center in Seattle, WA.

Grocery Shopping
◆ Check "sell by" and "use by" dates and do not use items that are out of date.
◆ Do not buy or use any bulging, damaged or deeply dented cans.
◆ Make sure frozen foods feel solid and that refrigerated foods are cold.
◆ Do not buy cracked or unrefrigerated eggs.
◆ Store groceries promptly after shopping.
◆ Do not buy bulk foods from self-service bins.

Food Preparation
◆ Prepare food on surfaces that have been thoroughly washed in hot soapy water. You can clean cutting boards in a solution of 10 parts water mixed with 1 part household bleach.
◆ Use separate cutting boards for cooked foods and raw foods.
◆ Do not use raw, unpasteurized eggs in uncooked foods, since raw eggs are the perfect medium for the growth of bacteria such as salmonella.
◆ Discard eggs, egg mixtures or prepared egg dishes left at room temperature for more than an hour.
◆ Wash the tops of cans and the can opener before use.
◆ All meats should be cooked until well done and should have no remaining pink color.
◆ Foods should be cooled inside the refrigerator rather than outside. A good way to do this is to divide large amounts of hot food into small, shallow containers

for quick cooling in the refrigerator.

◆ Do not eat perishable foods that have been left out of the refrigerator for more than two hours.

◆ Do not eat foods that have been sitting in the refrigerator for more than three days. A helpful way to keep track of the number of days prepared foods and other perishable items have been sitting in the refrigerator is to write a date on them once they have been opened. It is also helpful to refrigerate only the amount of food that you will eat in two or three days and freeze the rest.

◆ Thaw meats and fish in the refrigerator.

◆ Throw away food that has any mold on it.

◆ Never taste foods that look or smell strange.

◆ Wash and rinse fruits and vegetables thoroughly before eating them.

The following foods are more likely to carry infection-causing organisms. In addition to the foods listed here, there may be other foods that your transplant center recommends that you avoid. To get a full list of foods to avoid, discuss food safety guidelines thoroughly with your dietitian or medical provider.

Foods to Avoid

◆ Free food samples.

◆ Foods at potluck meals where you don't know how food was prepared or how long it was sitting out of the refrigerator.

◆ Food from sidewalk vendors, delicatessens, smorgasbords, buffets and salad bars.

◆ Soft ice cream, milkshakes and frozen yogurt from yogurt machines.

◆ Sushi, raw fish, smoked fish.

◆ Raw eggs, Caesar salads containing raw egg, mayonnaise and foods containing mayonnaise, custards and other dishes that may contain raw or partly cooked eggs.

◆ Well water, unless it has been tested and found to be safe.

◆ Unpasteurized honey, milk, cheese and yogurt.

◆ Unrefrigerated cream.

◆ Unroasted nuts or nuts in the shell.

◆ Aged cheeses such as certain sharp cheeses.

◆ Moldy cheeses such as brie and blue cheese.

Nontraditional nutrition supplements such as herbal preparations should be avoided, as they may contain toxic impurities or infection-causing fungi, yeast, molds or bacteria. These can be life threatening for a person with a weakened immune system. Unsupervised high-dose vitamin and mineral supplements should also be avoided, as they may interfere with medications or may be harmful to major organs, especially the liver and kidneys.

Smoking/Alcohol/Drugs Your risk for lung damage post-transplant will considerably increase. It is therefore recommended that you avoid smoking before, during and after your transplant. You should also avoid second-hand smoke.

The damaging side effects of alcohol are greatest post-transplant. For this reason, you should avoid alcohol for the first six months post-transplant. If you are still taking medications six months post-transplant, do not drink alcohol until you have discussed the matter with your physician.

Do not take any over-the-counter medications without consulting your BMT doctor or clinical nurse specialist.

Work/School Avoid work and school for at least three to six months after an autologous BMT. The time you take off depends on the kind of work you do and the degree of fatigue caused by work. A computer consultant working at home, for example, may be able to return to work much earlier than an elementary school teacher. Give yourself time to take care of yourself and fully recover. You deserve it!

Sexual Activity Generally, sexual activity is considered safe as long as both you and your partner are healthy, follow good hygiene and have no sexually transmissible diseases. Before beginning sexual activity, however, talk with a member of your transplant team to see if there are any restrictions that pertain to your particular case.

Some transplant centers recommend using a condom post-transplant, whereas others maintain that a condom is not necessary if you are in a mutually monogamous relationship and neither of you is suspected of having a sexually transmissible disease. If one of you has a sexually transmissible disease, it is recommended that you refrain from sexual activity, since a condom may not provide a sufficient barrier during the time of immunosuppression. Some BMT centers recommend refraining from unprotected oral-genital sex during the time of immunosuppression; others maintain that it is safe as long as oral hygiene is good and there are no oral lesions, genital lesions or mucositis. Anal sex should be avoided until platelets have stabilized at a level above 35,000 and there is no evidence of diarrhea, anal lesions, bleeding or hemorrhoids.

The extent to which the transplant affects one's sexual life varies from person to person. Some people resume an active and highly satisfying sexual life shortly after transplant, whereas others find that their sexual life is greatly disrupted.

Changes in body image or sexual desire post-transplant can disrupt old behavior patterns or lead to insecurities about starting new relationships. Often the physical toll of the transplant and the resulting side effects such as nausea and lower energy levels may reduce the desire for sexual activity. In other cases, worry, depression or nervousness about one's ability to "perform" and to be sexually attractive post-transplant may also result in loss of desire.

If your sexual drive post-transplant is reduced, explore other forms of intimacy such as touching, holding hands, hugging and kissing. At this time, communicating with your partner is key to modifying your sexual routine in a way that will meet your needs for love and intimacy. Recognizing that your feelings of concern about resuming an active sexual life may be shared by your partner is a good starting point for discussion. Once you begin sharing your feelings, you may find that your partner has been holding back because of apprehension about appearing to be overeager or insensitive or hurting you physically in some way.

One suggestion to reduce nervousness when you first resume intimate physical contact is to set limits on sexual activity. You and your partner, for example, may choose to devote an evening to all-over body touching, where each partner takes a turn touching and being touched. If this feels comfortable, then you can try adding some genital touching during the next session. If lack of sexual desire persists, androgens, which are sometimes referred to as male hormones, can be taken by both men and women to increase sexual energy.

For patients who are not in a relationship, finding a partner and resuming sexual activity post-transplant may provoke a great deal of anxiety. Although the sad reality is that some potential lovers may reject you because of infertility or because you have had cancer, try not to limit yourself by not dating at all. After all, almost everyone with and without cancer can get rejected for a multitude of reasons. Although you may avoid rejection by not dating, you may also miss the opportunity to build a happy and rewarding relationship. (*See also* Chapter 24, "Sexuality and Cancer.")

Women and Sexuality Sexuality post-transplant can be affected by the effects of early menopause, which can result from chemotherapy and radiation treatment. The symptoms of early menopause include hot flashes, vaginal dryness and tightness, as well as mood shifts and irritability. Not all women become menopausal. In some rare cases, women have regained ovarian function post-transplant and in some very rare instances, women have also regained fertility and given birth to healthy babies.

For the majority of women who do experience early menopause, hormone replacement therapy alleviates many of the symptoms. It also reduces some of the risks associated with early menopause, such as osteoporosis (weakening of the bones) and heart disease. For women who have had breast cancer, however, hormone replacement therapy is not an option, as it may increase the chance of recurrence. In such cases, estrogen creams applied directly to the vagina can improve vaginal dryness without having systemic effects.

Women who experience vaginal dryness post-transplant may also find a water-soluble lubricating jelly helpful.

Exercise Regular exercise is an important part of the recovery process. By improving your stamina, muscle tone and muscle strength, you will feel better not only physically but also emotionally. Exercise can help counteract problems such as stiff joints, breathing problems, poor appetite and psychological lows. Seeing improvement in your physical state can be a real boost, particularly when you are adjusting to the stresses and difficulties of returning to a more normal lifestyle.

Initiating an exercise routine if your energy level is low and you are not feeling well may be difficult. A good way to begin exercising is to take walks outside or to visit the outpatient physical therapy department in your hospital where a physical therapist can work with you in selecting appropriate exercises and building your strength and stamina. You may

also be able to get your doctor to write you a prescription to buy an exercise machine such as a stationary bicycle. Your insurance plan may cover a portion or all of the cost. A doctor's prescription may also save you from paying sales tax on the purchase.

Exercise is particularly important if you are taking prednisone. Prednisone may cause muscle wasting and weakness, and thus regular exercise can be instrumental in maintaining muscle mass and strength. If you are taking prednisone, choose low-impact exercises to minimize stress on your joints, since prednisone can cause joint damage.

When exercising, pay attention to the messages your body gives you. You should challenge yourself, but you should also stop or slow down if you are experiencing pain. Between a scale of very light to very arduous, an optimal level of exercise is one that you would rank as moderately hard. The best way to regain strength is through regular exercise suited to your level of physical conditioning that builds slowly to progressively higher levels of activity. (*See* Chapter 21.)

Nutrition After the transplant, your body will require many nutrients to regain strength and to recuperate. Your nutritional requirements will vary depending on your medical condition, the type of transplant you had and the medications you are on. Your nutritional needs post-transplant may increase, requiring you to take mineral and vitamin supplements. During this period it is important to consult a dietitian about food choices to ensure that your nutritional needs are met.

If you are nauseated and find eating and drinking difficult, it is helpful to eat and drink small amounts throughout the day rather than eating three large meals. Have a wide variety of appealing snacks at hand for the times that you do feel hungry. Eating in a pleasant setting or having an attractive food arrangement may also make eating easier. During this time, you may need to increase your fluid intake to prevent dehydration and to help flush the drugs and their residues from your bladder and kidney. (*See* Chapters 16 to 20.)

RECOVERY

For some people, the recovery process is smooth and easy and entails few adjustments. For others, the period of recovery is long and difficult, requiring perseverance and patience.

PHYSICAL CHANGES POST-TRANSPLANT

There is considerable variation among bone marrow transplant survivors in physical, psychological and social functioning post-transplant. Some patients recover fully, returning to their old activity level several months after the transplant. For others, the recovery period is slow, and they never return to old levels of vigor and health. The extent of difficulty entailed in the recovery process is often closely tied to the degree of physical difficulties post-transplant. Having repeated infections or chronic graft-versus-host disease can contribute to stresses and difficulties in returning to normal activities. Some of the problems that survivors may experience are fatigue, decreased strength, muscle cramps, difficulty concentrating, memory problems, sleep disturbances, numbness in hands and feet, cataracts, skin and joint problems, dry eyes or mouth, frequent infections, and kidney or other organ dysfunction. Keep in mind that only some people experience these problems. Generally, the problems resolve themselves with time, and most people return to productive and fulfilling lives.

Some of the physical and mental changes may occur as a side effect of some of the drugs. Many of the drugs taken post-transplant can affect organ function, immune function, physical appearance and psychological well-being. Knowing that many of the changes are temporary can be helpful for everyone involved.

EMOTIONAL ADJUSTMENT POST-TRANSPLANT

Going through a bone marrow transplant changes us in many ways, requiring us to re-evaluate many aspects of our lives. Give yourself time to deal with the emotional effect of the transplant. Often people expect you to be over the experience in a month or two. In reality, recovery may take much longer. Recovering from the transplant not only entails a physical process but requires also a mental shift from seeing yourself as sick to seeing yourself as healthy.

Some people experience recurring memories of the transplant that conjure up feelings of vulnerability, anxiety or depression. You may find yourself going over the decisions you made, questioning the reasons for the transplant and reliving the difficult times you had. Fear of relapse or complications are also not uncommon.

If these fears cause a major disruption in your life or cause sleep disturbances, consider seeking outside help. Often speaking to a professional therapist or joining a support group can help you put the experience in perspective and move on. Keeping in touch with someone who had a transplant at the same time you did can allow you to compare notes, exchange information and tips and also reduce your sense of isolation.

The transplant may also have a strong positive effect on your emotional well-being. Many people find that they emerge from the experience strengthened, more resilient and better prepared for the challenges of life.

Changes in Self-Esteem Making it through the transplant is a heroic accomplishment. However, many people, upon emerging from the hospital, tend to compare their performance to their previous levels of activity or to the activity levels of their friends and colleagues. The inability to accomplish as much as before or to be self-supporting may dash your self-esteem. As you begin the recovery process, set realistic goals for yourself and adapt your activities to your energy level instead of berating yourself for not being able to do more. Respect your need for rest and relaxation. In the months after the transplant, you and your family have to adjust to your new role and new capacities.

Changes in Family Ties and Relationships
The transplant experience can often result in changed relationships among family members. Often these changes in roles bring families closer, but in some cases the changes exacerbate tensions and lead to additional strains.

Friendships may also change or take on new meaning as you reflect on the people who were supportive of you during the transplant and those who were not. Some friendships will be enhanced and enriched, whereas others may dissolve under the pressures of the transplant.

Recommendations for Coping During Recovery Although it is difficult to know ahead of time how the transition period from the hospital to the outpatient phase will be for you, keep in mind that recovery is a long-term process that does not always proceed in a smooth, linear fashion.

Celebrate Landmarks Often during the ups and downs of recovery, it is difficult to see the bigger picture and to appreciate how far you have come. Marking special dates such as your six-month or one-year anniversary with celebrations can serve as an important reminder of your progress. Another way to mark your progress is to give yourself a special treat at the end of a designated period.

BEYOND THE TRANSPLANT

Regardless of how long or how difficult the transplant process is for you, it is important to remember that the majority of people return to a normal and active lifestyle post-transplant. Survivors often report that the quality of their lives post-transplant is similar to or better than before the transplant. Others have some lingering effects, but do not experience significant deterioration in quality of life. A small minority of people suffer from more significant handicaps, resulting in the need to change their profession or to stop working altogether.

Every patient, without exception, is changed as a result of the transplant experience. Through the transplant, people are forced to look at themselves, their lives and their priorities. Those who undergo a transplant will inevitably suffer losses, but they probably will also gain new strength and insights. By becoming aware of the frailty of life, we also uncover many treasures and learn to live our lives more fully. It is my hope that by reading this chapter, you will be better able to face the road ahead. I wish you all a safe journey.

If you would like to obtain an expanded version of this chapter that includes the experiences of former transplant survivors, please send your name and address along with your check to:

National Bone Marrow Transplant Link
29209 Northwestern Hwy. #624
Southfield, MI 48034

◆ Price List (price includes shipping)
1 to 4 books: $9 per book
5 to 10 books: $8 per book
11 or more books: $7 per book

5
SIDE EFFECTS: CAUSES AND TREATMENT

Ernest H. Rosenbaum, MD, and Isadora R. Rosenbaum, MA

———————◇———————

Radiation therapy may damage normal tissues. The kind of side effect is determined by the tissues involved. For instance, hair loss may result from radiation to the head, whereas loss of taste and problems in swallowing can occur with radiation to the head and neck. Nausea, vomiting and diarrhea are often the result of radiation passing through the abdomen's gastrointestinal tract on the way to the targeted tumor. The skin may become red, itchy and dry.

In chemotherapy, it is virtually impossible to attack cancer cells without affecting normal tissues as well. The normal cells in the body are also dividing, and those that divide the fastest are more susceptible to drug damage. Fast-dividing normal cells are found in the lining of the digestive tract, in the hair follicles and in the bone marrow that makes blood cells. Damage to these cells from chemotherapeutic agents leads to side effects such as hair loss, nausea, vomiting and lowered blood counts. Each drug has its own side effects.

Fortunately, these side effects are not permanent. Proper nutrition can be used to help with the following common side effects of chemotherapy and radiation therapy, including loss of appetite, weight loss, nausea, vomiting, diarrhea and constipation. Information on reducing these side effects is found in Chapter 17, "Nutrition Problems: Causes and Solutions."

Many people have heard frightening stories about side effects. Such stories can inspire more fear of therapy than of cancer; but such fears are largely unwarranted. Through today's sophisticated diagnostic and therapeutic techniques, major pain, suffering and treatment side effects can be reduced, alleviated or prevented altogether. New drugs have been developed that can prevent nausea and vomiting or decrease the toxicity of chemotherapy drugs.

Tolerance to a particular drug or combination of drugs varies with each patient. Psychological support from family, friends and the medical team is always important. We do not like to overemphasize the possibility of side effects because we believe that anxiety about discomfort has produced in some patients stronger reactions than they might otherwise have had. Conversely, we are convinced that other patients experience fewer side effects because of their attitude toward chemotherapy. At one time the philosophy of medical therapy was that to be effective a medicine had to make you sick. There does not appear to be a direct correlation between the degree of discomfort from drug treatment and the degree of its medical effectiveness. The most toxic therapy may be ineffective, whereas favorable results may be obtained with minimal side effects.

NAUSEA AND VOMITING
Medications are available to combat nausea and vomiting. These include

Compazine (prochlorperazine)*, Benadryl (diphenhydramine), Dramamine, Inapsine (droperidol), Reglan (metoclopramide), Zofran (ondansetron) and Kytril (granisetron). Marinol is also effective. The FDA has approved Marinol, the active ingredient in marijuana, in capsule form. Many patients obtain marijuana from private sources and add it to brownies, cookies or other food, brew it as tea or take it in gelatin capsules by mouth or in rectal suppositories.

TRANSFUSIONS

When the bone marrow is damaged by chemotherapy drugs, red blood cell, platelet and white blood cell transfusions can be given. The need for red cell transfusions is determined by the blood cell count (hemoglobin), which is monitored frequently during treatment. The bone marrow returns to normal usually about 10 to 20 days after receiving chemotherapy.

OTHER MEDICATIONS

Medications such as Neupogen (G-CSF, or granulocyte-colony stimulating factor), which helps to increase production of white blood cells, and Procrit and Epogen (erythropoietin), which help increase production of red blood cells, will help the patient to tolerate further chemotherapy. Neumega (oprelvekin) is a new growth factor for platelet production.

REDUCE YOUR RISK OF INFECTION

During chemotherapy or radiation therapy, there may be a decrease in your blood counts—white blood cells, red blood cells and platelets. Neutropenia is the term used to describe a lack of special white blood cells called neutrophils or polys,

which are blood cells that fight infections caused by bacteria, fungi and viruses. Therefore, patients with neutropenia are more susceptible to serious infections. When the absolute neutrophil count (ANC) is less than 1,000 cells/mm^2, the risk for an infection is greater.

1. Hand washing is the number-one priority. You should wash your hands before meals, on awakening and after using the toilet. All visitors should wash their hands when they arrive.
2. Get adequate sleep.
3. Eat frequent meals with high amounts of calories and protein (make an appointment with a dietitian if you need guidelines). For more specific recommendations, *see* "Food Safety" in Chapter 4 and the special diet for neutropenia included in Chapter 19.
4. Persons having a cold or sore throat or other infections should not visit the patient.
5. Short visits should be the rule to allow patients time for adequate rest.
6. Do not use rectal thermometers. Rectal examinations, suppositories and enemas should be avoided.
7. Avoid constipation. (*See* Chapter 17.)
8. Monitor fever (temperature above 100°F/38.5°C) three times a day or when you feel hot.
9. Drink plenty of fluids (six to eight glasses a day, more if you have a fever).
10. Report any sores, infections or new symptoms to your nurse or doctor. These include hot or flushed skin, fever, shaking chills, rapid heart rate, cough, cloudy urine, skin infections, rashes or ulcers.
11. Avoid contact with stagnant water. Common sources are denture cups, soap dishes and flower vases. Check humidifiers, irrigation containers and respiratory equipment.

Note: Throughout this book the brand name is capitalized and the generic name is lower case.

12. Use a soft-bristle toothbrush.
13. Skin care
◆ Shower or bathe daily using soap.
◆ Use skin creams and emollients (skin barrier creams) to avoid dryness.
◆ Massage skin daily.
◆ Use an electric razor to avoid skin cuts.
◆ Use a special pressure-relief mattress to prevent skin breakdown or pressure sores and ulcers.
◆ Keep skin around the anus clean and dry. Use special creams as needed to reduce risk of perirectal infections.
◆ Care for hemorrhoids with sitz baths and special medicated creams.
14. Report any mental changes to your nurse or physician. These include headaches, irritability, restlessness, mental confusion, a change in mental status, sleepiness or decrease in level of consciousness.
15. List the drugs you are taking—especially antibiotics.

HAIR LOSS

Losing your hair (alopecia) can be an upsetting experience. It is one of the most visible side effects of cancer treatment. The amount of hair loss varies from hair thinning to baldness. You may find it helpful to have your partner, a close friend or a relative with you when you talk to your doctor about hair loss.

Chemotherapy stops cell division of the more active cells in the body, including those of the bone marrow, the gastrointestinal lining and the scalp (hair) cells. About 85 to 90 percent of hair cells are in the growth phase at any one time and therefore can be affected by drugs. Many drugs, including bleomycin, Cytoxan, Adriamycin, etoposide (VP-16), vincristine, Velban, 5-fluorouracil, methotrexate and Taxol, can cause partial or total hair loss.

Scalp tourniquets and ice caps have been used with limited success, especially for drugs that remain in the circulation for many minutes or hours. However, because these methods reduce the delivery of drugs to the scalp, cancer cells in the scalp are not treated and the cancer could recur locally.

Hair loss usually occurs about two to three weeks after the beginning of treatment. Hair may come out in large clumps. Hair regrowth usually begins about four to eight weeks after chemotherapy ends, and sometimes hair begins to grow back during treatment. The new hair may have a changed color or texture.

How to Care for Your Hair Gently shampoo to avoid drying out the hair and scalp. Avoid overbrushing or overcombing. Use a wide-tooth comb or a vent-style hairbrush gently to avoid pressure or damage to the hair roots. Also avoid heat-generating hair appliances such as dryers, hot rollers and curling irons. Use styling aids such as sprays, mousses and gels to give the appearance of fullness and volume.

Although many patients avoid permanents and coloring, no relationship between hair loss and perms or coloring is proven. But it is wise to avoid permanents and hair coloring early in chemotherapy, since if hair loss occurs, you have wasted money.

Wigs Wigs can boost your morale, improve your appearance and improve your self-confidence. Purchase a wig before you start treatment so that a good match to your natural hair color and texture can be found. Synthetic wigs are less expensive than natural hair wigs and are easier to clean, care for and style. Wig care includes soaking the wig in a cleaning solution (such as Woolite), drying it in a towel and then keeping it on a wig-form so it can be styled and brushed. A purchased wig can be styled and shaped to fit your personality and may be individualized.

Wig prescriptions are not always covered by health insurance, and some synthetic wigs cost about $200. Cancer Care gives wigs away free.

PAIN

Wendy R. Robbins, MD, *and Robert W. Allen,* MD

Many patients with cancer fear that they will suffer pain. In fact, at some point during the course of the disease, 60 to 90 percent of patients will require a pain-relieving therapy. But not all cancers produce pain equally, and some cancers, even when advanced, may not cause pain at all. Cancers that are more typically painful include tumors of the bone (either primary or through spread) and the organs of the abdomen. Cancers of the blood system, such as leukemias or lymphomas, often never cause pain.

Pain can have a terrible effect on a cancer patient's life. It can lead to depression, loss of appetite, irritability, withdrawal from social interaction, anger, loss of sleep and an inability to cope. If uncontrolled, pain can destroy relationships with loved ones and the will to live.

Fortunately, pain can almost always be controlled. What is needed is an understanding by caregivers of the nature of the pain, of what causes it and of the appropriate treatments for the type of pain involved, as well as a commitment to relieving it. The oncologist is usually well equipped to handle most types of pain. For more unremitting pains, patients may be referred by their doctor to a specialist who will help to sort out the cause and treatments for symptoms.

Pain is a complex phenomenon. It has physical, emotional and psychological components. How each person responds to pain is also complex. The extent of disease and the nature of the discomfort contribute to a person's experience of pain. But pain is also modified by remembrances of past painful episodes, the special meaning of pain to each individual, the expectations of family and friends, religious upbringing and personal coping skills and strategies. Cultural beliefs also influence the pain experience. Certain cultures teach tolerance of pain or that the outward expression of pain is inappropriate. People from these cultures bear their pain without complaining or even expressing their needs. Externally, they may appear to have a higher threshold or tolerance to pain while in fact suffering quietly. Other cultures readily and outwardly express painful experiences, and people from those cultures may appear to have a lower threshold or tolerance.

TYPES OF PAIN

◆ *Somatic Pain* from the cancer itself may come from a bone broken because of tumor invasion or from an obstruction in the intestine or urinary tract. Pain from bone involvement is often described as achy, dull, localized and brought about by activity of the surrounding muscle groups or movement of the limb or spine. Obstructions in the intestine or urinary tract typically are described as crampy and more diffuse. They may be associated with inability to eat or to pass stool or urine.

◆ *Neuropathic Pain* from nerve involvement is either related to direct tumor spread, such as the spread of colon cancer into the pelvis where the nerves to the legs or pelvic structures reside, or is secondary to irritating substances that tumors secrete near nerves. Neuropathic pain may also result from pressure on the nerves, as when spinal tumors pinch or press on nerves to the arms or legs. Neuropathic pain is often described as sharp, burning, electrical, shooting or buzzing. It typically occurs in the area that the injured nerves serve.

◆ Surgery may cause both somatic and neuropathic pain. Pain from direct surgical injury is somatic and usually responds to opioid medications. Surgical injury to nerves may respond to opioids, antiseizure or antidepressant medications.

◆ Chemotherapeutic drugs act like poisons to tumors and may act the same way on some vulnerable nerves. Drugs such as antiviral agents or vincristine, cisplatin, carboplatin, Taxol and Navelbine can cause peripheral neuropathy, which is often felt as a burning in the hands and feet. This requires drugs specific for neuropathic pain or some other intervention for relief. The sore mouth (mucositis) that is sometimes a side effect of these drugs is one example of somatic pain from chemotherapy.

◆ After radiation therapy, pain may be due to skin reactions to the radiation, breakdown of mucous membranes or even scarring of the nerves (fibrosis), which can produce a neuropathic pain.

EMOTIONAL SOURCES

Pain is made worse by worry and fear of death, suffering, deformity, financial disability or isolation. The onset of pain or a new pain may trigger fears about the spread of the disease or of impending death. All these fears can be magnified when a kind of spiritual pain accompanies the fear. This might be triggered by surroundings, low levels of emotional support or feelings of loneliness and desperation. How one approaches the problems of life makes a big difference to the perception of pain. Also, whether pain is adequately controlled makes a big difference.

THE TREATMENT PLAN FOR PAIN

Treating and controlling pain is a primary concern for all members of the health care team, including your doctors, nurses and the hospital and home care team. According to the World Health Organization committee on cancer pain, 90 to 95 percent of all cancer pain can be well controlled using a special set of guidelines. These guidelines separate pain into levels of intensity and suggest tailoring the strength and potency of prescribed pain-relieving medications to the intensity. Not all cancer pain requires strong narcotics. But strong pain requires strong medications.

The guidelines suggest that

◆ mild pain be treated with nonnarcotic medications such as aspirin, acetaminophen (Tylenol) or other aspirin-like drugs called nonsteroidal anti-inflammatory drugs (NSAIDs);

◆ moderate pain be treated with a combination of NSAIDs and weak narcotics such as codeine (Tylenol with codeine), hydrocodone (Vicodin or Lortab), Percocet, Percodan or propoxyphene (Darvon), and

◆ severe pain be treated with strong opioids such as morphine, Demerol, Dilaudid, fentanyl (duragesic patches) or methadone in combination with an NSAID.

The guidelines also suggest adding an adjuvant medication to these narcotic and nonnarcotic medications when appropriate. These medications—which include steroids, bone-forming, antidepressant and anticonvulsant medications, antihistamines and sedatives—are often useful in treating opioid-resistant pain. For whatever reason, they do relieve pain, although they are not usually labeled as pain relievers.

Simple measures such as aspirin or Tylenol, with or without codeine, or ibuprofen may do the job well enough. But when pain is severe, the dosage has to be increased or the drug has to be taken more frequently. If these simple measures don't help, then it is important to increase the strength or potency of the medication.

Sometimes, just the addition of an adjuvant medication is all that is needed.

Side Effects Of Pain Medications Not all people tolerate all drugs equally. Some people are allergic to various medications. Some develop side effects from medications that others taking the same drugs do not share. Some people tolerate one specific drug in a class of drugs but do not tolerate others in the same class. Some do not tolerate any drugs in a particular class. Everyone is an individual.

While 90 to 95 percent of patients receive adequate pain control using the WHO guidelines, there are still 5 to 10 percent of patients who do not achieve adequate pain control. Certain direct interventions by specialists can modify or block pain information from reaching the central nervous system. These interventions include nerve blocks with local anesthetics or nerve-destroying agents, alternative delivery systems such as administering narcotics under the skin (subcutaneous) or into the spine, spinal local anesthetics or other therapies that destroy nerves causing the pain. These invasive, interventional therapies require the expertise and skills of a pain specialist.

Morphine remains the gold standard of medical practice. Morphine and other options can be taken in a variety of ways. Most methods control pain very effectively.

MYTHS ABOUT NARCOTICS AND CANCER PAIN CONTROL

A lot of cancer patients want to avoid taking opioids. Many fear that they will become addicted to these medications, and some feel that narcotics should be used only as a last resort for fear that they will not be effective when they are really needed. Doctors may also share some of the myths about opioid medications.

These myths form barriers to good and effective relief of cancer pain. These myths need to be recognized and addressed by patients and their caregivers.

◆ Myth 1. People given opioids for pain control are always doing worse or are near death.

Just because a person is placed on a narcotic does not mean that he or she is gravely ill. Opioids are highly effective medications that can be used at any stage in the disease when severe pain requires strong medication.

◆ Myth 2. All patients getting morphine or other opioids will become addicts.

Addiction is a psychological need for a drug and rarely, if ever, develops in people using narcotics for pain control. Physical dependence, however, always occurs in patients taking narcotics for a long time. Physical dependence is a problem only when a patient is suddenly taken off the drug. If this happens, a physical reaction, called withdrawal syndrome, takes place. If a disease becomes cured during therapy and opioid medications are no longer needed, they can be withdrawn slowly so that the withdrawal syndrome does not develop. (However, sometimes chronic opioid medications are still needed, because of the previous tissue destruction that the tumor or therapy caused.) The bottom line is that physical dependence does not equal addiction.

◆ Myth 3. Patients who take opioid medications develop tolerance and always need more and more medicine.

There are many reasons behind the need for increased doses of an opioid medication. One is spreading disease or a change in the type of pain, such as a new neuropathic pain problem developing with tumor spread. Another reason is tolerance, which means the need for an increasing dose of a drug in order to achieve a desired result. Tolerance, if it develops at all, does not develop suddenly, and doctors can respond to its development by increasing the dose.

Opioid medications are safe even at very high doses if given correctly. If a patient no longer experiences pain relief at one dose level, the dose can be safely increased again and again.

◆ Myth 4. Opioids are dangerous because they can make breathing harder for a terminally ill patient.

Morphine and other opioid drugs are not dangerous respiratory depressants in patients with cancer and pain. Doses are gradually increased and tolerance to the respiratory-depressant effects of these drugs usually develops before tolerance to their pain-relieving effects.

◆ Myth 5. People taking opioids must get it by injection since opioids are poorly absorbed by mouth.

Most opioids are absorbed very well when taken orally. However, a fair amount of the dose taken by mouth is "lost" to nontarget body tissues and therefore wasted, so larger dosages of the drug are required than the doses needed for shots. The pain equivalency between oral and intramuscular (shots) or intravenous morphine is 3 to 1 when taken over time, meaning that 30 mg of oral morphine is equivalent to 10 mg of intramuscular or intravenous morphine.

SUPPORTIVE

TECHNIQUES OF PAIN CONTROL

It is important to look after the emotional and psychological components of pain too. Psychological counseling can help in many ways: finding sources of emotional support, reducing any sense of loneliness and isolation, and coming to terms with your situation or planning for the future. Talking with clergy or other trusted spiritual advisers may also reduce anxieties and fears that contribute to your pain.

Anything that helps you relax can help your efforts at pain control. Relaxation exercises, massage, transcutaneous nerve stimulation, biofeedback, acupuncture and acupressure may all be of help.

Perhaps surprisingly, one very effective pain control device may be as close as your stereo. Music has been rated to have an analgesic effect twice that of a plain background sound. So listen to your favorite musical works and artists. Music can help you relax, raise your spirits, give you great joy—and help you control your pain.

FATIGUE

Barbara F. Piper, RN, OCN, DNSc

Fatigue is the most common symptom seen in cancer and cancer treatment. In many patients, quality of life and the tolerance of and effectiveness of cancer therapies will be adversely affected by fatigue. Yet little is known about what causes fatigue and how best to treat it.

Everyone gets tired. This is a universal sensation that is expected to occur at certain times of the day or after certain types of activities. Tiredness usually has an identifiable cause, is short-lived and is easily dissipated by a rest or a good night's sleep. In contrast, the fatigue experienced by people with cancer—both in and out of treatment—is often described as an unusual or excessive whole-body tiredness that is unrelated or disproportionate to exertion and that is not easily dispelled by sleep or rest. Fatigue is very subjective—it is hard to classify and it is a very personal phenomenon. It is often described as having "no energy."

Fatigue may be short-term (acute), lasting less than one month. Or it may be more long-term (chronic), lasting anywhere from one month to six months or longer. Whether acute or chronic, fatigue can have a profound negative effect on the quality of life.

Fatigue interferes with the ability to perform the kinds of activities and roles that give meaning and value to life. So fewer activities are undertaken and those that are undertaken may require more effort and take longer to complete.

As fatigue begins to change what cancer patients can do for themselves, family members and other caregivers begin to assume many of the roles the patients used to perform for themselves. These increased demands can lead to fatigue in family members and to social isolation for both patients and their families.

Fatigue is often not mentioned during the visit to the doctor and, often, physicians do not ask about fatigue. You may accept tiredness as part of the cancer and not ask for a treatment plan that may include diet, vitamin and mineral supplements and suggestions on how to save energy.

WHAT CAUSES FATIGUE?

No one knows exactly why people with cancer and other chronic illnesses experience this unusual fatigue. Age, sex and genetics, socioeconomic and environmental factors, and prior experiences with weakness and fatigue have been implicated in fatigue, as have sleep disturbances and depression. But with cancer, many other factors involved in both the disease and its treatment may also contribute.

◆ Changes in energy production and the lack of availability of nutrients may cause fatigue. The tumor itself may make the body function in an overactive, or hypermetabolic, state. Tumor cells compete for nutrients, often at the expense of normal cells' growth and metabolism. Weight loss, reduced appetite and fatigue are often the result.

◆ Disease complications and treatment side effects such as anemia, infection and fever can create additional energy needs that your usual food intake cannot supply alone. Nutritional supplements and therapy may be needed.

◆ Also associated with fatigue are diagnostic tests, anesthesia, surgery, radiation therapy, chemotherapy, biotherapy and drugs used to control symptoms and side effects such as nausea, vomiting, pain and insomnia.

◆ Eighty to 96 percent of all chemotherapy patients experience fatigue, which is perceived to be more distressing and disabling than nausea and vomiting. Fatigue will vary in part depending upon the type of cancer, its location, its duration and the chemotherapy drugs used.

◆ Drugs such as vincristine, vinorelbine and vinblastine may cause fatigue because of their toxic effects on nerves (neurotoxicity). With cisplatin, low magnesium levels, along with neurotoxicity, may cause fatigue.

◆ Fatigue that increases over time (cumulative fatigue) occurs in radiotherapy patients regardless of the part of the body being treated. This usually improves within one month, but may last up to three months after treatment stops.

◆ Fatigue may become so severe during biotherapy that treatment dosages may need to be limited.

◆ As cancer cells die in response to therapy, they release substances that may contribute to fatigue. More attention has recently been paid to the possible role of cytokines in the development of fatigue. Cytokines are natural cell products or proteins, such as the interferons and interleukins, that are normally released by white blood cells, lymphocytes and macrophages in response to infection. These cytokines carry messages that regulate other elements of the immune and neuroendocrine systems to control cancer growth. In high amounts, these cytokines can be toxic and lead to persistent fatigue.

◆ Changes in the patterns of activity and rest can play a significant role in the prevention, cause and relief of fatigue. Unnecessary inactivity, prolonged bedrest and immobility contribute to loss of muscle strength and endurance. Muscle that is not exercised loses its ability to use oxygen, so more effort and more oxygen are required for the same amount of work performed by conditioned muscles. This is one of the reasons why aerobic endurance exercise, such as walking three or four times a week for 20 to 30 minutes, is often prescribed for patients and family members.

◆ Lack of restful or adequate sleep at night can lead to fatigue and increased sleepiness and napping during the day. (Sleep disturbances such as insomnia, multiple awakenings and early waking are common symptoms of depression.)

◆ Anxiety can contribute to sleeplessness, increased energy demands and fatigue.

◆ Surgery and anesthesia can lead to postoperative fatigue.

WHAT CAN BE DONE?

The best way to combat fatigue is to treat the underlying cause. Unfortunately, it is not always easy to know what the exact cause is. Many factors may be involved and require treatment, particularly if the fatigue has become chronic. All possible causes must be thoroughly assessed.

If fatigue is related to anemia, for example, blood transfusions, supplemental oxygen and medications designed to increase red blood cell production (Procrit or Epogen) may be prescribed. Other causes can be managed on an individual basis. This management may include physical therapy and strength training, changes in nutrition and support and psychological counseling.

To treat fatigue:
1. Avoid too much rest, as it can cause physical deterioration and increase fatigue.
2. Exercise regularly. This can be as simple as a 20-to-30-minute walk three times a week. Chapter 21 has other suggestions for regular exercise.

3. Maintain good nutrition (see Chapters 16 to 20).
4. Control emotional fatigue (see Chapters 12, 13 and 14).

Ways to Conserve Energy
◆ Use aids to improve movement and save strength. These aids are detailed in Chapter 22.
◆ Whenever possible, have someone drive you door to door.
◆ Use ramps rather than stairs.
◆ Use an electric wheelchair, if necessary.
◆ Wear comfortable athletic or walking shoes.
◆ Plan your outfits ahead of time to avoid the stress of having to dress quickly.
◆ Use dressing aids.
◆ Dress sitting down as much as possible.
◆ Use grooming and bathing aids.
◆ Wear a terry robe after bathing to help you get dry.

It is essential to combat fatigue because it affects how you live, how well you tolerate cancer therapy, and your overall quality of life. Fatigue can rob you of your ability to live a fuller life to your best level. This advice applies equally to your family and caregivers, as they can also become fatigued.

Sleep and Pain Quality sleep and relief of pain are both essential to the healing process, but one or both elude some cancer patients. Often patients are so worried about their therapies or have such extended fears that they are unable to obtain quality sleep.

In addition to the standard methods of treatment for fatigue, effective approaches to pain relief are meditation, relaxation and hypnosis. Hypnosis appears to work by increasing relaxation and by preventing pain from entering one's consciousness. A reduction of pain can in turn lead to a reduction in insomnia.

LYMPHEDEMA

John P. Cooke, MD, PhD

Lymphedema is a swelling caused by a buildup of fluid (lymph) in the soft tissues of the limbs. This buildup often occurs after surgical removal of lymph nodes or radiotherapy to lymph nodes (because of blockage of the lymphatic system) and sometimes after chemotherapy. (It also occurs often after infections.) Gaps in our understanding of lymphedema have limited treatment, but recent advances in surgical techniques and imaging—x-rays, scans, ultrasound lymphangiography—as well as insights gained from physiologic studies, hold promise of more definitive therapy.

Occasionally lymphedema becomes a chronic problem and it may be permanent. Where cancer is involved, lymphedema is most often seen after breast surgery or radiotherapy, with malignant melanoma, testicular or prostate cancer, and after surgical lymph-node dissection and radiotherapy.

Chronic lymphedema may result in minor swelling and discomfort. Occasionally it leads to a grave disability and disfigurement. It is more difficult to reverse than acute lymphedema, which is often short-term. With chronic lymphedema, skin infection, even after a minor cut or bruise, can often be controlled only with short- or long-term antibiotics.

To prevent lymphedema:

1. Avoid limb injuries, especially cuts and bruises.
2. Keep skin lubricated with creams or oils.
3. Protect your fingers. For example, wear gloves to avoid injury when gardening or doing manual work.
4. Avoid cutting your cuticles and use extra care when cutting your nails.
5. Avoid the use of blood pressure cuffs or having needles in a limb with lymphedema.
6. Take care of cuts or injuries to the limbs; see your physician if you have any questions.

TREATMENT

Emotional problems associated with lymphedema are not uncommon and are often neglected by physicians. The need to address the psychological aspects of long-term disfigurement, especially with adolescent patients, cannot be overemphasized. In discussing these issues with the patient, the physicians should be realistic about the possibility of progression but should emphasize the patient's ability to modify the course of lymphedema by careful attention to the details of the medical program.

Some patients become sedentary in response to uncomfortable or heavy sensations in the affected limb. Reduced physical activity at work and at home leads to apathy and malaise; these can be avoided by encouraging physical activity with proper support hose. Regular exercise appears to reduce lymphedema as long as elastic support (or hydrostatic pressure) is applied. Swimming is a particularly good activity because the surrounding hydrostatic pressure of the water means compressive support isn't needed.

Elastic support hose should be fitted to the patient's limb after the edema has been reduced as much as possible by compression and elevation. This is important, because the stocking does not reduce the size of the leg but only maintains the circumference to which it is fitted. If the limb is fitted for a stocking while in a swollen state, it will be maintained by the stocking in a swollen state.

To reduce the swelling to a minimum may take several days of elevation and bandaging unless a pneumatic compression device is used. Pneumatic devices intermittently compress the limb.

1. Take antibiotics as needed and prescribed by your physician.
2. Use special pneumatic compression machines to "milk" lymphedema out of affected limbs. Special compression stockings and sleeves or ace bandages help keep the lymphedema under control. An alternative approach to mechanical pumps is decongestive physiotherapy, which uses massage, exercise and bandaging. This technique is at least as effective as mechanical pumps, and less costly if you learn how to perform the therapy yourself.
3. Have physical therapy in conjunction with exercise, such as riding a bike.
4. If lymphedema persists, it may be useful to be seen at a center for the treatment of lymphedema. Specialized massages and bandaging techniques will improve your condition.
5. Use a cream to lubricate and soften your skin.
6. If you have lymphedema affecting a leg, make sure that any fungal infection of your toes is treated.

6

ALTERNATIVE AND COMPLEMENTARY THERAPIES

Barrie R. Cassileth, PhD

———◇———

A striking characteristic of "alternative" medicine throughout the twentieth century is its inconsistency. During the early decades of the century, all-purpose health tonics and a variety of "cancer cures" were widely available, sold from town to town in horse-drawn wagons, in stores and through newspaper ads. "Energy" cancer cures, reflecting the growing capability and interest in radio waves, predominated during the 1920s. Competing mainstream therapies for cancer at the time included surgery, which had been used to remove tumors for many centuries, and radiation therapy, which had been discovered around the turn of the century. When chemotherapy was first developed, following World War II, popular alternatives included Koch's glyoxylide and then Hoxsey's cancer cure. Dr. Ivy's Krebiozen predominated during the 1960s, and Laetrile achieved prominence in the 1970s.

These popular unproved therapies were given many names, including "unorthodox," "questionable," "fraudulent." They were attacked as quackery, said to be doing more harm than good and to be robbing people of their money in exchange for worthless nostrums.

During the next decade, a new collection of unconventional approaches emerged. A return to the nineteenth century emphasis on self-care occurred in the form of an angry backlash against an increasingly technologic, specialized and proficient medical system. Although medicine cured more illnesses than ever, the system was said to be impersonal, focused on disease rather than on the patient. It was criticized for lacking a "holistic" emphasis, and for failing to care for the individual as a social and spiritual being. This movement occurred for medicine in general, including specialties such as oncology.

Starting gradually around this time, unproved or unorthodox medicine took on a different and broader meaning. It incorporated not only regimens and therapies promoted outside of mainstream medicine but also many approaches concerned with people's emotional and spiritual life. The resurgence of self-care meant that folk remedies and the family's favorite home treatments belonged under the newly popular umbrella term "alternative," along with the old unproved, unorthodox methods and the soothing efforts aimed at the person behind the disease.

THE CONFUSION OF TERMINOLOGY

The space under the "alternative" umbrella became crowded, filled as it was with a large collection of disparate healing products and techniques. "Alternative medicine" also became home to the views of new as well as existing extremist groups. These individuals and organizations claimed and continue to believe that a conspiracy-ridden medical establishment deliberately withholds "cures," meaning treatments offered commercially despite the absence of scientific evidence that they work. The reason is economic, they say: if major serious illnesses such as cancer were abolished, the medical establishment, the National Institutes of Health, the American Cancer Society and all the other groups involved in medical care would be out of business.

On several grounds, including the fact that health care professionals and advocates are no more immune to cancer and other serious illnesses than are other members of the general public, that contention seems far from rational or believable in this writer's view. Nonetheless, it persists as a no-longer-covert theme among radical believers.

At the other extreme of the continuum of therapies under the "alternative" umbrella, we see an assortment of approaches and techniques aimed not at curing major diseases but at reducing symptoms and enhancing quality of life. These techniques are used to sustain good health as well as to lessen the symptoms of serious illness. These include spiritual, psychological, social and physical approaches as well as remedies contained in bottles or capsules. They are typically called complementary therapies in Europe and other parts of the world. In North America, we still use the term *alternative*, or sometimes *alternative and complementary*.

These general terms are unfortunate because they mask crucial differences among very varied approaches: helpful, noninvasive therapies; unproven, harmful treatments; useless time and money wasters, and foolish and fraudulent methods. It is virtually impossible to judge whether one approves of alternative therapies without asking, "Which ones?"

To bring some clarity to this dissimilar collection of therapeutic techniques, it is helpful to look at the promoted purpose of a method and thereby separate "alternative" from "complementary" therapies. The former category includes treatments

recommended for use instead of mainstream care. These therapies are sold literally as "alternatives" to conventional medicine. Complementary therapies, in contrast and as the term literally implies, serve a supplementary role. Complementary therapies accompany mainstream treatment or are used as part of wellness and health maintenance programs. They include regimens that are part of preventive medicine and supportive care. In distinction to alternatives, they tend to be noninvasive, inexpensive and widely helpful.

Admittedly, this is a simplistic and imperfect dichotomy. How and when a remedy is applied, as much as what the remedy is, can categorize it as complementary and appropriate or as alternative and potentially dangerous. Thus, some therapies would be considered "alternative" under a particular circumstance and "complementary" under another. Aromatherapy is an example of how a single regimen can be either alternative or complementary, depending on how it is promoted or used. As a soothing fragrance in the bath or during massage, aromatherapy can be pleasant and calming. However, some books and advocates claim that aromatherapy can cure disease, and its use for that alternative purpose could be harmful by delaying needed treatment. In other examples, a relaxation program known to lower anxiety becomes alternative when it is applied to cure disease rather than used as an adjunct to conventional medical treatment, and mainstream chemotherapy drugs become alternative when used in dosages that exceed or fail to meet accepted standards.

CURRENT ACCEPTANCE OF COMPLEMENTARY THERAPIES

The idea of separating alternative from complementary medicine, despite its occasional drawbacks, is generally useful. Further, the apparent change of attitude among patients, the public, doctors and other health care providers toward the use of unconventional methods is due in large measure to the inclusion of complementary therapies under the "alternative" rubric. When reference is made to "alternative" approaches, frequently the therapy under discussion is actually "complementary."

The growing acceptance of complementary therapies today is evidenced in many ways, including the broad availability of information to the general public through every means of communication, including the Internet. Alternative and complementary therapies represent an international phenomenon. They abound not only in North America, but also in Europe, Australia and Asia.

Unconventional medicine has made unprecedented inroads into the major institutions of mainstream medicine: medical schools, academic medical research centers, peer-reviewed medical literature, insurance companies and the federal government. Many countries and institutions have developed research centers for alternative medicine.

In 1992, the United States Congress mandated the creation of the National Institutes of Health Office of Alternative Medicine (OAM). Some members of Congress had positive personal experiences with unconventional medicine and lobbied for approval and funding of the OAM. The purpose of this office is to facilitate the evaluation of alternative and complementary approaches, to determine their effectiveness and to help integrate effective therapies into the medical mainstream.

The OAM performs two roles in furthering research on alternative and complementary therapies. First, it logs and maintains interest in the numerous alternative medicine research projects funded over the years by the National Institutes of Health (NIH). Current support from the 17 institutes of the NIH totals more than $13 million. The National Institute of Drug Abuse and the National Heart, Lung and Blood Institute spend more on alternative and complementary therapy research than each of the other health institutes.

Second, the OAM funds research under its own auspices, usually in conjunction with a relevant institute. To date, OAM has funded 42 pilot studies for approximately $30,000 each. Seven of the funded pilot studies concerned cancer. Because these were pilot studies, results did not provide definitive data. They simply indicated which of the projects seemed promising and worthy of more careful investigation. The OAM also has funded 11 university-based centers where research in alternative and complementary medicine takes place. Each center focuses on a specific problem or disease, such as pain, women's health, cancer or AIDS. Research results are not yet available from the centers.

The National Library of Medicine (NLM) activity represents another example of greater federal acceptance of unconventional medicine. A meeting of NLM staff and OAM council members increased researchers' access to articles about complementary medicine. In 1995, the NLM expanded its number of key words and included additional journals related to alternative and complementary practices. The NLM now contains more than 60,000 citations for articles about alternative and complementary therapies.

Numerous medical schools and hospitals have developed programs or departments for the study of complementary therapies. At least 27 medical schools in the United States offer courses on alternative and complementary medicine, including Georgetown, Columbia, Harvard, Maryland and Wayne State

University. Many others provide occasional lectures or ongoing informal programs.

The First Annual International Congress on Alternative and Complementary Medicine in the United States was held in 1995. In addition, dozens of meetings are held throughout the United States on specific approaches, such as homeopathy, herbal medicine, Ayur Veda and spirituality. Medical doctors and others attend and speak at these conferences, which cover virtually every type of unconventional medicine.

Journals and books devoted to alternative and complementary medicine intended for health professionals or the public abound. Many are proponent-driven rather than objective, and therefore cannot necessarily be accepted at face value. This major drawback lies behind the emergence of a journal in England and another in the United States that take a scientific look at this field, evaluating the quality of research and trying to differentiate between therapies that are worthwhile and those that are useless or little more than quackery.

In another example of mainstream acceptance of complementary medicine, some insurance companies now offer plans that reimburse practitioners of complementary therapies, such as chiropractors, acupuncturists and massage therapists. These plans often are met with great public interest. The AlternaPath pilot program of Blue Cross gave subscribers access to acupuncturists, naturopaths and homeopaths, and quickly was fully subscribed when first offered on a pilot basis. (Acupuncture is a good example of a former alternative therapy that, for researched problems such as pain and substance abuse, is now widely accepted in mainstream medicine.) The American Western Life Insurance company offers a "wellness plan" using naturopaths, rather than conventional physicians, as gatekeepers. The plan emphasizes naturopathic remedies as first-line treatment and calls upon mainstream medicine only when necessary.

A further sign of acceptance of complementary medicine is the behavior of physicians. More than 60 percent of physicians in one survey referred their patients to alternative practitioners; primary care physicians were most likely to do so. Many complementary therapy practitioners are physicians; a 1984 study found that 51 percent were medical doctors. They tended to be family practitioners, generalists and psychiatrists almost exclusively.

ALTERNATIVE CANCER THERAPIES POPULAR TODAY

To bring structure to the wide and quickly changing universe of alternative therapies, the Office of Alternative Medicine groups them into the seven categories summarized below.

Diet and Nutrition Anticancer diets and nutritional supplements represent enduring alternative cancer treatments. Many alternative cancer clinics in Tijuana and elsewhere include special diets as part of their overall treatments. Up to 61 percent of British cancer patients use unconventional diets. It is true that the consumption of fruits and vegetables and fiber and avoidance of excessive dietary fat can reduce cancer risk. However, alternative anticancer diets go further, with proponents often claiming that a certain diet can cure cancer. Extending claims beyond what is supported by research is a hallmark of many alternative treatments. Although healthy diets are important in preventing some cancers, no diet has ever been shown to cure cancer or extend remissions.

Today's most popular dietary cancer cure is probably macrobiotics. The popularity of the macrobiotic diet can be traced to the efforts of Michio Kushi, a tireless proponent. Once nutritionally deficient, the macrobiotic diet has since been enhanced and now derives 50 to 60 percent of its calories from whole grains, 25 to 30 percent from vegetables, and the remainder from beans, seaweed and soups. The diet avoids meat and certain vegetables and promotes soybean consumption. Miso, a product of the fermentation of soybeans, is claimed to be the crucial ingredient of the macrobiotic diet "cure."

The OAM recently funded a pilot study of the cancer-preventive effects of the macrobiotic diet. The principal investigator was Lawrence Kushi, ScD, a researcher on the faculty of the University of Minnesota School of Public Health and the son of Michio Kushi. Furthermore, scientists at the University of Alabama at Birmingham and the National Institute of Diabetes and Digestive and Kidney Diseases are investigating the potential anticancer properties of genistein, a substance in soybeans, as a possible explanation for the lower rates of breast and other cancers in Asian compared to American women. An article in the *New England Journal of Medicine* concluded that soy versus animal protein significantly decreases total cholesterol, low-density lipoproteins (LDL) and triglycerides. Possibly the lower fat intake associated with dietary soy products relates to a decreased incidence of breast cancer, which may be elevated by fat intake.

Mind-Body Techniques The notion that we can influence health with our minds resonates well within the individualism of U.S. culture, and mind-body medicine is extremely popular in the United States. Some mind-body interventions have moved from the realm of the unconventional into mainstream medicine. This category includes prayer. Good documentation also exists for the effectiveness of meditation, biofeedback and yoga in stress reduction and the control of particular physiologic reactions.

Some proponents argue that patients can use mental attributes and mind-body work to prevent or cure cancer. This belief has great appeal. It ascribes to the patient almost complete control over the course of illness and suggests that the will of the individual or mental toughness can overcome malignancy. Studies suggesting that mental factors or prayer influence the course of cancer are widely publicized, although they may involve small numbers of patients or remain unreplicated. Examples include a 1989 *Lancet* article showing that women with breast cancer who attended weekly support group sessions had double the survival time of women who did not attend. (A replication of this study has been under way for almost a decade, but no results have been reported.)

Another well-known example is the San Francisco intercessory prayer study, a prospective, randomized, double-blind study of 393 patients, one-half of whom were randomly selected to be prayed for by people at a distance. Results were significant, suggesting that intercessory prayer had beneficial therapeutic effects, although there were no differences in length of hospital stay according to whether patients were prayed for or not.

Stories of individuals who successfully prayed to be healed or who experienced miraculous cures from cancer and other illnesses are frequently reported. Bernie Siegel, MD, a former cancer surgeon and author of *Love, Medicine and Miracles* and other bestsellers, is a leading and popular proponent of the link between mind and cancer. Siegel organized groups of what he termed "exceptional cancer patients" based on his observation as a surgeon that attitude influenced survival time. He encourages patients to maintain positive attitudes and to assume responsibility for their own health. He asks them to consider why they might "need" their cancer. The implication is that cancer results from unhealthy emotional patterns.

However, a study coauthored by Siegel found no difference in length of survival for these patients compared with similar others. Had these results been positive, the study would have received publicity similar to that afforded Siegel's bestselling books. Because the results did not confirm more than 12 years of public statements, the study received no media attention and even failed to alter proponent claims.

Attending to the psychological health of cancer patients is a fundamental component of good cancer care. Support groups, good doctor-patient relationships and the emotional and instrumental help of family and friends are vital. However, the idea that patients can influence the course of their disease through mental or emotional work is not backed up by study and can evoke feelings of guilt and inadequacy when the disease continues to advance despite patients' spiritual or mental efforts.

Bioelectromagnetics Bioelectromagnetics is the study of living organisms and their interactions with electromagnetic fields. Bioelectromagnetic therapies use the low-frequency portion of the electromagnetic spectrum. Proponents claim that magnetic fields penetrate the body and heal damaged tissues, including cancers. Wolfgang Ludwig, SCD, PhD, director of the Institute of Biophysics in Horb, Germany, asserts that magnetic fields can cure a wide variety of ailments, including malignant diseases. However, no peer-reviewed publications support any cancer-related claims regarding bioelectromagnetics.

Traditional and Folk Remedies This category includes ancient systems of healing that often are based on concepts of human physiology different from those accepted by modern Western science. Two of the most popular healing systems are traditional Chinese medicine and India's Ayur Veda, popularized by bestselling author Deepak Chopra, MD.

Traditional Chinese medicine is distinguished by its focus on *chi*, the life force said to flow through energy channels known as meridians. Traditional Chinese medicine relies on exercise techniques such as qi gong and tai chi to strengthen and balance *chi*. Traditional Chinese medicine also uses acupuncture, acupressure and a full herbal pharmacopoeia, with remedies for most ailments, including cancer. Chinese herbal teas, philosophy and relaxation techniques are soothing and appealing to many patients with cancer who use them as complementary therapies. Many studies are under way to evaluate the benefits of Chinese herbal remedies.

The term Ayur Veda comes from the Sanskrit words *ayur* (life) and *veda* (knowledge). Ayur Veda's 5,000-year-old healing techniques are based on the classification of people into one of three predominant body types. There are specific remedies for disease and regimens to promote health for each body type. Ayur Veda has a strong mind-body component, stressing the need to keep consciousness in balance. It uses techniques such as yoga and meditation to do so. Approximately 10 Ayur Veda clinics in North America served an estimated 25,000 patients over the past 10 years. The number of cancer patients among them is not documented.

Pharmacologic and Biologic Treatments This class of treatments remains highly controversial. Pharmacologic treatments typically are invasive and costly, and tend to encourage patients to try them and ignore or delay mainstream therapy.

A well-known pharmacologic therapy today is antineoplastons, developed by Stanislaw Burzynski, MD, PhD, and available at his clinic in Houston, Texas. As well as laboratory investigation by a respected scientist who concluded that antineoplastons do not even exist, clinical evidence evaluated under the National Cancer Institutes of both the United States and Canada failed to support the potential worth of this regimen.

Public interest remains high, elevated perhaps by publicity received not only from television appearances by Dr. Burzynski and his patients but also from the headline-producing indictment of Burzynski in late 1995 following a U.S. Postal Service and FDA raid of his Houston clinic. Dr. Burzynski recently initiated a plan to obtain follow-up information on his patients and maintain data on their progress. Such information has not been available previously and will be welcomed.

Immunoaugmentative therapy (IAT) was developed by the late Lawrence Burton, PhD, and offered in his clinic in the Bahamas. Burton's therapy is based on balancing four protein components in the blood. This injected therapy, as with antineoplastons, relies on strengthening the patient's immune system, although in both cases no evidence supports those beliefs. According to proponent literature, Burton claimed that IAT was particularly effective in treating mesothelioma. Documentation of IAT's efficacy remains anecdotal. The clinic has continued to operate since Burton's death but seems to have declined in popularity, possibly because of the rise of other alternatives, such as shark cartilage.

Interest in shark cartilage as a cancer therapy was spurred by a 1992 book written by I. William Lane, PhD, *Sharks Don't Get Cancer*, and by a television special that displayed apparent remissions in patients with advanced cancer treated with shark cartilage in Cuba. The televised outcome was strongly disputed by oncologists in the United States. Shark cartilage advocates base their therapy on the discovery by Harvard's Judah Folkman, MD, of a cartilage-based protein that inhibits angiogenesis, the creation of new blood vessels. (Tumors require a vigorous blood supply to thrive.)

According to mainstream scientists, however, the molecules of active ingredients in the "food supplement" shark cartilage sold at heath food stores are too large to be absorbed. They decompose into inert ingredients and are simply excreted. Despite lack of positive evidence, shark cartilage pills and suppositories are widely publicized (as arthritis as well as cancer cures) and are available in health food stores throughout the United States. Bovine cartilage is also under study for its potential anticancer properties. Although finding a way to kill cancer cells by cutting off their blood supply remains a major research focus, there is little scientific hope that shark or bovine cartilage can be helpful.

Another biologic remedy, Cancell, is especially popular in the midwestern United States and in Florida. Proponents claim that it returns cancer cells to a "primitive state" from which the cells are digested and rendered inert. FDA laboratory studies revealed that Cancell is composed of common chemicals, including nitric acid, sodium sulfite, potassium hydroxide, sulfuric acid and catechol. The FDA found no basis for claims of Cancell's effectiveness against cancer.

Popular metabolic therapies are readily available in Tijuana, Mexico, and elsewhere in North America. One of the best-known Tijuana centers is the Gerson clinic, where treatment is based on the notion that toxic products of cancer cells accumulate in the liver, leading to liver failure and death. Gerson's treatment aims to counteract liver damage with low-salt, low-fat, high-potassium diets and coffee enemas. The hills around Tijuana are dotted with similar cancer clinics, each offering its own version of metabolic treatment.

Manual Healing Methods Manual healing includes a variety of touch and manipulation techniques. Osteopathic and chiropractic doctors were among the earliest groups to use manual methods. Hands-on massage is a useful adjunctive technique for cancer patients and others for its stress-reducing benefits.

One of the most popular manual healing methods in North America is therapeutic touch, which, despite its name, involves no direct contact. In therapeutic touch, healers move their hands a few inches above a patient's body to remove "blockages" to the patient's energy field. Developed by a nursing professor emeritus at New York University, therapeutic touch is taught at most U.S. nursing schools. Although numerous critics in mainstream medicine deride its fundamental premises, therapeutic touch is widely practiced and usually appreciated by patients. It is likely that psychological benefits are achieved by a caregiver's presence and concern.

Herbal Medicine Herbal remedies typically are part of traditional and folk healing with long histories of use. Some form of herbal medicine is found in all areas of the world. Although many herbal remedies are claimed to have anticancer effects, only a few have gained substantial popularity as cancer therapies.

Essiac is one of the most popular herbal cancer alternatives in North America. It was popularized by a Canadian nurse, Rene Caisse (Essiac is Caisse spelled backwards), but developed earlier by a native Canadian healer. Essiac comprises four herbs: burdock, turkey rhubarb, sorrel and slippery elm. Research at the National Cancer Institute and at Memorial Sloan-Kettering Cancer Center in New York has found that it has no anticancer effect. It is illegal to distribute Essiac in Canada, although under a special arrangement Canadian patients may receive it from a supplier in Ontario. A problem with

Essiac is that Caisse never revealed its formula, so several competing firms sell different versions, each claiming to have the true formula. It is widely available in U.S. health food stores.

Combinations of Chinese herbs to treat cancer have been used for hundreds of years. Herbal combinations are still used by some people who do not have access to modern therapies, and some herbal remedies are used in Asia along with modern mainstream cancer care. Chinese herbal remedies, particularly teas, are prized for the comfort patients feel that they bring.

Iscador, a derivative of mistletoe, is a popular cancer remedy in Europe, where it has been used as folk treatment for centuries. Iscador is available in many mainstream European cancer clinics. European governments fund ongoing studies of Iscador's effectiveness against cancer, but no definitive data support proponent claims.

The FDA does not examine herbal remedies for safety and effectiveness, and most have not been formally tested for side effects. There have been recent reports in the medical literature of severe liver and kidney damage from a limited number of herbal remedies, including chaparral tea. These reports underscore the fact that "natural" products are not necessarily safe or harmless.

THE PREVALENCE OF ALTERNATIVE AND COMPLEMENTARY CANCER MEDICINE

Complementary therapies are popular with the public, with better-educated people using them more often than others. A national telephone survey found that 34 percent of Americans visited alternative practitioners in 1990, spending $13.7 billion on these visits. Americans made more visits to alternative practitioners (425 million) than to primary care physicians (388 million).

There are few studies on the use of alternative therapies for cancer in North America. The investigations that have been conducted found that substantial proportions of cancer patients use complementary therapies. A smaller percentage of cancer patients use alternative medicine. One study of the prevalence of alternative cancer therapy use in the United States found that the percentage of cancer patients using questionable methods (alternatives were not differentiated from complementary therapies) ranged from a low of 6.4 percent in the South Atlantic region to a high of 14.7 percent in the Rocky Mountains.

Studies conducted in other countries reveal a similar range of usage rates. In both England and the United States, patients using alternatives are more likely to be women, younger and affluent. An investigation in Poland discovered that more than one-fourth of cancer patients use unconventional treatments, whereas 66 percent of 235 Canadian patients with rheumatologic diseases, 46 percent of children with cancer in South Australia and 15 percent of 949 cancer outpatients surveyed in the Netherlands used alternative or complementary therapies, typically in conjunction with conventional care.

The majority of physicians who practice alternative medicine are family practitioners or psychiatrists; very few oncologists or other medical specialists do so. Most oncologists are not familiar with the alternative and complementary therapies used by many of their patients.

COMMUNICATING WITH PATIENTS

A small minority of cancer patients use alternative therapies, although it appears that many more adopt therapies such as massage, acupuncture or herbal teas for strictly complementary purposes. It is vital that you, the patient, and your family feel comfortable talking with your oncologist about alternative and complementary therapies. You can teach your oncologist about complementary methods and learn together what can be done in addition to mainstream treatment and following completion of mainstream treatment.

The possible harms, benefits and interactions of therapies require evaluation. Physicians also need to understand patients' motives for using alternative or complementary therapies. Inadequate pain management, for example, which remains a problem in cancer treatment, may be helped by nonsedating techniques such as acupuncture.

Access to psychosocial support services can be essential for many families and patients in improving quality of life, and psychosocial support services should be a routine component of cancer care. Providing such access also should help in counteracting the perception that alternative practitioners have cornered the market on caring and concern for patients as people.

One of the most difficult situations arises in terminal illness when some patients make last-ditch efforts to find a cure. These patients are most susceptible to quackery. They also risk emotional distress, false hope and wasted money. In addition to failing to experience the promised "cures," patients are not likely to find enhanced quality of life. The combination of good communication between oncologist and patient and assiduous use of appropriate complementary therapies should reduce patients' frustration and dissatisfaction with oncologic medicine and encourage them to continue conventional care. The soothing attention of complementary practices, including psychosocial care, along with the technologic expertise of oncology practice is a merger that can greatly enhance patients' quality of life and satisfaction with care.

GROWING INTEREST AND ACCEPTANCE

The substantial interest in alternative cancer therapies appears to stem from several sources. The sheer numbers as well as content of mainstream and alternative therapy magazine articles, books, media, patient reports and so on suggest that the public is frustrated with establishment medicine's inability to treat many cancers effectively. The public is distressed by the absence of substantial treatment gains for the major cancers despite the decades and billions of dollars spent fighting this collection of diseases.

Chemotherapy and its side effects have become increasingly intolerable to a public focused on the appeal of natural products and wanting, as we all do, gentler as well as more effective substitutes for standard cancer treatments. Public distrust and dissatisfaction with establishment medicine and related institutions remain. The FDA is seen not as protective but as obstructive. The pharmaceutical industry is viewed as intent on maintaining prohibitive pricing, hindering access to promising products even for dying patients and, despite commercial efforts to display a contrary image, ignoring natural products in favor of high-technology, high-priced drugs.

In many respects, alternative cancer therapies represent the antithesis of the perceived values and actions described above. Patients are simultaneously drawn away from mainstream medicine and toward competing types of care. A major reason for today's public and professional interest in complementary therapies is dissatisfaction with what is perceived as the technologic and impersonal nature of modern medicine. Patients complain about insensitive, limited and hurried interactions with oncologists in every setting, from small suburban hospitals to the top-notch comprehensive cancer centers.

Patients complain that frequently provisions are not made to relieve the anticipated side effects of chemotherapy, and sometimes patients are not even told to expect these effects. Patients often feel helpless and ignored. Many fail to understand why oncology medicine does not include the nontoxic complementary techniques that control pain, reduce stress and alleviate symptoms (see below) that are standard in other countries. The United States is approximately two years behind most European countries in establishing government-level offices of complementary medicine and in offering complementary therapies to augment mainstream cancer care.

Practitioners who provide alternative and complementary therapies are viewed as more caring, as treating the whole person and as providing more emotionally satisfying, communicative relationships. Typically they are able to spend more time talking with their patients than can conventional physicians. This is especially true today in the U.S. under managed care. For this reason, conventional physicians often are termed disinterested and "reductionistic," focused only on the disease, whereas practitioners outside of the mainstream are considered "holistic," concerned with the whole person. Some patients seek alternative care for its more egalitarian approach, for better practitioner-patient relationships or for enhanced opportunities to make therapeutic decisions and play a major role in their own health care.

One can only hope that a more balanced position will emerge for alternative and complementary medicine, one that avoids irrationality and acceptance of therapies on the basis of anecdotal reports, rejects attacks against science and accepts only methodologically sound research. Optimally, a balance can be forged between the science and technology of cancer medicine and the comfort that the best of complementary medicine can bring.

COMPLEMENTARY THERAPIES TO EASE CANCER TREATMENT AND FOLLOW-UP CARE

Alternative and Complementary Treatments for Cancer, a new publication from the American Cancer Society, information on the ACS web site and publications such as those listed in Resources detail these and other interventions that help relieve symptoms and enhance quality of life for cancer patients.

Important interventions such as individual and group therapy are not included in the list below because they are considered mainstream, as opposed to complementary, therapies.

The complementary therapies listed below have been studied, primarily in Europe, and found to be effective for the purposes noted. They are inexpensive and easily accessible. Most of these remedies can be prepared or administered by the patient or a family member. Because some herbal and other ingested remedies may possibly interact with prescription medications, it is important to discuss with your oncologist any therapy that you take on your own.

For Anxiety and Stress
◆ Acupressure
◆ Aromatherapy
◆ Meditation and other relaxation techniques
◆ Therapeutic massage
◆ Valerian tea
◆ Yoga

For Colds and Flu
◆ Garlic
◆ Echinacea

◆ Eucalyptus or peppermint oil
◆ Ginger
◆ Iceland moss and plantain tea
◆ Watercress tea
◆ Zinc lozenges

For Constipation
◆ Cascara or buckthorne bark
◆ Plantago seed
◆ Pureed rhubarb
◆ Water and fiber

For Depression
◆ Hypericum or St. John's wort
◆ Light therapy
◆ Meditation and yoga
◆ Tai chi

For Headache
◆ Acupressure
◆ Evening primrose tea, sunflower seeds. Garlic and onion relieve headaches too.
◆ Feverfew tea
◆ Progressive relaxation or massage

For Indigestion
◆ Peppermint or chamomile tea

For Muscle Aches
◆ Capsicum cream
◆ Hydrotherapy
◆ Massage
◆ Volatile mustard oil

For Nausea
◆ Acupressure
◆ Cinnamon or peppermint tea
◆ Ginger

For Chronic Pain
◆ Acupuncture
◆ Biofeedback
◆ Various herbs
◆ Hypnotherapy
◆ Massage

For Sleep Problems
◆ Lavender oil-scented bath
◆ Lemon balm herb tea
◆ Massage
◆ Meditation
◆ Other herbal teas

PART II:
THE MIND

7
THE WILL TO LIVE

Ernest H. Rosenbaum, MD, Isadora R. Rosenbaum, MA, and Andrew W. Kneier, PhD

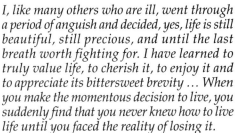

I, like many others who are ill, went through a period of anguish and decided, yes, life is still beautiful, still precious, and until the last breath worth fighting for. I have learned to truly value life, to cherish it, to enjoy it and to appreciate its bittersweet brevity … When you make the momentous decision to live, you suddenly find that you never knew how to live life until you faced the reality of losing it.
—William Cohen, MD, a 42-year-old patient and physician

Physicians are always fascinated with the power of the will to live. Like every creature in the animal world, human beings have a fierce instinct for survival. The will to live is a force within all of us to fight for survival when our lives are threatened by a disease such as cancer. Yet in some this force is stronger than in others, determined by the innate character and personality of the individual, the quality of his or her current life, and whether there is a purpose to life.

Often when cancer patients have prolonged or unexpected remissions or cures, we have felt that the added critical factor was the will to live. We have often seen how two patients, similar in age, diagnosis, degree of illness and treated with the same therapy, can experience widely different therapeutic results. Each case is unique, and of course the biology of a cancer often dictates the course of events regardless of the patient's attitude and fighting spirit. Nonetheless, in many cases the strength of a patient's will to live appears to be an important factor for those who obtain an unexpected remission.

We are constantly impressed by the spirit and grace with which people cope with chronic disease or disability, even under the threat of death. We have observed how they refuse to let physical debility or discomfort affect their enjoyment of family and friends or prevent them from going to work or pursuing outside interests. Inspired by their fortitude, we asked several of our patients how they were able to transcend their problems and what factors they considered essential to their will to live. Their stories touched on many different elements: hope, faith, perseverance, optimism, courage, goals, love, supportive family and friends, purpose, fear of dying, strong coping skills and a feeling that it was their destiny to endure and survive. Whatever aspect patients focused on, continuing to live was essential to their inner drive.

It seemed that the most critical ingredient of their will to live was having something compelling to live for. They set goals and they did whatever they could to get the most out of life. After an initial period of feeling devastated, they decided to make the most of each day.

This spirit was exemplified by Maria, who had a mastectomy at age 29. After nearly 18 years of chemotherapy, radiotherapy and hormonal therapy, she died recently after 26 years of living with her illness.

She always led an active and productive life as a wife, mother and realtor. When she first learned of her diagnosis, Maria began throwing bricks through a window of her home. When asked how many windows she broke, she replied, "A lot. Sometimes one a day. They really got rid of a big thing inside."

Her will to live was one of the strongest we had ever seen. "I got out of bed every morning as if nothing was wrong," she said. "I knew I was going to have to face things and that I could feel sick during the day, but I got out of bed that way. There was a lot I was fighting for—I had a three-year-old child. I had a wonderful life and a magical love affair with my husband."

Maria's story is similar to the so-called Christmas syndrome, wherein a person summons the will to live until a specific occasion or to meet a desired goal—the birth of a grandchild, a final birthday or Christmas. In Maria's case, she lived to raise her child and to be with her husband. After her child was grown and her husband died, she finally let go.

Many of our patients told us that facing the uncertainties of living with cancer makes life more meaningful. The smallest pleasures—eating dinner by the fire, walking the dog, the smell of fresh-cut grass—are intensified. Much hypocrisy is eliminated. When bitterness and anger begin to dissipate, there is still a capacity for joy.

Some patients have written about what it is that makes them so determined to live. "I love living, I love nature," wrote one. "Being outdoors, feeling the sun on my skin or the wind blowing against my body, hearing birds sing or breathing in the spray of the ocean."

Another patient also wrote about this: "I don't think I perceive color, sound, all the senses more deeply, but I do relish them more. I really wallow in a good sunset, but I don't think, 'This may be my last sunset.' I try to be honest with my emotional reactions instead of overdramatizing them."

These and many other patients have shown that success and victory have many definitions. For them, victory consisted of trying their best to achieve the best quality of life possible under the circumstances, no matter how difficult. As Theodore Roosevelt wrote: "It is hard to fail, but it is worse to never have tried to succeed." Milton, though blind, wrote

great poetry. Beethoven, though deaf, wrote beautiful music he would never hear. "Oh how would it be possible to admit the deficiency of a sense that I ought to possess to a more perfect degree than anybody else?" he wrote. "What a dejection when someone next to me heard a flute, and I did not hear anything, or when somebody heard the shepherd sing, and I could not hear even that. Such incidents made me desperate, and I was not far from putting an end to my life. It was only my art, my art that restrained me. Oh, I felt unable to leave this world before I had created what I felt had been assigned to me."

A strong will to live when critically ill is easier said than done. Depression, self-pity and despair are understandable. Experiencing these emotions is part of being human. If you are feeling low enough, your first decision may be whether you want to live. It is natural to have moments of not caring whether you live or die, but in our experience, when the chips are down, most people choose life.

The question that arises, however, is how to live passively as a person who is resigned to fate or actively as someone who is ready to make the best of one's fate and surmount bad luck. At some point you will probably begin to look for ways of regaining control and living as normal a life as possible. Even if the medical crisis passes and we are either cured or reach a long-term compromise with a chronic medical problem, the lesson is not lost.

A threat to our existence typically triggers us to make an objective appraisal of our lives: the kind of people we have become, what is important to us and how we want to live in the future. And it renews our appreciation of the importance of life, love and friendship, and of all there is to enjoy and learn. We begin taking risks we haven't had the courage to take in the past.

Sudden ill health or disability is a rude reminder that our time on earth is limited. Such circumstances can be likened to being hit by a Mack truck. All of a sudden, your entire life is changed. Everything you took for granted, even the things you complained about, suddenly belong to another life that you'd give anything to reclaim. And yet we are often able to survive a crisis because of the way we have coped with a traumatic situation in the past. At our lowest ebb there is a small flame, an inner strength that makes us try again to take an active role in life rather than a passive role.

THE FOUR HORSEMEN CHALLENGE TO THE WILL TO LIVE

The biblical Four Horsemen of the Apocalypse—conquest, war, famine and death—were sent to ravage the earth in preparation for its final destruction. A similar analogy can be applied to the threats to one's will to live that come with a life-threatening and debilitating illness. Just as the will to live can be nurtured by a positive attitude, so can it be undermined by fear, anger, loss of self-esteem and alienation. These are common responses to the diagnosis of cancer. If allowed to go unresolved, they lead to feelings of depression, helplessness, futility and resignation and loss of the will to live. This may lead to premature death by giving up early rather than fighting for your life.

Fear Cancer is the most feared of all diseases. In fact, the word *cancer* is one of the most feared words in the English language. After questioning many newly diagnosed cancer patients, we have found that much of the disproportionate fear associated with this disease is due to the anticipation of prolonged periods of suffering and disability. There is a belief that

little can be done to control the malignancy or relieve its symptoms. Nothing could be further from the truth.

Some patients react to the diagnosis of cancer in much the same manner that people in primitive societies react to a witch doctor's curse—as a sentence to an inevitable and ghastly death. Being "scared to death" is a well-known consequence of bone pointing, an ancient custom attributed to the Papua New Guinean and Australian Aborigines and other South Pacific cultures. A group of natives sits in a circle and spins a bone on the ground. The person the bone points to receives a tribal curse. Death could take place in a few weeks. Of course, such a curse is effective only if the person believes in its power.*

In modern medical practice, a similar phenomenon may occur when a patient believes the diagnosis of cancer to be a death sentence. For instance, a physician may tell a patient that the surgery or other treatment has been unsuccessful and that nothing more can be done. Such patients may simply accept the idea that they are going to die and extinguish their will to live. Such patients can die rapidly, long before their disease has progressed enough to cause death by itself.

Cancer is the most curable chronic disease. It is important to know that 50 percent of persons diagnosed with cancer can be cured. The cure rate climbs to 75 percent when good preventive and diagnostic medicine routines are followed. These include mammograms, yearly physical examinations, colorectal sigmoidoscopy and digital (finger) rectal examinations, blood tests and medical follow-up. As well, people should follow a healthy lifestyle—exercise, quit smoking, reduce alcohol consumption and eat less red meat and more grains, vegetables and fruits.

Sometimes a doctor says to the patient,

*References for the studies cited in this chapter are available on request from Keren Stronach, Cancer Resource Center, UCSF/Mount Zion Cancer Center, 2356 Sutter Street, San Francisco CA 94143-1705.

"I'm sorry, Mrs. Jones, but you have advanced cancer and there is no cure." Although the surgeon may feel sympathy and empathy, and may even cry with the patient, all Mrs. Jones hears is, "I can't be cured. I'm dying." How different the outcome might be if the doctor had added, "But we have treatment for you that can treat your cancer to help you continue to live. We will soon work out a therapy plan for you."

It is impossible to predict longevity for an individual patient before therapy. Even after therapy has begun, some time is necessary to assess the response. Until the response to therapy has been established, no projection is feasible. Furthermore, even if one therapy is unsuccessful, another may still be possible. There is always hope that you may outlive any average projection by many months or years.

When a physician makes the effort to explain carefully the nature of cancer, and the anticipated problems and future tests, most patients are surprised to find that their ideas about cancer were considerably more pessimistic than the facts warrant. They find that most of their fears can be resolved by understanding the problems to be faced and the treatments and other supportive measures, and by having a reasonable estimate of the discomfort and inconvenience to be expected. Then they are able to adopt a positive attitude and to accept the compromises that come with the disease and the treatment.

One patient whom we have been treating for advanced cancer for the past six years has taken meticulous precautions to ensure that most of her closest friends do not discover her illness. She does this to protect herself from their possibly negative reactions. Your own fears may be under control, but having to deal with the fears of well-meaning friends can drain emotional energy and cause depression. However, rather than hide your disease, you may feel better including close friends, as well as family, in consultations with your doctor so that they may be able to function as part of your informed support team.

Every patient runs the risk of encountering fear, pessimism, or other destructive attitudes on the part of doctors, nurses, family, friends, or acquaintances. Patients will also be overwhelmed at times by their own fears, discouragement, or sadness. This is normal. Nevertheless, the patient who is willing to fight and to accept guidance and support in his fight for life will have the basic confidence and equanimity with which to confront the ignorant and the fearful. Although fears and fantasies don't disappear, they are put into a manageable perspective. The individual is free to do more than engage in solitary battle with self-made phantoms.
—Ellen, *Living with Cancer*, 1982

Anger Much of your reaction to the diagnosis of cancer depends on your personality and how well you have adapted to life's problems in the past. Some people have difficulty coping with any adversity. Every time they meet a problem they ask, "Why me?" When such people develop cancer, they may spend all their emotional energy being angry that the disease is happening to them. To the person with a positive attitude toward adversity, cancer is a problem that can be attacked in the same way as other problems, with the determination to make the best of it.

When people ask me, "How could God let it happen to me? What justice is there from such a God?" I tell them that God is not doing something to hurt them. Illness or death before one's time is a malfunction of nature just as much as an earthquake or a hurricane.
—Rabbi Joseph Asher, *Living with Cancer*, 1982

Anger is a normal reaction and a way of grieving during the initial period of shock following the diagnosis of cancer.

In fact, if anger cannot be felt or expressed, it may turn into depression. If anger remains unresolved, it takes away energy that could be channeled into coping with the disease and living life as fruitfully as possible.

To be able to resolve anger, you must first recognize that you are angry. Often the anger and bitterness about one's disease are displaced; people make major issues out of minor events, like complaining about someone being late, the dinner not being satisfactory or finding fault with a friend or mate. This displaced anger may be self-defeating: it can alienate people when you need family and friends most.

By recognizing your anger for what it is, you will be setting your mental attitude to cope with it. Letting the anger out by talking about it, even screaming, punching a pillow or throwing things, can further help to release its hold on you. In the end, you can focus the energy of your anger and apply it in a positive direction by putting it to work to fight against your disease.

Maria also addressed this topic:

Cancer is devastating. At first you can't even think about it. You're smacked hard and all the wind goes out of you. You don't begin to think about yourself and your family and your reasons for living. I have seen people destroy themselves with their attitude in all kinds of situations, and, although I don't believe your attitude can cure your disease, I do believe it can help you. Therefore, I reject my negative thoughts. It sounds insane, but it keeps me healthy. Negative thinking breaks down my energy level. Although my drive and my will and my pace are basically the same as they were before, I have changed in one way. I no longer fly off the handle over unimportant matters. My priorities are being alive and loving my family. I've always loved life, and the biggest pain is that I hadn't had enough of it when this thing happened. So I said, "Screw you, world! I just ain't leaving."

Loss of Self-Esteem The very idea of having cancer may itself threaten your self-esteem. Old superstitions still cling to the word *cancer*. Some feel that it is a supernatural punishment or a disgrace. These are only superstitions; having cancer does not mean that you are bad or less worthy, or that you are guilty of some terrible wrongdoing. The disease can happen to anyone; in fact, one out of every two men and one out of every three women in the United States will develop cancer.

Cancer can take away or change the particular things that have given you your sense of self-esteem: body image, independence, the ability to work and provide for your family.

Changes in body image that result from surgery, radiation therapy or chemotherapy may have a devastating effect on your self-esteem, particularly if the changes are visible to others. You may experience the loss of body parts, voice changes, scars or other skin changes, hair loss or weight loss. Patients undergoing ostomy surgery (the creation of an artificial opening connecting the bowel to the skin) may feel humiliated because they must wear a bag to collect body wastes. Surgery affecting the genitals or reproductive organs may cause loss of self-esteem because one thinks that one is not "really a man" or "really a woman" any longer.

Communicating with other cancer patients who have experienced similar body changes will help to remind you that, just as you can relate to them for who they are, so others can relate to you for who you are. Volunteers from various organizations and support groups (*see* Chapter 28 and Resources) can help you to adjust emotionally, and, in turn, you may be able to reciprocate and be of value to them.

A major problem affecting self-esteem is the loss of independence and control. Until illness deprives us of normal responsibilities, we may not realize how much our sense of self-esteem is related to accomplishment, productivity and the ability to "pull our weight" and care for ourselves and others. At the outset, disease and therapy make you dependent on the medical system for your very life. In the hospital you are dominated by the medical system. Tests are carried out, therapy is given. When you eat, bathe, eliminate, walk or even sleep may all be determined by others. You may feel humiliated by having to use a bedpan or by having your body exposed to doctors, nurses and other hospital personnel. Later, you may not be able to return to work or to carry out former responsibilities at home. You may have to depend on family, friends or social service agencies for personal care, household help or financial needs. You may feel guilt at being a burden and feel that you are of no value to others.

Your feelings of independence and self-esteem can be increased by taking responsibility in areas that you can handle. Eating a nutritionally adequate diet, exercising regularly to increase your strength and mobility and performing as many self-care tasks as possible can help accelerate your recovery. Keeping progress notes on your improvement can help enhance your sense of accomplishment.

Involve yourself in supportive programs, such as patient support groups, or special group counseling for cancer patients. Other examples may include meditation, yoga, tai chi or biofeedback. If there are no support groups in your community, enlist the aid of a social worker, counselor or clergy, or find other cancer patients and begin one yourself. At home, choose the tasks you can do yourself. Caring for a pet, growing plants or giving to family members in thoughtfulness and attention what you may not be able to give in physical effort can be outlets for your ability to nurture and will give you a sense of self-esteem.

If work and former interests must be put aside, find new ways of being pro-ductive, such as writing, art, music, sewing, knitting, crocheting or crafts. You may find talents that you have not had the time to explore before.

Alienation Nothing can be as destructive to the will to live as alienation, the feeling of being cut off from life. Isolation and loneliness can cause some patients to lose their will to live and to give up and die very rapidly because they have lost their connection with other human beings. Cancer patients may experience isolation because of physical circumstances, hospitalization, loss of employment or confinement to the home. You may feel socially isolated because of the attitudes of other people, and you may also experience alienation from within because of your own attitudes.

Hospitalization removes you from the mainstream of life—from family, friends and all the daily habits and contacts that make you part of society. Although a hospital is full of people, they are busy strangers, and you may feel very lonely. When you return home, if you're unable to go back to work or must be confined to home, your isolation there may be greater than in the hospital. In the hospital you were at least part of a community. Now you may be alone: you may live alone, your family may be gone during the day or there may be no one to visit you.

While our society espouses rehabilitation of the disease, in reality we often tend to shut people with chronic diseases out of employment. A patient who has had cancer and who is able to work may not be able to return to a former job because the employer is afraid that he or she may not be able to carry responsibilities or that the patient may relapse. If the patient does return to work, fellow workers may avoid him or her because they are afraid cancer may be contagious, or because they do not know how to relate to their coworker. Although laws such as the 1990 Americans with Disabilities Act protect patients' rights, there is still leeway for employers to get around such problems, and unfortunately, some do.

Family and friends sometimes inadvertently isolate the cancer patient. They may at first be sympathetic and attentive, but with time they may drift away; they have their own problems and their own lives to live. They may also find it difficult to carry on a normal conversation with someone who is ill or dying, and they may not know how to relate to you. Then you feel you're being abandoned by those you thought cared most.

A case that exemplifies the problem of alienation involves a patient, physicians and the medical staff. During the last few weeks of life the patient constantly reminded the hospital staff of his existence by saying "good morning" and would tell them, "Please do not skip me on rounds. I'm not dead yet."

Loneliness and alienation may exist for the cancer patient even when the patient is not physically or socially isolated. The uncertain and the life-threatening nature of the disease puts us in touch with the essential aloneness with which we all must face death. Even the patient who is surrounded with family and friends may feel alone, and perhaps lonely in this awareness.

In fighting their disease, some patients turn so much of their energy and attention inward upon themselves that they lose contact with the rest of life and create an isolation and loneliness that they may not recognize as self-inflicted. Other patients withdraw from their connections with the outer world because their focus is on grieving and feeling sorry for themselves. Patients who regard cancer as an automatic death sentence may unconsciously cut their ties with life and live as though they already belong to the dead.

When isolation is thrust upon you from the outside, when old connections to life are broken, you must learn to make new bridges. Loss of independence may encourage you to "wait for things to happen." You may feel frightened or pessimistic about taking any steps toward making a new life; yet we all have the capacity to alter our direction, make changes and rearrange our strategies.

Getting involved in rehabilitation programs and support groups made up of other cancer patients and their families can be your first step (*see* Chapter 28). You will be aiding your recovery as well as making connections with people who share your experience.

Do not let pride prevent you from asking for help or from admitting your need for other people. And do not be ashamed to express emotions. Sharing with others can deepen and strengthen relationships. The closest bonds are made in times of crisis.

Your nurse, social worker, clergy, counselor, doctor and patient support groups are there to hear you and to help you. Expressing what you feel and discussing your feelings with others can give you distance and new perspective, as well as heal the alienation that comes from living in a separate emotional world. You will not be abandoned.

REGAINING CONTROL

In the face of a disease and treatment effects that are both largely beyond your control, you may feel vulnerable and helpless. Feeling a lack of control, patients often have a sense of "why bother?" Although they want to live, and they have a desire to fight for their life, they feel that it may be futile to even try. These feelings can be offset by finding ways of regaining control.

We try to help patients do this by involving them as active participants in combating their disease. In this way, they no longer perceive themselves as helpless victims, but instead become active partners with their medical support team in the fight for improvement, remission or cure. We have found this is the best action we can take to strengthen a patient's will to live.

Many patients develop their own programs for taking control of their lives. One patient, Joanna, who was diagnosed with breast cancer 10 years ago and ovarian cancer 5 years ago, created her own regimen for handling fatigue and depression that she calls "recharging her batteries." Her program includes "juicing" (drinking a blend of fresh-squeezed apple, cabbage, carrot and parsley juices every day) and a diet that includes organic produce and hormone-free meat.

I also try to exercise regularly, which really has a good effect. It relaxes not only my body but also my mind, especially when I come back from the office after a stressful day. I love the ocean, and when I feel depressed I walk out to the beach and sit there until I feel better. When I can't get outside, I put on one of my nature tapes with rainfall, the surf and storms and lie on the floor with my eyes closed listening to them. Classical music has a very calming effect on me, too. If I am really unnerved or depressed, I read one of my favorite spiritual books. Whenever I feel discouraged, I think about one of the survivor stories I've read. I'm not saying it can save you, but it really helps you through the whole mental process.

Each person must find his or her own ways to regain control and thereby strengthen the will to live. Still, there are some essentials, which we have outlined below. Although the purpose of this list is to try to direct the course of your illness toward health by mobilizing your will to live, our experience has been that a significant benefit to the people who use these 11 suggestions is an improvement in the quality of their lives. This is reason enough to give them serious consideration.

1. *Choose a physician you can trust with your care.* Find a physician who projects hope, optimism and confidence—someone you can talk to. Remember, the choice of doctor is yours, although if your medical insurance coverage is the HMO type, your choice may be restricted. You and your physician should have a mutual goal: your getting well, regardless of the diagnosis. As one of our patients said:

The physician is the most important person in a seriously ill patient's life and has the most telling effect on the kind of life the patient leads. No one—parent, child, husband, lover or best friend—can take the physician's place. Having had cancer for more than two years, I know what a doctor can mean in liberating one to live actively during the remaining time of one's life.

A doctor should recognize that by his own courage and respect for the patient, he can relieve terror. If he shows confidence that he can remain in control of the disease and the pain, it removes an enormous burden from the patient's life. This is the approach my doctors have taken with me. It was never spoken, but they communicated it in their actions and manner. It has been a wonderful feeling. Instead of seeing each setback and loss of time as a defeat, we turn it around. Each day, week and month that we pass—particularly if I am free to enjoy life during that time—is a victory.

If a doctor can add to the quality of his patient's life, if he can let the patient live more fully, there is no greater gift.

2. *Become partners with your physician.* Be an active participant with your physician and find out everything you can about the nature of your problem and your potential treatment. Try not to see yourself as a victim.

The partnership between you and your physician must be based on honesty and open communication about therapy options and rehabilitation.

You and your doctor must also develop a program to help you maintain healthy nutrition, appropriate physical exercise and proper mental attitude. Becoming well-informed about your medical problem is also an important step. Take advantage of medical libraries and hospital resource centers. Learn as much as possible about your condition. If you have any questions about your cancer or treatment, ask your doctor or seek a second medical opinion.

3. *Make plans for the future and set goals.* People don't plan for the future if they believe there will be no future. You may find it helpful to come up with a list of short-term and long-term goals. Making plans in itself is a pleasant and positive experience. Why not enjoy yourself while giving yourself hope for the future? As one of our patients told us, "I'm too busy to die."

4. *Seek psychological support.* The powerful emotions released by a serious illness—fear, despair, anger and guilt—fade with recovery, but anxieties can accumulate with an illness that's chronic and possibly fatal. You may worry so much that you lose sight of the possibility of recovery. On the other hand, you may also become so hopeful and confident that you lose sight of reality and fail to follow medical advice. You need to find a balance between undue pessimism and unwarranted optimism.

Choose your support systems carefully. Support groups with skilled leaders can provide a safe atmosphere in which to ventilate your feelings and learn from the experiences of others. The groups not only seem to enhance their members' sense of control over their lives and ability to cope with their illnesses; they also may have positive biological effects.

The best way to judge if a support group is right for you is to attend a meeting. You may find too many people there who are so depressed they may ruin your ability to cope and keep a positive attitude. If you feel a group is not helping you, don't go back. You may have to visit several groups or find that you have to seek other ways of getting support. Many people need one-on-one contact for their support.

5. *Use some method of relaxation and stress reduction.* The "relaxation response" is the name used to describe a physical state that can be achieved through acupressure, meditation and directed visualization, yoga, biofeedback, tai chi and other methods. The relaxation response is important because, when that state is achieved, the immune system may be temporarily enhanced. This may have a beneficial effect on the course of your illness.

Choose a method that works for you and use it regularly. Herbert Benson, MD, author of *The Relaxation Response*, pioneered studies on the effects of transcendental meditation on health. Dr. Benson found that people who meditate using a simple prayer, word or phrase show dramatic physiologic changes, including a decrease in oxygen consumption, respiratory rate, heart rate and blood pressure. Symptoms for a variety of diseases diminish as well.

6. *Try to control negative emotions.* Anger, depression and loss of self-esteem are normal reactions, as are feelings of isolation and loneliness. You need to use all the means at your disposal to combat them. Allowed to fester, they can destroy hope and lead to a wish to die.

Most important, you should not always believe the statistics concerning your illness. They give you only an average percentage, derived from large population studies on illness and treatment similar to yours. A statistic can give you only a general idea of what the odds are for you to get better or have a recurrence of disease. Even if your odds seem poor, your real chances are anywhere between 100 percent (success) or zero (failure).

7. *Find ways to bring joy back into your life.* Positive emotions not only bolster the will to live, they also stimulate the production of natural morphine-like chemicals in the brain called endorphins, which can decrease depression. Even daily walks, enjoying nature, creating art, reading and writing poetry or stories, watching funny movies, getting a massage or helping others can produce endorphins.

Gardening is also a life-affirming activity. One patient told us, "I had never gardened before, but I was going to be home a lot, so my husband put in a garden and I became a gardener. Nothing makes me happier now than to be out in the backyard when the sun is out and plant my bulbs or prune my flowers or just sit out there and read."

If you're an animal lover, consider adopting a dog or cat. Pets have been scientifically proven to be more than just good company. They have been found to act as a natural sedative, lowering the blood pressure of their owners and promoting wellness.

We frequently encourage our patients to take trips. Most people return rejuvenated because they have had a chance to rest, reflect, reassess and step out of their daily lives.

8. *Avoid social isolation.* Spending time alone is important to the healing process. It is normal to want to be alone. However, too much solitude can lead to depression. Nothing can be as destructive to the will to live as the feeling of being cut off from life. Feelings of alienation, isolation and loneliness are often due to physical circumstances—hospitalization, loss of employment or confinement to the home—but also may arise because of the attitudes of other people toward your illness.

Tell your friends and family what you want and expect of them. Be open and honest about when you need their help and about what you want or don't want to talk about. When you are feeling physically or mentally low, many people will try to raise your spirits by saying, "Don't worry, everything will be fine." This is a common, socially acceptable statement, but the true message seems to be, "Don't tell me that you don't feel good. Tell me you're okay." When you aren't feeling all that great, this isn't what you want to hear. What you want to hear is, "I'm sorry you're feeling down and I'm here for you."

9. *Be open and honest.* One of the most important realizations is that you have everything to do with how others perceive you and treat you. If you can discuss your disease and medical therapy in a matter-of-fact manner, people will respond without fear or awkwardness. Remember, you're in charge.

10. *Be open to making compromises.* The key to compromise is learning how to adjust to symptoms and treatments while returning to as many of the normal activities of daily living as possible. Maybe you won't be able to take a planned vacation. Maybe you won't be exercising as vigorously or as often as you did before or working as hard at the office. Then again, maybe you will.

You need to continue, adopt or create a lifestyle and an attitude that will let you function physically and emotionally. But whatever compromises you make, you will find that your intellectual and emotional potential have not diminished. On the contrary, they will probably have been enhanced. Illness can be an opportunity to redirect your life in new and productive ways.

In *Creativity and Disease*, Phillip Sandblom, professor of surgery at the University of Lund in Sweden, relates the story of the artist Henri Matisse, who was a lawyer when he was suddenly afflicted by acute appendicitis. This was before the era of successful surgery, so Matisse was treated conservatively and spent over a year recovering from the many complications. During his convalescence, his mother provided him with art materials as a diversion. He became infatuated with colors and through courage and boldness became a very inventive artist.

As Sandblom notes, "Had Matisse lived in our current era, he would have been hospitalized for a few days and then discharged to continue his career as a lawyer rather than one of the great artists of our time."

11. *Seek inspiration from others with a similar condition who have either recovered or are living full lives.* Physicians and other medical staff will often introduce new patients in the early stages of diagnosis or treatment, and who may be frightened and apprehensive, to those who have had a similar experience. Someone who may be starting a course of chemotherapy and is afraid of losing his or her hair, for instance, may benefit from meeting someone who has already gone through that ordeal.

Finally, try not to let illness dominate your life.

HOW HOPE HELPS PATIENTS LIVE FULLER LIVES

Because of illness, body function is generally reduced, and idleness is often forced on the patient. This forced idleness promotes depression and reduces the will to live. Thus the mind, which can be a powerful ally, is not allowed to fulfill its positive function in the struggle with the illness. Hope promotes recovery.

There is no medicine like hope
No incentive so great
And no tonic so powerful
As the expectation
Of something better tomorrow
            —*Orison Swett Marden*

Hope is an essential part of your will to live. Hope can be maintained as long as there is even a remote chance for survival. It is kindled and nurtured by even minor improvements, and when crises or reversals persist it is maintained by the positive attitude of family, friends and the health support team.

But primarily hope will come from yourself, if you are willing to do everything you can to improve your health and if you are willing to fight for your life.

Self-motivation and what you can do for yourself is critical. By helping yourself, you gain control over your life, thus strengthening your will to live.

Hope is the emotional mental state that motivates you to keep on living, accomplish things and succeed. It is the expectation when you awaken that today will be a good day. It is what motivates you to get out of bed in the morning. It is a driving force for positive living, which can be damaged or decreased by frustration, anxiety, depression, pessimism or distractions.

Hope can be increased or improved by having good things happen and by enjoying more of life each day with positive activities, such as going to a concert or football game or enjoying your family and friends. Some of the "good things" come from sheer luck; but you too can help make "good things" happen.

When hope is diminished, a patient can lose the will to live. This is the time when "living proof stories"—how others courageously dealt with a similar problem—can be a great help. These stories may be necessary at the time of diagnosis, when everything seems bleak and the future has not yet been imagined.

Hope can last for a long time, or it can be felt during a short burst of activity or thought. You will need to increase your motivation and compliance with whatever task you are undertaking or with treatment to help maintain a state of hope and not give up. For example, the anticipation of getting well or having a pleasurable event decreases pessimism and anxiety and also gives a sense of control over the future. It also can increase the sense of aloneness and increase the feeling of helplessness and even pain.

Sometimes, just supportive care by physician, family and friends can help maintain a person during this most difficult time in life.

One of the major themes of this book is that you must become an active partner in the treatment of your illness. You must consider yourself an integral part of the medical team. You should know what is happening in your medical treatment, for with knowledge your role is supported. In this way, your will to live can be channeled into action.

Even when you are very ill, you still have physical and emotional reserves that you can draw on. These reserves will help you to survive yet another day and will become the foundation of your recovery program.

When exhausted soldiers march home after a rigorous day, they sometimes begin to march and sing together. They have a revival of mood and spirit, and find new energies and strength. And you can muster reserve energies too, even when you feel exhausted by disease and illness.

Each of us has the capacity to live each day a little better, but we need to focus on purposes and goals and then set into action a realistic plan that will help us achieve our goals. Only by using the power of the will to live, nourished by hope, can you achieve the sublime pleasures of knowing and experiencing the wonders of life and appreciating its meaning through vital living.

Those resources are the foundation of the will to live.

To heal sometimes
To relieve often
To console always
—*Sir William Osler,* MD

8
STRESS AND CANCER: AN OVERVIEW

Mark J. Doolittle, PhD

The cure of many diseases is unknown to physicians … because they are ignorant of the whole. For the part can never be well unless the whole is well.

—Plato

◇

In recent times there has been a substantial shift in health care toward a recognition of the wisdom of Plato's creed—namely, that mental and physical are not separate, isolated and unrelated but are instead vitally linked elements of a total system. Health is becoming increasingly recognized as a balance of many parts—physical and environmental factors, emotional and psychological states, nutritional habits and exercise patterns.

As a part of that balance, the role of stress is well established as the cause of a broad range of disorders.

For example, it is now generally acknowledged that for heart disease—the nation's leading cause of death—emotional stress is a major risk factor equal in importance to such other recognized risk factors as hypertension, cigarette smoking, elevated serum cholesterol level, obesity and diabetes. Stress also has been recognized as an important risk factor in high blood pressure, ulcers, colitis, asthma, pain syndromes (e.g., migraine, cluster and tension headaches, and backache), skin diseases, insomnia and various psychological disorders. Most standard medical textbooks attribute anywhere from 50 to 80 percent of all disease to stress-related origins.

The role of stress in cancer is unclear. Although stress may influence the onset and progress of many illnesses, most important for patients is that the reduction of stress may very well improve your chances for recovery—as well as improve the quality of your life and give you an opportunity for greater participation in your total treatment.

It should also be emphasized that stress is only one element of the mind-body balance that determines your well-being. Like a river with many tributaries flowing into it, health depends on the contribution and equilibrium of many factors. There can be no doubt that exposure to harmful substances (carcinogens) increases the incidence of cancer; but there is also evidence that genetic predisposition, exposure to radiation and a poor diet contribute.

THE NATURE OF STRESS

We often speak casually of "stress" as if its meaning was well established, but scientific study has continued to provide new meaning for the concept and new importance for its role in health and disease. While the word may imply a purely mental reaction, research has shown that virtually every part of the body is involved.

Most research has focused on the so-called fight-or-flight response that the body has to threats and on the long-term effects of chronic stress, in which the body is subjected to repeated arousal.*

*References for the studies cited in this chapter are available on request from Keren Stronach, Cancer Resource Center, UCSF/Mount Zion Cancer Center, 2356 Sutter Street, San Francisco CA 94143-1705.

The fight-or-flight response has been shown to produce a wide variety of mental and physical changes. For instance, when a car swerves toward us on the highway, we may consciously feel afraid, anxious and angry. Internally our body is literally reverberating from head to toe with all the aspects of the stress response: a part of the brain called the hypothalamus stimulates the pituitary gland, which in turn activates the thyroid and adrenal glands, which quickly flood the bloodstream with adrenalin, cortisone and other stress hormones. The entire body is affected: heart rate increases, blood pressure rises, breathing becomes faster, body muscles tighten, facial muscles constrict, pupils dilate, hearing becomes sharper, sugar is secreted into the bloodstream, blood flows to the brain and muscles and away from the stomach and intestines, bowel and bladder relax, brain wave activity quickens, palms sweat, and hands and feet become colder as blood flows away from the skin to the brain and muscles.

This complex response was well designed as a survival mechanism for our distant ancestors. Danger would arise suddenly, be either fought against or fled from and life would return to normal.

In addition to its usefulness for physical survival, the fight-or-flight response carries with it an emotional safety valve: by discharging the internal tension, either in physical struggle or escape, the body first releases the built-up pressure, then eventually goes to a post-stress let-down phase and finally returns to a neutral nonstress state.

What worked in other societies or times often does not work in ours. Recent research has shown that the fight-or-flight response can, ironically, become a threat to our health and survival. The nature of civilization makes this response inappropriate in many situations. For example, being stopped by a police officer may arouse the fight-or-flight response, but to

fight or flee would only make matters worse. We therefore stifle those responses for the sake of personal survival and social harmony. But as the number of similarly charged situations increases and tension is not discharged, a state of chronic stress can develop, with the risk of resulting health problems.

It is not difficult to understand how modern life increases the chances for arousal of the stress syndrome: living conditions become more crowded, noisy and polluted; the pace and intensity of life increases; mass media remind us constantly of the deaths, injuries and threats all around us; sources of information proliferate and then become increasingly confusing.

When the world around us is itself increasingly and chronically stressful, the tendency is for the fight-or-flight response to be chronically activated. If the body is unable to regularly let down, the pendulum tends not to swing back to its neutral nonstress point but to be pulled more and more toward a chronic stress response. The result is a slowly rising level of internal pressure.

This prolonged buildup of tension and excessive arousal can lead to a host of disorders. Many researchers have found that chronic stress can wear down our body's defenses, lowering our immune response and making us more vulnerable to all sickness, including cancer.

Some researchers have attempted to clarify to what degree stressful life events are related to sickness. After long research, Drs. Thomas Holmes and Richard Rahe developed a scale based on 43 common stressful experiences, in the order they were found to be related to illness. By checking the items that have occurred in the last year, you will arrive at a total score that indicates your supposed level of vulnerability to illness.

This scale clearly reflects the fact that change, whether *positive or negative*, tests our ability to adapt. However, the scale

SOCIAL READJUSTMENT RATING SCALE

Rank	Event	Value	Your Score
1	Death of spouse	100	
2	Divorce	73	
3	Marital separation	65	
4	Jail term	63	
5	Death of close family member	63	
6	Personal injury or illness	52	
7	Marriage	50	
8	Fired from work	47	
9	Marital reconciliation	45	
10	Retirement	45	
11	Change in family member's health	44	
12	Pregnancy	40	
13	Sex difficulties	39	
14	Addition to family	39	
15	Business readjustment	39	
16	Change in financial status	38	
17	Death of a close friend	37	
18	Change to different line of work	36	
19	Change in number of marital arguments	35	
20	Mortgage or loan over $10,000	31	
21	Foreclosure of mortgage or loan	30	
22	Change in work responsibilities	29	
23	Son or daughter leaving home	29	
24	Trouble with in-laws	29	
25	Outstanding personal achievement	28	
26	Spouse begins or stops work	26	
27	Starting or finishing school	26	
28	Change in living conditions	25	
29	Revision of personal habits	24	
30	Trouble with boss	23	
31	Change in work hours, conditions	20	
32	Change in residence	20	
33	Change in schools	19	
34	Change in recreational habits	19	
35	Change in church activities	19	
36	Change in social activities	18	
37	Mortgage and loan under $10,000	17	
38	Change in sleeping habits	16	
39	Change in number of family gatherings	15	
40	Change in eating habits	15	
41	Vacation	13	
42	Christmas season	12	
43	Minor violation of the law	11	
	TOTAL		

Source: Holmes, T.H., and R.H. Rahe. "The Social Readjustment Rating Scale." *Journal of Psychosomatic Research* 11 (1967): 213–18.

needs to be interpreted cautiously; the higher the score, the higher the probability that a person will become sick. But high scores (above 300) do not necessarily mean a person will get sick, only that the risk is greater.

For instance, in one study using this scale, the 30 percent with the highest scores had 90 percent more illnesses than the 30 percent with the lowest scores. In another study, 49 percent of the high-risk group (scores above 300) became ill; 25 percent of the medium-risk group (200–299) became ill; but only 9 percent of the low-risk group (150–199) became ill.

The life-change scale, though, also shows that there is nothing necessarily health-threatening about life changes. For example, in one of the studies, 51 percent of the high-risk group did not get sick—pointing up the fact that stress exists not in the event but in the reaction to it.

When difficult and threatening events occur, it is how we perceive and respond to them that determines the intensity of the stress. As any sailor knows, it is not the direction of the wind that determines our course so much as how we set the sails—in sailing parlance, known significantly as the "attitude" of the sails. Our attitude about what we feel we should be and our imagined punishment if we fail determine how we see and react to events.

In a classic study of heart-disease patients, Dr. Nanders Dunbar noted the recurring trait of compulsive striving: the patients would rather die than fail. The study showed clearly how attitude can create a chronic life-threatening situation where no real threat exists.

Failure is not death, and it is certainly not worse than death. But as long as we believe that it is, our bodies will respond with the fight-or-flight response just as if we were being attacked; coming events that might be handled with relative ease instead create the constant burden of chronic stress—with the ironic possibility of creating an actual life-threatening illness if the pressure is not removed.

On the positive side, it is equally true that by altering our attitudes and tension-producing habits, we may tip the scales in a more healthful direction. Recent research in areas such as biofeedback and meditation has shown that we can become aware of our stress responses and can influence them.

STRESS AND CANCER

The possible role of stress-related factors in the onset and course of cancer (*see* Chapter 9 for a fuller discussion) is certainly not a new or radical notion. As far back as the second century CE, the Greek physician Galen noted that melancholy women appeared more likely to develop cancer than cheerful ones. Eighteenth- and nineteenth-century physicians frequently noted that severe life disruptions and resulting emotional turmoil, despair and loss of hope seemed to occur before the onset of cancer. In 1870, Dr. James Paget emphasized that emotional disturbance was related to cancer: "The cases are so frequent in which deep anxiety, deferred hope, and disappointment are quickly followed by the growth and increase of cancer that we can hardly doubt that mental depression is a weighty additive to the other influences favouring the development of the cancerous constitution."

In 1885, Dr. Parker made the mind-body connection in a prophetic way by emphasizing the physical results of emotion: "There are the strongest physiological reasons for believing that great mental depression, particularly grief, induces a predisposition to such disease as cancer, or becomes an existing cause under circumstances where the predisposition had already been acquired."

Despite the consistent trend of these observations, the interest in more physical interventions—such as radiation, surgery and chemotherapy—drew medical attention away from the emotional contribution. Furthermore, the lack of tools for dealing with stress understandably has led to a reliance on these medical interventions.

Emotional Life-History Pattern of Cancer Patients Recent exploration of the role of stress and emotions in cancer, led by the work of Lawrence LeShan, has aroused new interest. A quarter-century ago, LeShan studied the lives of over 500 cancer patients, many of whom he worked with in psychotherapy. He found a distinct emotional life-history pattern in 76 percent of the cancer patients but in only 10 percent of a control group that did not have cancer.

This pattern had four distinctive features:
◆ The person's childhood was marked by extreme difficulty in establishing warm, satisfying relationships. Usually, because of death of a parent, divorce, chronic conflict or prolonged separation from one or both parents, the child developed a deep sense of isolation and loneliness, with a hopeless view of ever gaining lasting, fulfilling relationships. The child tried to please others first in order to win affection.
◆ In adulthood, the person found strength and meaning in a relationship or career and poured a great deal of energy into this vital source of support.
◆ When this key source was removed—through death, divorce, disillusionment or retirement—and the childhood wound reopened, the person again experienced that sense of loss, despair, hopelessness and helplessness.
◆ Feelings, especially negative ones like anger, hurt and disappointment, were constantly bottled up; in fact, others viewed the person as "too good to be true." But this superficial saintlike quality was a reflection of a deeper inability to express hostility and an overcompensation for feelings of unworthiness.

The pattern described by LeShan in *You Can Fight for Your Life* has been found with remarkable consistency by other researchers. However, it is important to understand that this research identifies emotions as only one possible factor in the development of cancer—not the only one.

Positive Role of the Emotions Research can be seen as suggesting that there is a positive role for the emotions in cancer. For, just as an attitude of hopelessness and helplessness may hurt a person's chances for health or recovery, so an attitude of determination, hope and fighting back can help lead to a positive outcome. If bottling up emotional expression and holding a reservoir of tension inside can create a dangerous load of chronic stress, so can learning to let go reduce that burden and its risk.

This perspective has led many physicians and patients to recognize that a comprehensive approach to cancer includes dealing with the emotional and stress-related aspects of the disease. Even physicians who are skeptical of the role of stress in the onset of cancer generally speak of the will to live as an important element of treatment. Adding counseling and stress-reduction techniques to traditional medical care is becoming more common.

Cancer treatment is beginning to focus on the "whole" person, as Plato put it, and on how the patient may actively join in the rehabilitation effort.

COPING WITH STRESS
It is much more important to know what sort of patient has a disease than what sort of disease a patient has.

> —Sir William Osler, MD

The importance of attitudes, feelings and beliefs has been revealed by various studies.

The Placebo Effect First, it is well known, though perhaps not well understood, that if a person has faith in the treatment and believes that it will work, the chances are greatly increased that the treatment will work—even if the treatment has no known therapeutic value. In science this is described as the placebo effect, and it is one of the most powerful tools available to the health practitioner.

The power appears to rest solely on the strength of the patient's positive beliefs and expectations; the placebo effect is stronger if the doctor also believes that the treatment is effective.

The more severe the pain, the more effective the placebo. And the placebo effect goes beyond pain relief to actually changing the state of disease.

For example, two groups of patients with bleeding ulcers were given the same medication, but one group was told by a physician that the drug would undoubtedly produce relief, while the second group was told by a nurse that the drug was experimental and its effectiveness was unknown. In the first group, 70 percent showed significant improvement; in the second group, 25 percent improved. The sole difference was the positive expectation created in the first group.

In another intriguing study, 150 patients were divided into three groups. The first group was the control group and received no medication. The other two groups were told they were going to receive a new drug that would increase health and longevity. One of these groups received a placebo, and the other group the actual drug. After years of follow-up, the first group showed a normal amount of illness and mortality; the experience of the placebo group was significantly better than the first group, and the third group displayed about the same amount of additional improvement over the placebo group as the placebo group had over the first group. Thus, while the drug reduced illness and prolonged life, so did the placebo.

How the power of belief affects the body remains a mystery. Recent research suggests that the placebo may relieve pain by releasing the body's own natural painkilling chemicals. But whatever the mechanism, the fact remains that attitude and belief can play a vital role in the success or failure of any treatment. To ignore or neglect the power of positive expectations and beliefs is to abandon one of the most valuable tools known to medicine.

Biofeedback Another area that confirms the influence of mind on body is biofeedback, which involves showing a person, through the use of sensitive electronic devices, activities of the body that used to be considered involuntary and beyond conscious influence—for example, heart rate, brain wave activity and skin temperature. The startling finding has been that if people can "see" their internal biological activity, they can generally learn to exercise some conscious influence over that activity.

Although the study of biofeedback is still in its early stages, it has already proven effective for a broad range of stress-related problems, including heart disorders, high blood pressure, migraine and tension headaches, asthma, ulcers and chronic pain. The range of applications keeps expanding. Epileptics have been able to reduce seizures by using biofeedback to control their brain wave activity.

Meditation Recent research into meditation has shown that simple periods of daily deep relaxation can have important and lasting effects on a wide variety of stress disorders, perhaps most notably high blood pressure.

Yoga Yoga can help a person react to potentially stressful situations in healthful and productive ways by counteracting many of the body's natural responses to stress.

Many yoga practices activate the parasympathetic nervous system to bring relaxation and restoration to the body by stabilizing blood pressure, lowering heart rate and the body's demand for oxygen, slowing breath rate, increasing lung capacity, improving digestion, increasing feelings of calm and tranquility and bringing about a measurable immune improvement.

In a yoga class for cancer patients, students are encouraged to extend themselves gently into their own immediate personal experience at the physical, emotional, sensory and thinking levels. They practice a slow, deliberate yoga that they adapt to their own needs and limitations. Attention to breathing and a focused awareness of the movements and the stillness of each yoga pose characterize this particular style of yoga.

As the body gains flexibility and the breath deepens, the mind and emotions settle into greater ease and balance. In quiet times of deep relaxation and meditation, habitual patterns of thinking and behaving may become more obvious and lend themselves to change.

Yoga practices include yoga postures and stretches, breathing practices, imagery, meditation and progressive relaxation. While each technique has its own specific purpose, all have the common aim of helping to develop a focused awareness of what is happening in the body and mind—emotionally, physically and spiritually.

CHANGE

Given the research described earlier and these additional findings, the conclusion seems inescapable: For a person facing cancer, learning to cope with stress in a self-nourishing way can be an important factor in aiding the treatment process, increasing chances for recovery, helping to prevent or minimize flare-ups and maximizing the quality and length of life.

Coping with stress is only part of a comprehensive treatment program, but it is the part perhaps most influenced by the patient.

It is often possible, even necessary—though undoubtedly difficult—to see a major illness as an opportunity rather than a tragedy. To become hopeless and feel helpless only makes the situation worse; to go to the other extreme with a denial of feelings and a "business as usual, everything is fine" facade also does nothing about the internal load of stress. Between blindly giving up and blindly charging on is another option—self-examination and change. The key elements of change are:

◆ Analyzing and restructuring your lifestyle
◆ Practicing and developing enjoyable techniques for reducing stress.

Both these tasks are easier said than done. The first is no doubt the more difficult and requires real motivation. The key questions you must ask if you are going to alter your stance toward life are:

◆ What do I want out of life?
◆ What is important to me?
◆ What are my priorities, and where has my own health and happiness been on the list?
◆ What chronic habits do I have that may have helped lead to the illness?
◆ Are they worth dying for?
◆ What realistic steps can I take to change?

Answering these questions may require the involvement of professionals, family, a number of close friends and, perhaps, a support group. To establish new priorities and develop realistic ways to reach them takes time, communication and honest self-analysis. Changing is not easy. But by making a concentrated effort to alter your pattern of stressful life events and the way you respond to stress, you can influence the pace and intensity of your life.

In conjunction with that goal, you may want to seek professional help in developing useful stress-reduction techniques, especially if you feel that tools such as biofeedback may have value for you. In any event, the following relaxation technique will provide a good beginning.

AN EASY INTRODUCTORY RELAXATION METHOD

1. Sit or lie down and get comfortable. Let your arms rest at your sides, and don't cross your legs. (Initially, it's useful to eliminate as many distractions as possible. A quiet, darkened room helps. As you practice, letting go becomes easier and easier, even in less than ideal settings.) Squirm and stretch your muscles a little until you feel more relaxed. Then let your eyes gently close.

2. Take a slow, deep breath in through your nose, feeling your lungs fill up and your stomach expand. When your lungs are full, hold the air in for just a second, then slowly let the air go, feeling yourself letting go all over. When you feel the air exhaled, don't hurry to inhale, just slowly take another smooth, deep breath, feel yourself filling up, hold it for a second, then slowly and completely let it all go and feel yourself relaxing even more. Let the exhale be longer than the inhale, and really let go. Get lost and absorbed in simply listening to your breathing and feeling your body letting go. Do this for a few more breaths, then breathe naturally, without trying to take especially deep breaths. Make sure you are breathing deeply and not shallowly (as in just from the chest).

3. Now let your attention drift down to your toes. Slowly and gently tense the muscles in your toes. Become aware of how the tension feels, then let the toes relax and feel the difference. Notice the sensations you feel in the toes as you let them relax.

4. Repeat this cycle of tensing and relaxing with each major muscle group as you move up your body—your calves,

thighs, hips, stomach, back, shoulders, arms, neck, jaws, eyes and forehead. Just as you became absorbed in your breathing, get lost in feeling and enjoying the sensations you produce in directly relaxing all your muscles.

5. After going through each muscle group separately, stretch your arms and legs out and tense up all your muscles at once (or as many as you can). Then let your body go limp.

Take a few deep, slow breaths. If you notice any residual tension in any part of your body, repeat the tense-and-relax cycle there to see if you can loosen up that area.

6. Finally, before opening your eyes, take a brief journey around your body, sensing how it feels to be more deeply relaxed. Become familiar with the feeling. Then, when you are ready, take another deep breath and slowly open your eyes.

Slow, deep breathing and overall muscular relaxation are perhaps the two easiest and most direct ways to calm down. Most of us breathe 16 to 20 times a minute; with slow, deep breathing we cut that in half or more.

Combined with muscular relaxation, the ultimate effect is to slow down heart rate, lower blood pressure, relax muscles, increase blood flow to the hands and feet—in short, to produce the opposite of the stressful fight-or-flight response.

This relaxation technique can be modified in many ways. One helpful maneuver is to silently repeat a sound, word or phrase in rhythm with your breathing, such as, "I am …" (as you breathe in) "… relaxed" (as you breathe out).

As the often-quoted Buddhist saying goes, "The mind is like a drunken monkey." It wanders and rambles all over the place. Thoughts run past in random fashion, like the chatter of several radio programs. Images flash across the internal mental screen like a movie.

The key to stopping these distracting

thoughts and images is to have a simple focus, a home base to return to when you are aware you've been wandering or getting distracted by external stimuli or internal chatter. Then you simply take another deep, slow breath, let the word, phrase or sound repeat itself in rhythm with your breathing, and let go again. The possibilities for a control focus are endless—music; self-suggestions (such as "My arms and legs are warm and pleasantly heavy"); simple words such as "calm," "peace," "serene," or traditional mantras like Om, Shum and Mu. One pleasant technique is to imagine yourself in a peaceful, pleasurable setting—a warm beach, a lush green meadow, a refreshing mountain lake or floating on a soft white cloud.

The key is to keep it simple and enjoyable. If the process isn't enjoyable, chances are good it won't be effective and eventually it won't be done. Making it into a chore will only tend to maintain tension. Stress reduction should be viewed along with food, sleep and exercise as a vital element in maintaining health and resisting disease.

POSITIVE ATTITUDE

Perhaps the most noted and controversial proponents of the importance of stress in cancer treatment have been Carl and Stephanie Simonton. In addition to providing traditional medical care, they have emphasized a full-scale treatment of the psychological aspects of cancer. Their perspective emphasizes mobilizing the positive attitude of the patient as part of the treatment.

The Simontons reason that, if chronic stress increases the probability of cancer, reducing stress and encouraging the will to live should improve the chances of recovery and enhance the quality of life. To that end, they employ relaxation imagery techniques and intensive counseling in addition to the usual medical treatments. They write: "Essentially, the visual imagery process involved a period of relaxation, during which the patient would mentally picture a desired goal or result. With the cancer patient, this would mean his attempting to visualize the cancer, the treatment destroying it and, most importantly, his body's natural defenses helping him recover."

The Simontons believe that a positive attitude toward treatment is a better predictor of response to treatment than the severity of the disease. Although the extent of "mind over matter" is not known, dealing with stress and encouraging the will to live are undoubtedly important in extending the length of life and enhancing its quality. To what extent we can actually influence our immune system and help it fight cancer remains to be explored.

To have suggested 20 years ago that people with epilepsy would today be stopping their seizures through control of their own brain waves would have been considered sheer nonsense; yet that, and much more, is now a reality. The importance of mobilizing the mind as a positive ally cannot be questioned. Cancer is a dreaded disease, perhaps the most frightening diagnosis a person can face. Helping the person facing it to cope with that fear is clearly an essential element of any complete treatment.

The perspective emphasizing the relationship between stress and cancer carries with it a new role not only for doctors and other health practitioners but for patients as well. No longer can patients be seen, or see themselves, as passive recipients of treatment, helpless bystanders awaiting the outcome. In many ways the patient's motivation, attitude and behavior can be the key elements that shift the scales from a poor outcome to a good one.

In this light, one anecdote from medical history seems particularly relevant. Louis Pasteur is a well-known name in science: he was the pioneer in exploring the microbe, dispelling the myth of "spontaneous generation" and helping to eradicate such diseases as diphtheria and typhus that ravaged the world in the nineteenth century. Less well known is his colleague, Claude Bernard, who insisted, somewhat in opposition to Pasteur, that it was not so much the presence or absence of microbes, bacteria or viruses that determined health, but the overall equilibrium of the entire organism. As he put it, "The constancy of the inner terrain is the essential condition of the free life." In other words, microbes hover around and inside us constantly, but it is only when our "inner terrain" is out of balance and vulnerable that they can take root. Pasteur's dying words were reported to have been, "Bernard was right. The microbe is nothing, the terrain, everything."

Both Pasteur and Bernard were right. A total treatment approach encompasses both the physical (the microbe) and the mental and emotional (the inner terrain) and recognizes their interaction. Major illness confronts us with what most of us would rather avoid—the inevitability of death. While death certainly has its tragic aspects, its blunt reality can be a spur to recognizing the importance of really living, here and now, and to re-evaluating (as even Pasteur did) our perspective. No matter what quantity of life is left to each of us, we all have a choice about its quality. Nurturing, enjoying and balancing our "inner terrain" is perhaps the best place to start.

9
DOES STRESS CAUSE CANCER?

Andrew W. Kneier, PhD, *and Ernest H. Rosenbaum,* MD

There is a widespread belief that emotional stress plays a role in the development of cancer. Many of our patients feel they were somehow "set up" to get cancer, and look back at some specific stressful event or situation (such as financial or marital problems) that may have brought on their disease. Sometimes patients cite the long-standing inner stress from some trauma in their life history (such as alcoholism in their family, or being abused when they were children). Patients have also felt that certain aspects of their personality (such as being too submissive or emotionally repressed) made them prone to cancer.

It would not be surprising if you have also wondered about these connections. Many claims about stress, personality and cancer have been made in the popular press and media in recent years. Patients are also routinely told to keep a positive attitude as if the stress of negative thoughts or emotions is bad for you. We have seen several books and magazine articles on these topics. Woody Allen once quipped that he never got angry, but just grew a tumor instead.

Does scientific evidence support these claims? Certainly the belief that stress can contribute to cancer is not without some basis in the scientific literature. However, many studies have also found no such connection.*

A CAUTIONARY NOTE

A recent review of a wide variety of studies over the last 25 years on the role of psychological factors in cancer incidence listed over 20 variables that have been associated with the onset of cancer. This list included stressful life events, depression, suppression of emotion, social isolation, excessive anxiety, inhibited sexuality, long-standing emotional conflicts, constricted personality type, rigidity, submissiveness and a facade of pleasantness. It would seem there was a mountain of evidence that such factors (which could all be subsumed under the heading "stress") played a role in the development of cancer.

However, many of the studies that show this connection have a serious flaw—they look at what cancer patients report about past stress, emotional states or personality traits after they have been diagnosed with cancer. What patients remember and report may well be distorted by the fact of their cancer.

For example, one study asked a group of women who had been diagnosed with lymphoma or leukemia to list the stressful life events that occurred during the four years before their diagnosis. The researchers found that the year just preceding the diagnosis was significantly more stressful for these women than the other three years, and they speculated that this increased stress may have contributed to the development of the cancer. It is easy to see that these women, like everyone,

*References for the studies cited in this chapter are available on request from Keren Stronach, Cancer Resource Center, UCSF/Mount Zion Cancer Center, 2356 Sutter Street, San Francisco CA 94143-1705.

probably had a better recall of stressful events during the more recent year; but in addition, the emotional impact of a cancer diagnosis can make a person see past events in a more negative light. Moreover, these women may have wanted to find an explanation for their cancer that would give them a feeling of control over the outcome: if stress caused the cancer, then reducing stress would help eliminate it.

(An additional methodological problem with this study, and one that afflicts most such studies, is that the cancers in question originated, in microscopic form, years before they could be diagnosed. Thus, the stress of the few years before the diagnosis was entirely unrelated to the onset of the disease at the cellular level.)

Some studies have sought to work around the problem by interviewing patients who have a suspicious symptom of cancer but have not yet been diagnosed. For example, 160 women who had undiagnosed breast lumps were given psychological tests before biopsies were performed. Those who turned out to have breast cancer showed significantly more emotional suppression (especially of anger) than the women who had benign tumors. But caution is still warranted in interpreting these results. There is evidence that patients are very good at predicting whether biopsies will come back negative or positive for cancer. And that the diagnosis of cancer, or the suspicion of having it, can cause a greater suppression of emotion, thereby raising questions about cause and effect.

As well, what is stressful to one person may not be stressful to another, and people also differ in how they cope with stress. Thus, many studies that look at stressful life events, or at personality traits that are supposed to create stress, have not determined whether the persons involved actually experienced these events or traits as stressful.

Evidence of a Stress-Cancer Link Even

though most studies have these or other flaws, there have been a few well-designed studies that have demonstrated an association between stress and the later development of cancer. These studies have been prospective (unlike the ones described above, which are retrospective); that is, they have obtained psychological information from a large number of people who are then followed over several years. Those who developed cancer are then compared with those who did not to determine whether there were any long-standing psychological differences.

For example, in 1957 the Western General Electric Health Study began with 2,020 middle-aged men, each of whom was given a standardized personality test and then followed for 17 years. Those who died of cancer during this period were found to have been significantly more depressed when they were tested at the beginning of the study. This stress–cancer association was unrelated to age, smoking, alcohol use, occupational status or family history of cancer. The researchers concluded: "The results are consistent with the hypothesis that psychological depression is related to impairment of mechanisms for preventing the establishment and spread of malignant cells." (It is also possible that depression resulted in poor diet, avoidance of regular medical checkups or ignoring early warning signs of cancer, any one of which could have increased cancer mortality.)

In the 1960s, nearly 7,000 adults were enrolled in the Alameda County Health Study. These participants are being followed for psychosocial and other factors that have a bearing on cancer incidence and mortality. After 17 years, women who were the most socially isolated and felt lonely had a significantly greater incidence of cancer. Socially isolated men, once they developed cancer, had a significantly shorter survival time. These findings suggest that the stress of loneliness may be a risk factor for cancer.

Another study interviewed 110 patients who had undiagnosed lung lesions about stressful events since childhood. The researchers used the results to predict whether biopsies would be benign or malignant. Eighty percent were correctly predicted to have benign tumors, and 61 percent were correctly predicted to have lung cancer.

Numerous studies have firmly established that stress can alter certain measures of immune functioning. Depression is associated with a decrease in the number and potency of natural killer cells, which respond to cancer cells. These changes occur because immune cells, through specific receptors, are sensitive to many of the hormones, neurotransmitters and neuropeptides affected by stress.

These immunosuppressive effects are relevant to the possible role of stress in the development of cancer. It appears that one role of the immune system is to recognize and destroy malignant cells when they develop (which may occur commonly in all of us, although we never know it, thanks to the success of immunological surveillance). It is therefore possible that a weakening of the immune system, caused by stress, could make someone more susceptible to cancer. This could represent an additional pathway by which stress could increase cancer risk.

Evidence That Stress Does Not Cause Cancer After 17 years, the Alameda County Health Study found no association between earlier depression and the later development of cancer. In another prospective study, looking at the association of depression and development of breast cancer, nearly 10,000 women were followed for 14 years. No association was found between depression and a subsequent diagnosis of breast cancer.

Although bereavement has been found to suppress certain immune functions, this suppression is apparently not relat-

ed to an increased risk of cancer. For example, 4,032 people who were widowed in Maryland between 1963 and 1974 did not have an increased cancer rate during a 12-year follow-up period. In Finland, nearly 10,000 people who were widowed in 1972 were followed for 14 years. This group showed no significant increase in cancer mortality.

In 1944, a total of 9,813 soldiers were discharged from the U.S. Army for psychoneurosis. They were matched with 9,942 controls, and the two groups were followed for 24 years. The discharged veterans had no greater cancer mortality than the control group during this period. In a similar study by the same author, approximately 10,000 soldiers who had been prisoners of war during World War II or the Korean War were matched with approximately 9,000 controls. The World War II vets were followed for 32 years and the Korean War vets for 20 years, during which time the former prisoners of war had no greater mortality from cancer.

In the Terman Life-Cycle Study, 1,528 participants have been followed since 1921–22 (when they were in elementary school) for various psychosocial factors and longevity. As of 1991, 663 had died of various causes. These deaths were associated with divorce of parents during childhood, childhood impulsivity and egocentrism, marital instability and poor psychological adjustment in adulthood. These associations (history of divorced parents, etc., and death) were independent of smoking and alcohol consumption. However, these factors were associated with subsequent death from a variety of causes; they did not predict a higher death rate from cancer.

WHAT CONCLUSIONS CAN BE DRAWN?
Obviously the scientific evidence neither proves nor disproves the role of stress as

a cause of cancer. Usually, most evidence suggests that there is no link. Remember, however, that most of these studies involve large groups of patients and are looking at stress–cancer associations in the group as a whole. If there is an association in some individuals within the group, but not in others, then the overall effect will not be significant—although the effect on those individuals will be significant. Thus, the evidence is compelling that stress can, and sometimes does, contribute to the development of cancer. That is, in some cases the immune system and/or DNA repair mechanisms are probably impaired enough by long-standing and severe emotional stress to produce malignant transformation of cells.

Given this, you might ask: "Did stress contribute to my cancer?" Based on the scientific evidence to date, we would answer: "Probably not." We would add that even if stress was a factor, its role was probably very minor compared to the other causative factors that we know exist. But we would also add that stress could have played a role, although it was not the cause itself.

The question is still worth asking, because your cancer diagnosis may help you to identify sources of stress in your life that deserve more attention and that you might be able to change. This process could be helpful to you: it could lead to a better attunement to your own feelings and needs, and help you to make positive changes in your lifestyle, health habits or priorities. Your emotional well-being would be enhanced, as well as your overall quality of life. This process might also help medically, by fostering a greater participation in your treatment regimen and by promoting an improved immune response to your cancer.

But reflecting on the role of stress in your own cancer may also be harmful if it causes you to blame yourself. The popular notion that stress and certain personality traits contribute to cancer often makes patients feel responsible or guilty for getting cancer. We have heard patients blame themselves for tolerating too much stress in their life, internalizing their emotions or being too submissive, as if this behavior had caused their cancer. Research indicates that such factors probably had nothing to do with the development of cancer.

The belief that stress contributes to cancer—and the self-blame that stems from this—derives in part from how we account for good fortune and misfortune. When things are going well for us—in our lives, our jobs and in our health—we tend to assume that we are doing something right, living on the right track, and must be deserving of our good fortune. The flip side of this assumption is that misfortune can lead to the thought that we were not so deserving of our good fortune after all, perhaps because of some flaw in our character, having the wrong priorities or living under too much stress. Therefore, it is not uncommon for people diagnosed with cancer to feel at fault and to search for causes (such as stress) in themselves or in their past. Although cancer is a biological disease, our culture tends to see it as a reflection of the cancer patient's character, personality or life.

Another reason for this view is the influence on our cultural attitudes of the Judeo-Christian view that disease and death are the result of sin.

The themes of domination, mastery and control are also powerful motifs in our culture, and are quite at odds with our vulnerability to the capriciousness of nature. Rather than accept that we are often victims of natural malfunctions and body processes beyond our control, we tend to think that such imperfections can be fixed with ample understanding and technological intervention. In this context, we look for causes of cancer that we can control. Stress is one of these.

10
DOES YOUR ATTITUDE MAKE A DIFFERENCE? PSYCHOLOGICAL FACTORS

Andrew Kneier, PhD, *and Ernest Rosenbaum,* MD

———————◇———————

The easy answer to the question posed by the title of this chapter is "Yes." Your attitude makes a difference to how you feel about your illness, how you cope with it and your overall psychological adjustment and quality of life. For example, patients who adopt a fighting spirit feel less vulnerable and depressed than do patients who have a helpless, fatalistic attitude. Your attitude also makes a difference to the side effects of medical treatments and your recovery from surgery. For example, patients who think of chemotherapy as strong and effective medicine are much less distressed over the side effects, and actually experience fewer side effects, than patients who regard chemotherapy as a dreadful poison.

The more complicated question is whether your attitude makes a difference to your medical outcomes—that is, whether a cancer recurs or progresses after treatments, the rate at which such progression occurs and whether the cancer is fatal.

The question is not only whether the course and outcome of your illness are influenced by your attitude but also whether they are influenced by your emotional state, stress level, coping style, personality traits and degree of personal support you get from others. (In this chapter, we will refer to all of these as psychological factors.)

The question is complicated because some studies indicate that psychological factors do influence medical outcomes in cancer, whereas other studies have found that they do not. Furthermore, we know of cases where certain positive aspects, such as a strong will to live and unshakable hope, appeared to make all the difference in the world; but sadly, we also know of cases where such aspects appeared to make no difference whatsoever.

The question is also complicated by the issue of how psychological factors might influence medical outcomes. It is often assumed that such factors affect cancer through psychoimmunological process-es—that is, that patients' emotional states (which are affected by their attitudes, coping behavior and social support) cause changes in their immune response, which in turn affects medical outcomes. As we will see, there is evidence to support this possibility. Eastern perspectives on healing, such as the Chinese focus on *chi*, emphasize the balance and flow of energy within the body to explain how psychological factors make a difference.

It is also possible that these factors affect how well a patient adheres to medical treatment, or whether the patient pursues an aggressive treatment approach, perhaps participating in an experimental protocol. Because patients differ on these matters, their medical outcomes could be affected.

Most cancer patients believe that a positive attitude makes a difference to their medical outcome; indeed, patients are often encouraged by family members, friends and health professionals to maintain a positive attitude and to never give up. This is not surprising. Claims are frequently made in the popular press and media about mind-body connections that affect cancer. If a new study shows some connection along these lines, it usually receives a lot of media coverage, whereas studies showing no such connection are ignored. Proponents of various mind-body approaches to cancer healing often overstate the proven effectiveness of such approaches.

In the discussion that follows, we review the scientific evidence—both pro and con—regarding the influence of psychological factors on cancer outcomes. First, we want you to know about some of the positive evidence to encourage you to pursue ways of coping with your illness that might make a difference, and to support you in the constructive efforts you might already be making. Second, we want to offer an objective review of the evidence to correct the claims that are often made in the popular press and media. By exaggerating the medical benefits of a "positive attitude," these claims can make patients feel that their normal "negative" emotions are somehow dangerous, and that it is up to them to deal with their cancer in the right ways. Consequently, patients often feel that the progression of their cancer is somehow a personal failure on their part. As we will see, it is actually healthy—psychologically and immunologically—to express an appropriate degree of fear or sadness when dealing with cancer. And there is no justification for burdening patients with the responsibility of their recovery from cancer.*

EVIDENCE THAT PSYCHOLOGICAL FACTORS AFFECT MEDICAL OUTCOME

Most of the studies in this area have a straightforward design: they assess the psychological differences among patients who have a similar cancer diagnosis and then follow these patients over time to see whether these differences are associated with differences in medical outcomes. It has been impossible for these studies to completely separate out the influence of the psychological factors from all the other factors that affect medical outcome (such as differences in medical treatments and tumor aggressiveness and whether the immune system is normal). Nonetheless, some intriguing findings have been reported.

One of the first noteworthy studies was reported in the *Journal of the American Medical Association* in 1979. To their surprise, the researchers found that women with metastatic breast cancer who were visibly angry and upset had significantly longer survival times than those who exhibited less distress. A related study in the same year found that newly diagnosed melanoma patients who acknowledged the adjustment difficulties they were experiencing had a lower incidence of recurrence than those who seemed to minimize their adjustment needs. A similar finding was reported with newly diagnosed breast cancer patients: those who exhibited and acknowledged the severe impact of the diagnosis had a lower incidence of recurrence than patients who appeared to be less distressed.

*References for the studies cited in this chapter are available on request from Keren Stronach, Cancer Resource Center, UCSF/Mount Zion Cancer Center, 2356 Sutter Street, San Francisco CA 94143-1705.

It is interesting that acknowledging anxiety may be healthy but that dwelling on it may not be. In one study, leukemia patients who had undergone a bone marrow transplant and who exhibited "anxious preoccupation" with their illness had poorer outcomes than those who were more successful in mastering their anxiety.

A number of studies have found that a patient's degree of interpersonal support, as opposed to social isolation, had an effect on medical outcomes. One such study interviewed 200 newly diagnosed breast cancer patients about their level of social support and then followed these women for 20 years. Those in the premenopausal group (age 15 to 45) and the postmenopausal group (age 61 to 90) who had high social involvement survived longer than those who had low social involvement. However, those in the perimenopausal group (age 46 to 60) showed no such differences in survival as related to their social involvement. To complicate matters further, a study involving lung, breast and colorectal cancer patients found that the benefits associated with social support were different depending on the type of cancer and extent of the disease.

Two widely cited studies found that patients who participated in a group intervention program had improved survival over control patients who did not participate. The best known is a Stanford University study. Women with metastatic breast cancer who participated in a weekly support group for one year (which involved sharing emotions, problem-solving discussions and self-hypnosis training for pain control) had significantly longer survival times than the control group. The other study involved newly diagnosed melanoma patients at the UCLA Medical Center. Patients who participated in a weekly support group for six weeks (which involved sharing emotions, teaching about melanoma and instruction in positive coping skills) exhibited several improvements over the control group. They coped more effectively with their illness, their emotional state was better, their natural killer cell activity and number was higher and their survival rates were better over the six-year follow-up period.

It is not known why these patients had improved medical outcomes, or whether these findings can be replicated. Perhaps the emotional benefits of a support group are translated into immunological changes that make a difference to outcome. Or perhaps patients in support groups take better care of their overall health through diet and exercise, pursue medical treatments more aggressively, cope more effectively with stress, make lifestyle changes to reduce stress or participate in supplemental approaches such as acupuncture, meditation and Chinese herbal medicine. Clearly, additional research is needed.

A study in the *British Medical Journal* compared the stressful life events of 50 women who had suffered a breast cancer recurrence with a matched group of 50 patients who remained in remission. Those who had a recurrence reported a significantly greater degree of stress in the years preceding the recurrence. A problem with this study is that the emotional effect of a cancer recurrence can distort a patient's memory of past events. Moreover, these patients may have wanted to find a causal explanation of the recurrence (i.e., stress) that would give them a greater feeling of control over the future.

There is a widely held belief among cancer patients, and among proponents of mind-body medicine, that stress contributes to the development of cancer (*see* Chapter 9). Insofar as this is the case, it would follow that stress would also influence the medical outcome after cancer was diagnosed.

PSYCHOLOGICAL FACTORS AND IMMUNE RESPONSE

There is considerable evidence to support the possibility that psychological factors affect the immune system, thus influencing medical outcome. For example, depression is associated with a decrease in the number and potency of natural killer (NK) cells, which respond to cancer cells. These kinds of changes occur because immune cells, through specific receptors, respond to many of the hormones, neurotransmitters and neuropeptides that are affected by stress. Enzyme levels necessary for the repair of mutated DNA have also been found to be lower under stressful conditions.

Although the immunosuppressive effects of stress could theoretically increase a person's susceptibility to cancer, and thereby contribute to the onset of cancer, no studies have demonstrated that this happens.

What about the role of immune suppression, as caused by (or at least associated with) psychological factors, on medical outcomes? The evidence here is more intriguing. As we saw above, the degree of social support and interaction has been associated with differences in medical outcomes. These connections could result from changes in immune responses that are related to social support. It would follow that separation and loss, such as divorce or the death of a spouse, would be associated with immunosuppression. Indeed, several studies have shown that this is the case.

In the UCLA study on melanoma patients, the patients who participated in the group intervention program showed a greater improvement in their emotional state than the control group, and this improvement was associated with an increase in certain types of NK cells and an increase in the tumor-fighting potential of NK cells. In their follow-up study,

the researchers found that these changes were in turn associated with improved survival.

With breast cancer patients, certain psychological factors (level of adjustment, degree of social support, energy level and mood) were associated with variability in NK cell activity three months after mastectomy. It was also found that patients who were most depressed had a greater decrease in NK activity and a higher number of lymph nodes testing positive for cancer involvement. It was not clear whether there was a causal connection between depression, immune suppression and number of involved nodes, or whether the nodal involvement caused the depression. In a follow-up study, the researchers found that the psychological factors they studied, as well as the variance in NK activity, were associated with the incidence and timing of subsequent recurrences.

EVIDENCE THAT PSYCHOLOGICAL FACTORS DO NOT AFFECT OUTCOME

The findings summarized above have been contradicted by a number of studies that have found no associations between psychological factors and medical outcomes.

A major study reported in the *New England Journal of Medicine* involved 359 melanoma and breast cancer patients. A number of psychological factors were measured, including social ties, marital history, job satisfaction, use of medication for anxiety or depression, general life satisfaction, hopelessness and amount of adjustment required to cope with the diagnosis of cancer. These patients were followed three to eight years after diagnosis, and none of the psychological factors were associated with differences in medical outcome—with one exception.

Patients who reported a moderate degree of hopelessness had longer disease-free intervals than patients who reported either a low or high degree of hopelessness. This is an interesting finding; it may indicate that denying or minimizing hopeless feelings, as well as feeling extremely hopeless, are both associated with poorer outcomes.

Other studies have failed to find a relationship between coping style and medical outcome. A mixed group of patients (92 with hematologic cancers and 47 with rectal cancer) were assessed when they were diagnosed and followed for six months. Coping style was not related to length of survival; nor were degree of depression or whether it was felt the disease came from within or without. A similar study with breast cancer patients, who were followed for three years after diagnosis, found no relationship between coping style and outcome.

Studies have also looked at the associations between marital status and outcome. In a large study in Denmark, 1,782 breast cancer patients were matched with 1,738 controls; no differences were found in the death rates of married as opposed to widowed patients. The *New England Journal of Medicine* study described above also found no association between marital history and outcome.

One study showed an association between stressful life events and breast cancer outcomes. However, another study, of 202 breast cancer patients, found no association between stressful events and recurrence during a 3.5-year period. Yet another study found no association between depression and breast cancer outcomes.

Two studies that examined the effectiveness of group therapy found no association with medical outcomes. In one, 34 breast cancer patients who participated in Bernie Siegel's intervention program (consisting of weekly peer support, family therapy, individual counseling and positive mental imagery exercises) were matched with 102 patients who did not participate. The patients were followed for 10 years, and no differences in survival time or ultimate survival were found. In the other study, some patients received weekly group psychotherapy and a control group did not. There were no significant differences between the survival times of the two groups. In a third study, 120 end-stage male cancer patients were assigned either to receive weekly individual counseling or to a control group that did not. The patients who received counseling showed an improvement in their quality of life, but did not differ from the controls in survival after one year.

The evidence thus far suggests that psychological factors sometimes make a difference to medical outcomes, but that they do not consistently do so. This conclusion would certainly explain the contradictory findings of these and other studies.

The studies in this area have investigated and measured the relationship of psychological factors and medical outcomes in large groups of patients. In order for a relationship to be found, it must be relatively consistent or uniform within the group. If the relationship existed in some patients within the group, but not in others, then these would cancel each other out and no consistent relationship would be found. The authors would conclude that there was no relationship of the psychological factors with the medical outcomes; but what they really mean is that no consistent relationship was found in the group being studied. Given the nature of statistical analysis, relationships must be consistent in order to be deemed "statistically significant." The rules for this are very strict: For example, if a relationship was found, but the analysis showed that there was a 10 percent chance that the relationship was due to chance alone, then the relationship would be dismissed as too inconsistent to be "significant."

In an individual case, a psychological factor will in theory influence a medical outcome only if a number of conditions are met. First, the psychological factor in question (e.g., an optimistic outlook) would have to be strong enough to affect the immune response. Second, the right effects on the immune response would have to occur. Third, these effects would have to be strong enough to affect the cancer cells, which in turn would have to be susceptible to the immunological changes that occurred as a consequence of the patient's optimism. Fourth, the effect on these cancer cells would have to be strong enough, and widespread enough throughout the body, to make a difference to the medical outcome.

These "links in the chain" between a psychological factor and cancer growth sometimes do occur, which is remarkable given the complex and intricate processes involved.

APPLYING THE EVIDENCE

As you go through your cancer experience, it is impossible to predict whether your attitude, emotions, coping style or degree of support will influence your medical outcome. Because these factors might make a difference, however, we believe you should act as if they will. In other words, give it your best shot in responding to your illness in ways that could improve your medical outcome.

But if, despite your best efforts and the best efforts of your doctors, your cancer gets worse, this does not mean that you failed to have the right attitude, that your will to live was not strong enough, that you did not cope as you should have or that you did something else wrong. It probably means only that the biological deck was stacked against you from the outset—that is, that the inherent biology of the tumor, the shortcomings of one's bodily defenses against it and the inadequacies of medical intervention all led to outcomes

that were beyond your control. However, no one knows that in advance, just as no one knows in advance whether your attitude will make a positive difference.

We therefore encourage you to respond to your cancer in ways that could make a difference. In every situation, there is a realistic possibility that the patient will achieve medical outcomes that are better than expected; in some cases, there is a realistic possibility that the patient will recover fully.

You can maximize your own chances of realizing these possibilities by, first of all, becoming involved in learning about your illness and pursuing the best medical treatments and follow-up evaluation. Make changes in your lifestyle and health habits that are associated with improved outcomes. In other words, become an active participant in the recovery process, as opposed to having a passive, fatalistic attitude.

Medical literature suggests that certain ways of coping with the stress of having cancer can affect the outcome. These include acknowledging stress and expressing the negative emotions that come with it, adopting a fighting spirit and reaching out for support from others. Participating in a cancer support group might also make a difference.

It is interesting that the belief that attitude makes a difference is so prevalent while the scientific evidence is much more ambiguous. This is also true of popular but unsupported claims about the mind-body connections that affect cancer outcomes. There are two sides to this coin: on the positive side, patients are often encouraged by these ideas to respond to their illness in positive and constructive ways; on the negative side, these ideas often pressure patients to have the right attitude, and they make patients feel responsible and guilty if their illness progresses.

If the scientific evidence is so contradictory, why is the belief that a patient's attitude makes a difference so widespread, and why is the focus in the media and popular press so one-sided? First, there is, as we have shown, good evidence that psychological factors can influence cancer outcomes, and case reports of spontaneous remissions in cancer underscore the remarkable power of these factors—especially the power of emotional catharsis, and the patient's total belief that a medical treatment or some other substance (even if it is biologically inert) will be a cure.

Second, most patients want to believe that how they respond to their illness can influence the outcome, as this helps to reduce their feelings of vulnerability and helplessness. Family members and friends also want to believe this and want the patient to act accordingly to reduce their own anxieties.

Third, the nature of cancer lends itself to the notion that it implies something about the person who has it. These cells—which have spun out of control and which, if left to their own devices, are ultimately destructive—are part of the person's body, originating from within, and it may seem that they are therefore evidence of some underlying personal pathology or dysfunction. Many patients feel that if they can fix whatever is wrong internally, or change their behavior, then the malignancy will go away.

These ideas stem in part from a fourth reason for the emphasis on the patient's role in beating cancer. Our culture places a strong emphasis on our controlling our destiny and in overcoming obstacles, even natural ones, that stand in our path. The fact that we are susceptible to natural processes beyond our control is not well accepted in our society. The late historian Richard Hofstadter addressed this issue when he wrote: "A great part of both the strength and weakness of our national existence lies in the fact that Americans do not abide very quietly the evils of life. We are forever restlessly pitting ourselves against them, demanding changes, improvements, remedies, but not often with sufficient sense of the limits that the human condition will in the end inevitably impose upon us."

To conclude, we want to return to the defining power of your attitude in shaping how you experience and respond to your illness. We offer the following reflection:

The longer I live, the more I realize the impact of attitude on life. Attitude, to me, is more important than facts. It is more important than the past, than education, than money, than circumstances, than failures, than successes, than what other people think or say or do. It is more important than appearance, giftedness, or skill. It will make or break a company ... a church ... a home. The remarkable thing is, we have a choice every day regarding the attitude we embrace for that day. We cannot change the past ... we cannot change the inevitable. The only thing we can do is to play on the one string we have, and that is our attitude. I am convinced that life is 10 percent what happens to me and 90 percent how I react to it. And so it is with you ... we are in charge of our attitudes.

— Charles Swindoll

11

COPING WITH CANCER: 10 STEPS TOWARD EMOTIONAL WELL-BEING

Andrew Kneier, PhD, Ernest Rosenbaum, MD, and Isadora R. Rosenbaum, MA

───────◇───────

Coping refers to the attitudes and behaviors that you use to maintain your emotional well-being and to adjust to the stresses caused by cancer. Different people cope in different ways, and some ways of coping are more successful in promoting a person's emotional well-being and psychological adjustment than others. Currently, you might be coping with treatments and their side effects. Perhaps you are also coping with a recurrence of your cancer or with pain and disability. Your life has been disrupted and perhaps altered by your illness, and you are dealing with the effect on your loved ones of all that is happening to you.

When someone had cancer 50 years ago, there was little discussion of how he or she was "coping." The person just dealt with it. In the last 25 years, however, the notion that patients are coping with their illness, in better or worse ways, has received an enormous amount of attention by health care professionals. Even the federal government got involved and, in 1980, the National Cancer Institute published *Coping with Cancer*. In the 1990s, over 2,500 articles on some aspect of coping with cancer have appeared in medical and mental health journals.

In this chapter, we attempt to summarize the vast amount of research on coping with cancer by highlighting 10 coping strategies that we believe may help you.*

We have also drawn upon the experience of the many patients we have cared for over the years.

"Coping strategies" reflects the process of coping and the ways of meeting goals and challenges. When you are dealing with cancer, you face many goals and challenges. Some of these are medical and physical, some are emotional, and others are interpersonal and spiritual. In one way or another, they all have to do with the quality of your life, which has been threatened and disrupted by cancer. You have adopted some strategies for pursuing your goals and meeting personal challenges that promote your recovery and enable you to remain emotionally intact. You are able to carry on, perhaps deepened and changed by your cancer experience. This is what coping is all about.

These coping strategies are not applicable to all patients. This is because the method of coping that works best for one person may not work so well for another. What works best for you depends on many factors related to your personality, your current life situation and how you have coped in the past. Moreover, the goals and challenges you are facing are personal to you, and many of these are dictated by the nature of your illness and the medical treatments. Thus, the coping responses that are warranted also depend on these individual matters.

Finally, coping with cancer is a process

*References for the studies cited in this chapter are available on request from Keren Stronach, Cancer Resource Center, UCSF/Mount Zion Cancer Center, 2356 Sutter Street, San Francisco CA 94143-1705.

that goes on over months and years, and patients use different strategies at different times, depending upon the changing situation within themselves and their relationships and with the stage of their illness. It is nonetheless true that research on the coping strategies used by large numbers of patients has found that some strategies, in general, are better than others. More often than not, these strategies are associated with an optimal degree of psychological adjustment.

The positive coping strategies we discuss below may also help to improve your medical condition. They can promote your emotional well-being when dealing with cancer, and thereby enable you to feel more energetic and resilient. These effects may also enhance your immune system's response against cancer cells. (*See* Chapter 10.)

The coping strategies suggested here are for all patients, whether you are newly diagnosed, undergoing medical treatment or dealing with the many stages of cancer, including terminal cancer.

1. *Facing the Reality of Your Illness* Patients respond in different ways to their diagnosis, the initial medical work-up, subsequent test results and the implications of all that is happening to them. Many patients respond by confronting the full reality of their illness. They ask pointed and brave questions about the seriousness of their condition and the pros and cons of the various treatment options. They read up on these matters on their own. They react as if they are strongly motivated to know what they are facing. This way of coping has been found to promote their psychological adjustment.

Other patients react as if the realities confronting them are too much to deal with and they therefore retreat into a state of denial. It sometimes seems that a patient in denial is saying, in effect, "I can't cope with all this." Yet the denial is a way of coping. It protects the person from being overwhelmed. But it can also prevent a person from coming to terms with their illness and getting on with other constructive ways of coping. It is therefore associated with a poorer psychological adjustment.

Denial is often a positive coping strategy because it enables the patient to gradually face the reality of his or her illness, in a piecemeal manner, without feeling overwhelmed, and feeling more supported by loved ones. In our experience, patients seldom remain in denial; it fades away over time, as indeed it should, at least for the good of overall adjustment.

As you read this, you might ask yourself how much you really know about your cancer and your individual case. Are there any relevant questions that you haven't ask? Have you avoided learning more about your illness by not reading about it? You might want to become more proactive in seeking information; the evidence indicates that this will help you.

2. *Maintaining Hope and Optimism* After facing the reality of your illness, it would be good to feel hopeful and optimistic about the future course of events. Not surprisingly, patients who are hopeful and optimistic show a better adjustment to their illness than patients who are pessimistic. It is important, however, that your optimism be realistic; otherwise it represents denial or wishful thinking. In most cases, there is a solid and realistic basis for a certain degree of hope and optimism.

Most patients tell themselves to be positive, but for many, this is easier said than done. There are several reasons for this, some of which may apply to you. Being optimistic means that you may feel lucky. However, you were unlucky enough to get cancer and may now feel that you are an unlucky person. You would not expect, therefore, that you would now enjoy the good fortune of a long remission or cure. You might feel just the opposite: that good luck is unlikely for you.

Optimism can also seem presumptuous: after all, other patients with your diagnosis have not done well, and you might think, "What right do I have to expect to recover?" Your optimism could also make you feel that you were not worrying enough about your cancer—that is, that you were not giving cancer its due, that you were acting too boldly or confidently in the face of it, and that you were therefore asking for trouble, as if the cancer might come back to teach you a lesson. Finally, if your prognosis is more favorable than for other patients with your type of cancer, you may feel that it is not right to enjoy this good fortune or to take advantage of it (that is, by being optimistic and going on with your life in a positive and constructive manner).

Despite these obstacles, you should try to feel as hopeful and optimistic as the medical realities of your case allow. This leads to our next point.

3. ***Proportion and Balance*** Your emotional response should not only be one of optimism and hope. It is also appropriate and helpful for you to be upset and worried, at least to a certain degree.

In most cases, the medical situation provides a basis for hope and a basis for worry. The statistics indicate a certain chance of survival, but also a certain chance of dying of cancer. Of course, the chance of survival and the risk of dying vary greatly from case to case. Ideally, your emotional response would take both aspects into account: you would experience a degree of hope that was proportional to the positive survival chances that applied to you, but you would also experience a degree of worry that was proportional to the mortality rate in similar cases. That is, you would not feel overly worried, upset or preoccupied, but neither would you feel overly cheerful, complacent or optimistic.

Your feelings should also be in balance. Your feelings of worry or upset should be reduced in intensity, or tempered, by feelings of hope and optimism.

Alternatively, the nature and intensity of your positive emotions should be tempered by, or take into account, the possibility of death. If you are ignoring this possibility, then your optimism involves a denial or minimization of this threat; in the long run, this will not help you. It is better to acknowledge this threat and to work through the negative emotions that stem from it. In short, it is best if your positive and negative emotions balanced each other out such that you would be neither overreacting nor underreacting to the medical realities facing you.

A number of studies have found that patients who maintain this kind of mixed emotional response—well-proportioned to the realities of their illness and well balanced—enjoy a better psychological adjustment than patients who feel too pessimistic or too optimistic. In our experience, patients who have told us of their mixed feelings not only appear well adjusted but it also feels that way to them. They feel that they are coping well with the uncertainty inherent in their medical condition, neither dwelling on nor denying their legitimate fears, and yet keeping their sights set on getting better. Again, all this is easier said than done.

4. ***Expressing Your Emotions*** People differ in the way they express and communicate how they feel, and in our society women are generally better at this than men. Take stock of how well you express what you are feeling about your illness. If you feel you are not doing well in this regard, we encourage you to do better. Many studies have shown that patients who express their emotions and concerns enjoy a better psychological adjustment than people who tend to suppress their feelings or keep quiet about them.

Emotional expression is usually helpful because it gives you an outlet for your feelings, a means of working through them and an opportunity to obtain better emotional support. It can be an enormous help just to know that your feelings are understood by others and seen as valid, but this requires open communication on your part.

If you tend to keep your feelings to yourself, it is probably because you have learned to do so. (You were not born with this tendency.) Your earlier experience may have taught you that sharing your feelings led to negative consequences. Perhaps your emotions were not validated by others, or you were criticized for expressing them ("Children are to be seen but not heard," "Big boys don't cry" and so on). You may have felt that your emotional needs were an imposition on others, and that your role was to take care of the feelings and needs of others rather than expressing your own. It is not uncommon for cancer patients to hide their true feelings as a way of protecting their loved ones.

Some people do not express their emotions because they are not very adept at even paying attention to what they are feeling. They seldom stop and check in with themselves and try to identify the feelings and concerns that are weighing upon them. Children need permission and encouragement to develop this skill, and then some practice and positive reinforcement. In this process, we learn that our emotions are important and valid and thus worthy of attention and expression. Some people just do not have much experience with this essential ability, and even regard it as pointless or self-indulgent. If you find yourself admitting, "Yes, this applies to me," then we encourage you to consider psychological counseling, which could be of great help to you.

As you probably know, cancer patients are consistently encouraged to "keep a positive attitude." This can make you feel that there is something wrong or dangerous about your "negative" emotions (fear, sorrow, anger). Research suggests just the opposite: experiencing and expressing such emotions is psychologically and immunologically healthy.

Finally, timing is important. The period after your diagnosis, when you are learning about your illness and undergoing the initial work-up and treatments, may not be the right time for you to be taking stock of all your emotions. Your plate is already very full. You may need to put your emotions aside for a while as you attend to everything else. Moreover, it will benefit you most to express your emotions with the right people and when their support is available to you.

5. *Reaching Out for Support* The amount of support available to cancer patients varies across the country, and patients themselves differ in how much they tend to reach out and take advantage of the support. Those patients who have at least a few loved ones available for close emotional support and who call upon their support or practical help show a better psychological adjustment to cancer than patients who are largely alone or tend to "go it alone" in coping with their illness.

Reaching out for support often means just expressing your feelings and concerns to others—which, as we saw, can be a challenge for many patients. It can also mean that you ask your loved ones for the type of support you need most, and this requires that you first ask yourself what that support might consist of. You will probably identify ways that people can help you that have not occurred to them.

For example, family members and friends often assume that they should provide encouragement and stress the positive (this is sometimes called the "cheerleading" role). Patients generally appreciate the positive intent behind this, yet it can put a damper on patients sharing their fears or sorrows. Often, patients would rather hear that others understand how they feel, regard these emotions as valid and will stick with them regardless of what happens. You might need to tell people that. On a more concrete level, you might ask others to accompany you during a medical appointment, pick up the kids after school, look up information for you (the Internet is a wonderful resource for this) or prepare a nutritious meal for your family.

If you find that you are not reaching out for the support that is available, reflect on the reasons for your stoicism. You may be minimizing your own needs for support, perhaps because you pride yourself on being independent and self-sufficient. It may seem to you that others would be bothered by your need for support or help and resent your imposing on them. More often than not, this is an assumption based on earlier experience. Perhaps you have found in the past that it is best to rely on yourself. While you should continue to draw upon your own internal resources, you should also realize that other people can and want to assist you in meeting the challenges of your illness, and you should give them a try.

Obtaining support often means joining a support group, and research has shown that such groups help patients to cope with and adjust to their illness. Support group members find that they have a great deal to offer each other in the way of mutual support and encouragement, discussion of common problems and ways of coping, and sharing of medical information. Groups also offer a safe and supportive haven for confronting one's fears. The American Cancer Society office or hospitals specializing in cancer treatments in your community will know of support groups that you could join. See also the Resources at the end of this book.

6. *Adopting a Participatory Stance* How much initiative do you take to actively participate in getting well? Some patients tackle their cancer head on. They have a strong fighting spirit, and they find ways of putting it into action. They go out of their way to learn about their illness and the options for treatment. They pursue the best treatments available and also consider alternative or holistic approaches. If you are like this, you would strongly agree with the statement "A lot depends on what I do and how I take part." Research has shown that patients who respond in this manner have less emotional distress than patients who respond in a more passive manner or try to avoid their situation.

Patients who adopt a participatory stance believe they can make a difference, and they put this belief into action. They therefore feel less helpless and vulnerable. This is a main reason why their emotional state is better. This belief in yourself as an active and effective agent is called self-efficacy, and research has consistently documented its positive emotional effects.

Patients who are coping in this way usually ask their doctors about treatment options and alternative therapies that their doctors had not mentioned. Instead of only following what their doctors say, they come up with ideas of their own. Also, they usually embrace some ways of promoting their physical well-being that go beyond the normal recommendations. These include dietary changes, increased exercise, stress reduction, vitamins, herbs, yoga, acupuncture, meditation, prayer, guided imagery and others (*see* Chapter 6). These patients often pursue new, experimental therapies that may offer additional hope. In all these ways, the patient is actively participating in an effort to recover fully or (if that is not realistic) to maintain the best physical health possible.

In contrast to those who feel they have an active role to play, some patients adopt a resigned, fatalistic attitude. One reason for this attitude is that it lets the patient off the hook for any extra effort that could make a difference. We have heard patients say, "What will be will be." The research on coping has consistently shown that this attitude is linked to a poorer psychological adjustment to one's illness.

7. *Finding a Positive Meaning* While the diagnosis and treatment of cancer is an awful experience in many respects, it can also be a challenge and even an opportunity for positive change in a person and in a person's life. In response to their illness, many patients step back and take stock of who they are and how they have been living. They reflect on their ultimate values and priorities, and often identify changes that are warranted (and perhaps overdue) in their lifestyle and personal relationships. This is often called the "enlightenment" or "gift" that comes with cancer, or the "wake-up call" aspect of cancer. Patients who embrace this aspect of their cancer experience have been found to be especially well adjusted and better able to deal with the many trials and disruptions caused by their illness.

It is often noted that growing old forces us to pay attention to what is important in life. The same can be said of a diagnosis of a life-threatening illness. What is important to a person often stems from their spiritual or religious beliefs. Even if you are not inclined toward spirituality, you probably have a basic philosophy of life and your life journey that highlights for you the importance of certain goals and values. These are important because of what they mean to your personal integrity and fulfillment.

To what degree does your lifestyle demonstrate these goals and values? This is a question for all of us, but it can become especially compelling if you are dealing with cancer. For many, their illness inspires them to pay more attention to what matters most. This could mean spending more time with family and close friends, making a greater contribution to the causes you believe in, showing more appreciation for all that you have and are, bringing forth aspects of your personality that have been suppressed, taking bet-

ter care of your physical and emotional needs and seeking to be more honest and true to yourself. In all these ways and in many more, your illness can become an impetus for positive change.

Sometimes that idea that there is a message or lesson in one's cancer implies that the person needed to get cancer and perhaps even got it for that reason. This kind of self-blame is completely unwarranted, and it fosters feelings of guilt and depression. A more psychologically healthy response was voiced by one of our patients when she said: "It's too bad that it took cancer to make me see things a bit more clearly, but you know, some positive things have come out of it for me."

8. *Spirituality, Faith and Prayer* Most people in our society have some fundamental spiritual beliefs, and these beliefs can be called upon for help in dealing with cancer. Patients who do so benefit in a variety of ways: they have a greater sense of peace, an inner strength and an ability to cope, and show an improved psychological adjustment and quality of life. These benefits derive especially from the perspective offered by your religious faith or spirituality and from the power of prayer and religious ritual.

All of us, whether we have cancer or not, are challenged at some point with the question of how to respond to our vulnerability to disease, suffering and death. For some, these realities lead to a kind of existential despair. Others embrace a perspective that goes beyond these realities, or that penetrates more deeply into them, to find meaning and value that transcends their individual existence or plight. This is the perspective offered, in one form or another, by the world's religious and spiritual traditions.

This perspective can help with the "Why me?" question. (*See* Chapter 13 for a fuller discussion of religious issues.) It is difficult to reconcile how an almighty, loving and just God could allow cancer to happen to a good person. Patients often believe that the illness is a punishment. In our culture, we often assume that what happens to a person is somehow linked to what the person deserves.

The emotional turmoil and doubt that stem from these issues can be soothed by themes of consolation and forgiveness that permeate the world's major religions. In the Judeo-Christian tradition, it is emphasized that God is with us in our suffering, providing the grace we need to endure rather than doling out suffering to those who deserve it.

Through prayer and liturgy, patients are able to connect to the core of their faith and to their religious community and derive the solace and fortitude they need to cope with their illness. Prayer can also have healing effects—most certainly in healing one's soul, but perhaps also in healing the body.

9. *Maintaining Self-Esteem* There are many ways that the experience of cancer can harm a person's self-esteem. One of these is the stigma of having cancer—that is, that it can imply something bad about the person who has it. In addition, many of the sources of your self-esteem can be threatened by cancer and the effects of medical treatments: your appearance, your physical abilities and activity level, personal attributes (such as being healthy and independent) and your role and identity within your family or in your work life. One of our breast cancer patients lamented: "I used to take pride in how I looked, and in being a good mother and working, helping to support the family. Now look at me."

These threats to your self-esteem pose a danger and an opportunity. The danger is depression and, with that, the weakening of the will to live and the resilience you need. The opportunity lies in finding additional sources of self-esteem within yourself. For example, you might take pride in the way you are coping with your

illness. You might have a new appreciation for how much you are loved—not because of what you do or how you look but because of who you are. Perhaps it has been difficult for you to depend on others because your independence has been overly important; you might now take pride in your ability to express your needs and ask for help. Perhaps your spirituality has been deepened by your cancer experience, and this can also help to renew your self-esteem. The overall emotional well-being of patients is enhanced when they discover or develop new sources for positive self-regard.

You can also protect your self-esteem by maintaining your normal activities and roles as much as possible. Your illness does not suddenly define you as a cancer patient, as if that is your new identity. Patients who continue to do the things that are important to them, to the extent possible, enjoy a better psychological adjustment than those who too quickly abandon these roles and activities or expect too little of themselves because they have cancer. One study specifically noted that patients need to "deal with the cancer" but also to "keep it in its place."

10. *Coming to Terms with Mortality* It may seem that a major challenge when dealing with cancer is to fight against the possibility of death rather than work on coming to terms with it. Certainly the philosophy and technology of modern medicine are preoccupied with this fight. The practitioners of alternative therapies also stress their healing potential. From all quarters, cancer patients hear that they must maintain hope, keep a positive attitude and try not to give up. It seems that everything revolves around getting better. And yet many patients die of cancer, and even those who do not are living with the possibility that they might. Very little support is offered to patients coming to terms with this possibility and reaching some sense of peace about it, and not feel-

ing that it is a failure and outrage to die.

We are not saying that you should accept the possibility of dying, and therefore not rail against it and do all you can to prevent it. Nor are we suggesting that if your cancer progresses, and death seems inevitable, that you should accept it then. Facing death is profoundly personal and inherently difficult: our survival instinct runs counter to it. The loss of life and everything that entails seems unbearable, and for most of us dying is almost too dreadful to think about. But it is possible to come to terms with death. And patients who do, enjoy the peace that acceptance brings.

The majority of newly diagnosed patients have a favorable prognosis. You might think that it would be better to confront death when the time comes. But even now, you are facing the possibility of dying of cancer and striving to prevent or delay it. This fight for your life is bound to be filled with fear, desperation and inner anguish if you are not also striving, in your own way, to come to terms with this possibility. This does not mean that you dwell on it; it means that you deal with it and then go on. It is always wise to review your personal and financial affairs. (*See* Part V, Planning for the Future.) Having done so, you will be all the better at living in the fullness of life, one day at a time, rather than in the dread of what could possibly happen.

The work of coming to terms with death can draw on our religious, spiritual or philosophical beliefs about what is important in life, and why. These beliefs can provide meaning and purpose to life, and therefore consolation when facing death. Many people have been able to feel, and to know, that their life has been about something important and of lasting value. This is one of the major ways that our religion or spirituality can help us.

We have found that most of our patients are struggling with these issues and longing for a sense of peace, but they are forced to do so quietly because they have so little support for this important inner work. Many patients abandon this effort, and come to feel hopeless about it. We encourage you to go forward, through reflection and reading in the religious or spiritual traditions that appeal to you. One book that many patients have found helpful is *The Tibetan Book of Living and Dying*.

THE BENEFIT FOR PATIENTS

The coping strategies we have discussed are not right for everyone, but there is good evidence that they are generally helpful to patients who are dealing with cancer. The bottom line is that they help patients feel better and stronger. Patients feel better because they are facing their illness squarely and working through its emotional impacts, and yet also keeping a perspective on it so that it does not define them or take over their life. Through all the trials and challenges that cancer can bring, they are keeping their wits about them and are able to carry on. They feel stronger because they have support, from other people and from within themselves. They have taken stock of their most cherished reasons for living, which strengthens and sustains them in their fight against cancer. And yet they also feel that their survival is not the only important objective; the quality of their lives and relationships, the values they live by and their spirituality also deserve attention and effort. They have the peace of knowing that their death from cancer, if it comes to that, will not obliterate the meaning, value and joy that their life has given to them and their loved ones.

ONE PATIENT'S WAY OF COPING

Diane Behar

I have been treated with chemotherapy for over six years and am now on my fifty-fifth course.

My current treatment is an experimental infusion that lasts 15 days each month. Almost immediately, I experience a nearly imperceptible ebbing away of my physical stamina and soon I prefer to walk rather than run, take an escalator instead of the stairs, sit down rather than stand. My life moves into slow motion. I gradually witness a change in my personality and the way I react to people and situations. What makes this experience so difficult and frightening is the loss of control that takes place—a transformation from a fully active and vital person into someone who can barely sit up and function effectively, which is overwhelming and disheartening.

Somewhere inside the deepest part of me, my truest self hides out under cover, and tells me that all of this is temporary and that I must just wait out these drug-induced episodes. This kind voice, along with my unwavering faith in God, enables me to conquer and think somehow I will be able to see my way into the clearing.

And so I go on. These are the coping mechanisms that work for me.

1. I try to live day to day. I focus my thoughts in the present tense and try to deal with matters close at hand.
2. I make myself "stupid" and I try not to think too much about the implications of what it means to have advanced cancer. Instead, I concentrate on concrete and practical things.
3. I try as best I can to compartmentalize the illness and not give it free rein over my existence. I perceive it as unwelcome and boring.
4. I live in a constant state of denial and keep my mind off the disease as much as possible.
5. I surround myself mostly with people and situations that bear no relationship to the illness.
6. I avoid reading or listening to too much about cancer or involving myself with people who are also fighting the disease. Although I am aware they can be beneficial and therapeutic, I avoid support groups in order to prevent myself from allowing any new fears and anxieties about the illness to enter my consciousness.
7. I internalize a belief system that everything I am going through is temporary and will come to an end. I say to myself that in spite of everything, everything will be all right.
8. I stand up to death with a courage I myself do not comprehend, and I do not permit myself to give in to a fear of dying.
9. I acknowledge that it is impossible for anyone to feel like a "normal person" after living with this illness for so many years, and accept the fact that it's okay to feel crazy and alienated some of the time—or even much of the time.
10. I remind myself that no one knows when their last day will be and that, so far, I have lived longer than many people predicted. I then think that maybe I'm doing something right after all and decide to continue to follow my prescription for coping.

12
COPING WITH DEPRESSION

Andrew Kneier, PhD

— ◇ —

If you are dealing with cancer, there are many reasons that you may feel depressed from time to time, or at least feel in danger of becoming depressed. Cancer confronts us with our mortality and all of the fears and losses associated with it. It can turn your world upside down, disrupting your life and threatening the roles, purposes and goals that give you meaning and satisfaction. Cancer therapies may have debilitating side effects and in some cases may cause irreparable damage to your body. Cancer affects not only you but also your loved ones, and much of your emotion is felt for them.

Many cancer patients have episodes of depression. Depression makes your entire experience with cancer more difficult, weakens your resilience and may hamper your overall adjustment. It can also undermine your will to live and compromise the courage, fortitude and determination that you need to face cancer and to endure the necessary medical treatments.

Depression is a serious threat to your ability to cope with cancer and to your will to live. It is the exact opposite of what you need: energy and stamina, a vision of a brighter future, hope that inspires and sustains you and the motivation and commitment to travel through the arduous road of cancer therapy.

Depression is therefore a serious threat for anyone dealing with cancer. Fortunately, you can protect yourself from depression, and there are effective remedies for it.

THE NATURE OF DEPRESSION

Most of us have been depressed at some time and know what it feels like. Three complaints are especially common:
◆ loss of interest in things you used to enjoy (even a simple pleasure, such as listening to your favorite music, could lose its appeal to you);
◆ feeling sad, blue or down in the dumps, and being tearful or crying easily, and
◆ feeling depleted of energy and overcome with a paralyzing fatigue. On some days, a depressed person may feel too drained or apathetic to get out of bed in the morning.

You might also feel pessimistic and hopeless, and begin to welcome death as a relief and to think of suicide. Depression can cause you to feel worthless and guilty, sometimes because of the self-loathing you have developed because of being depressed.

Some of the mental problems that accompany depression include difficulty concentrating, difficulty making decisions and forgetting things. Some of the physical complaints include loss of appetite, sleep disturbances, headaches, digestive problems and loss of libido.

CAUSES OF DEPRESSION

Depression can have psychological or biochemical causes. The psychological causes arrive from experiences and events that have a depressing effect; the biochemical (or clinical) causes involve imbalances in the neurochemistry of the brain.

Sometimes the psychological causes lead to depression because of these biochemical changes. Regardless of cause, depression is associated with biochemical change in the brain.

Life experiences may cause depression when they carry certain meanings for the person involved. For example, if you were abused as a child, you might conclude that you were undeserving of love or a happy life. Thoughts and feelings of being unworthy, whether conscious or unconscious, can then lead to depression. Other thoughts that commonly underlie depression involve the sense of being helpless, hopeless and a victim. These thoughts and feelings have their origin in traumatic events in the person's life (although the person may not remember these events). Not only do these events cause depressing thoughts, they can also bring about a biochemical imbalance in the brain, and this imbalance contributes to the depression.

Sometimes when you are depressed you can identify what you are depressed about or are able to identify depressing thoughts (e.g., "Nothing will make a difference"). However, sometimes depression may seem to come out of the blue. People have "come down" with depression in ways that feel similar to coming down with the flu, and they may not be aware why they are depressed. This is because the psychological factors are unconscious or because the depression is caused solely by changes in the neurochemistry of the brain.

CANCER AND DEPRESSION

Cancer patients often get depressed simply because having cancer can be a depressing experience. However, there is usually more to it than that. Most cancer patients are not clinically depressed. To varying degrees, they are frightened and upset, but this is not depression. When cancer causes depression, there are psychological or biological reasons for it. These causes are understandable, and they are treatable.

The experience of cancer can cause depression because of the various meanings that the illness takes on as a result of the circumstances or psychological background in which it occurred.

Cancer happens to you as a person, not just to your body. You therefore experience it as part of your personal life, as opposed to its being an isolated event that happened in a vacuum. The personal issues, themes, perceptions and feelings that are imbedded in your own personal history color your experience with cancer, giving it a certain meaning and feeling, or tone.

The clearest example is seen in the reactions to the diagnosis of cancer in people of various ages. In general, cancer patients in their thirties experience a feeling of incompletion about their life and a strong emotional investment in a long future; to them, the cancer may feel like a threat to that future and to all the goals and purposes that it holds. Patients in their eighties, on the other hand, generally bring some sense of life completion to their experience of cancer, along with an awareness that their future is relatively short; to them, the same cancer may feel more acceptable because of the long life they have already enjoyed.

Of course, chronological age is not the sole influence on how you experience having cancer or whether you become depressed. The following examples illustrate other ways that the psychological context in which you experience cancer can contribute to depression.

The feeling of sadness (for yourself and loved ones) evoked by a cancer diagnosis is not itself depression, but it can be magnified by other sorrows in your life, so that it does become depression. In this case, a sorrowful life history before your cancer is the context in which the cancer is experienced. The cancer, for example, can represent a kind of crowning blow to a long history of abuse, misfortune or frustration. It can therefore tap into or reactivate many old feelings. The depression that emerges stems partly from having cancer, but it also grows out of one's personal life history and its resulting emotional baggage.

Another example: suppose you had recently achieved an important life goal or were on the verge of doing so. Perhaps you had struggled for years to achieve this goal. Then, on the heels of this important accomplishment, you are diagnosed with cancer. You could therefore feel that you were being thwarted, that the deck was stacked against you or that you were having to pay a price for your ambition. These are the meanings that cancer could hold for you—derived from the context in which it occurred—and they can cause depression.

The medical treatment for cancer cannot help but cause some degree of physical suffering and damage to your body. The optimal goal of treatment, of course, is to restore your body to health, but this comes at some price. Sometimes the price is severe (such as a mastectomy, head or neck surgery, bone marrow transplant or skin damage from radiation therapy). Different patients feel differently about the bodily effects of cancer treatments, and one response is sometimes depression. Our feelings about ourself are to some degree dependent upon our appearance and our physical abilities. When these are compromised by cancer, the loss that we suffer (sometimes to our self-esteem, sometimes to our role and identity) can be deeply depressing.

Our culture often assumes that what happens to a person is somehow linked to what that person deserves. Unfortunately, this assumption, which is often very subtle, can involve cancer. When things are going well for us, we tend to assume that we are doing something right and deserve our good fortune. Misfortune—such as cancer—may make us think that we were not so deserving of our good fortune after all. It is not uncommon, therefore, for cancer patients to wonder where they went wrong. Some patients have felt that things were going too well for them, that their life was too easy or that they were enjoying more happiness than most people, and that cancer was a way of balancing things out, that they deserved to get cancer. One woman said of her cancer: "It's all of my repressed resentment and bitterness coming out." Another patient felt that it was an expression of his self-hatred. One referred to it as "a pathetic attempt for the attention I've never had." Such ideas can cause depression.

As already mentioned, there are also biological causes of depression in cancer patients. The emotional consequences of cancer can bring about biochemical changes in the brain. But biochemical changes can also be caused by chemotherapy drugs, hormonal treatments, anti-inflammatory drugs, pain medication and radiation therapy.

If you are depressed, it does not necessarily mean that you are not coping or adjusting as you should. It is often important and psychologically healthy for underlying feelings to emerge, as this may provide an opportunity for you to confront and work through the emotional traumas from past years.

Whatever the cause, depression is dangerous, especially to your quality of life and your will to live. There are steps you can take to alleviate it.

WHAT YOU CAN DO

Protecting Yourself There are four important ways to protect yourself from depression when you are dealing with cancer:

◆ First, try to become aware of your emotions, and then acknowledge and express these emotions with someone you feel close to. Depression often results from the suppression of painful and upsetting emotions. Research has shown that cancer patients who openly express their feelings and obtain support from others are much less likely to become depressed.

◆ Second, maintain close connections and frequent contact with your loved ones and reach out for their support. Studies have demonstrated that interpersonal support is a strong buffer against feelings of isolation and depression.

◆ Third, become an active participant in fostering your physical and emotional well-being. Discuss the treatment options with your doctors so that you are informed and can fully embrace the treatment plan, and consider supplemental approaches as well (such as acupuncture, better nutrition, herbal medicine, meditation and guided imagery).

Your active involvement in your recovery will help to counter the feelings of helplessness and passivity that often characterize depression.

◆ Fourth, try to obtain as much exercise as possible. The physiological and mental benefits of exercise help to offset the depressing effect of a serious illness. One reason for this is that exercise increases the brain levels of endorphins, which are natural mood elevators (*see* Chapters 21 and 23 on exercise and massage).

If you become depressed, try to identify what is bothering you. You might make a list of these problems and ways that you could address them. Discuss these problems and emotions with a relative or close friend.

Depression often results from suppressing our emotions, depriving them of the discharge they need. For example, when depression persists long after the loss of a loved one, it is often because the person's grief has not been adequately expressed. One theory is that unexpressed emotions build up internally and cause depression; another is that the mental energy required to contain such emotions

results in the kind of mental fatigue and lethargy characteristic of depression.

It is common to be unaware of what you are depressed about. You might feel that you have no good reason for being depressed, especially because others have had far worse problems or because you are grateful for the many blessings you have enjoyed. Try to push yourself beyond that: give yourself the benefit of the doubt—that you have legitimate reasons for your depression—and do some soul-searching to find out what these reasons are. Think about the many ways that cancer can cause depression, as discussed above.

Think especially about your life as a whole, and about the disappointments and sorrows that you have encountered along the way. These may be affecting you now more than you realize. Whatever you come up with in this self-exploration, talk about it with someone you feel especially close to, even if you think you are being foolish, shallow or self-centered. Permit yourself to feel what you are feeling, honor your reasons for feeling it and confide in someone about it. Even writing about these matters in a journal can have a relieving effect.

In this process, you might also think about why it is difficult for you to express your feelings. One common reason is not wanting to bother others with your feelings and needs. Some people have difficulty confiding in others because of an underlying belief that they cannot or will not be comforted by doing so. Confiding therefore seems like a setup for more letdown and hurt. Perhaps you let your parents know when something was bothering you, but they did not respond with the comfort or support you needed. Such experiences, over the course of your childhood, could cause you to feel that there was nothing to be gained by voicing your feelings, and that doing so only made you feel worse. While these fears are understandable, it is important to recognize that there is surely someone in your life now (a relative or close friend, a minister or rabbi, a doctor, a nurse, a therapist) who would support you in what you are going through.

One aspect of depression is that it may cause you to withdraw from others and to turn inward. This can make it all the more difficult to confide in others about your feelings and to obtain the support you need. A vicious circle can set in, wherein a person becomes depressed, withdraws, therefore has no emotional outlet or personal support and becomes even more depressed. It is essential that you break out of this cycle by finding some way of reaching out for help. If necessary, circle this paragraph, leave it for someone who cares about you to see, and write "Help me" in the margin.

Depression often involves feelings of despair, bitterness or lack of meaning, resulting in the painful cry of "Why me?" that often arises when someone is subjected to severe suffering. Your religion or spirituality can be a source of meaning and comfort for you, offering a perspective that can soothe the emotional anguish and mental torment that cancer sometimes causes. Chapter 13 discusses how religion and spirituality can help you deal with cancer.

TREATMENT FOR DEPRESSION

Psychotherapy Often the best help for depression is from a mental health professional. Research has shown that psychotherapy is an effective treatment for depression in the majority of cases. A therapist will help you to talk about difficult feelings and will create an emotionally safe environment in which to do so. He or she will also help you to explore all the factors that are contributing to your depression, including those that you may not be aware of. You will learn ways of mastering the thoughts that cause depres-

sion. In general, your therapy will consist of working through your depression and the life experiences that are related to it. It will not take your cancer away, and you may still feel upset and worried, but you will no longer be stuck in the deep, dark hole of depression.

Antidepressant Medication In many cases, antidepressant medication is warranted, especially in combination with psychotherapy. The best known of these involve the chemical serotonin, one of the main neurotransmitters. When a neural impulse reaches the end of a nerve cell in the brain, it releases serotonin in the junction (called the synapse) connecting this cell to the next, and this enables the impulse to be transmitted from one cell to the other. Sometimes the nerve cell sending the signal reabsorbs the serotonin too quickly, and an insufficient amount is left in the junction for the impulse to be transmitted effectively. This phenomenon is apparently associated with the experience of depression.

It is interesting that the mental slowness or lethargy of depression may reflect the state of the brain when serotonin levels are too low. Some antidepressants, called selective serotonin reuptake inhibitors (SSRIs), block the reabsorption of serotonin, and thereby relieve the symptoms of depression.

There are other types of antidepressant medication besides the SSRIs, and each of these works a little differently. Your physician or psychiatrist will prescribe the best medication for your individual situation. Still, it may take some trial and error to find the medication that works best for you and has the fewest side effects. It may take weeks for some antidepressants to reach their full potential.

The symptomatic relief provided by an antidepressant may be a godsend to a severely depressed person, even though it does not address what the person is depressed about. This relief is often essential in order for the person to even consider ways of addressing the psychological aspects of depression. Research has shown that the best treatment for depression in many cases is a combination of emotional support, psychotherapy and antidepressant medication.

STEPS TO OVERCOMING DEPRESSION

The depression that stems from cancer and its treatments can make you feel that you can't go on and that it's not worth the effort. But there are effective ways of combating and overcoming this depression:

◆ Do not blame yourself for being depressed.
◆ Identify what you are depressed about.
◆ Confide in someone you feel close to.
◆ Express your emotions.
◆ Engage in problem solving.
◆ Become an active participant in recovery efforts (do not give in to helplessness).
◆ Do things that enhance self-esteem.
◆ Exercise as much as possible.
◆ Talk with your minister or rabbi.
◆ Deepen your faith or spirituality (through prayer, reading, meditation).
◆ Obtain help from a therapist.
◆ Explore antidepressant medication.

13
HOW RELIGION AND SPIRITUALITY CAN HELP

Andrew Kneier, PhD, and Jeffery Silberman, DMin

———◇———

A life-threatening disease, such as cancer, confronts us with realities and questions that cause us to step back from our lives and reflect on the meaning and implications of the illness. Our perspective on these realities and questions emerges in large measure from our religious, spiritual or philosophical orientation, and it influences how we experience the illness—its meaning, how we feel about it and how well we come to terms with it. A religious perspective can help us as we grapple with these issues and seek to keep our bearing through the mental and emotional turmoil that comes with having cancer.

CANCER AND QUESTIONS OF MEANING

In order to discuss how religion and spirituality can help in dealing with cancer, we want first to review some of the religious and spiritual issues, questions and problems that cancer presents. These are questions of meaning—the meaning of our life and what is important, the meaning behind our personal affliction with cancer and finding meaning in our suffering.

Mortality The diagnosis of cancer confronts us with the fact that we are vulnerable to disease and suffering, that we are mortal and that our time is limited. When we are in good health, these realities often reside at the back of our minds; but when a serious illness strikes, they

surge forward and challenge us. They challenge us especially with the question of whether we are using our time wisely, and this question is linked to what our time is for—to what our life is all about. For many, these questions take on a central and compelling importance, which is why cancer is commonly referred to as a wake-up call.

Usually the most pressing priority when we are faced with the diagnosis of cancer is to regain our good health; if we succeed, the implications of our mortality might once again slip into the background. Sometimes the illness is regarded as only a temporary bump in the road of life, as opposed to a stark reminder of life's fragility. But more often than not, cancer has a way of capturing our attention, deepening our reflection on what is important and causing us to live with more awareness of ultimate priorities.

Patients who are fighting for their lives can be strengthened and sustained by a clear vision of what they want to survive for. Many talk of surviving for the sake of their families, to meet certain life goals and to fulfill certain inner potentials or strivings. Whatever a person's answer, it reflects deeply held religious, spiritual or philosophical beliefs about what is important and why.

As cancer patients reflect on their ultimate priorities, they often identify changes that they wish to make in themselves or their life. This is often referred to as the "enlightenment" of cancer or the "gift" of cancer. Countless patients have commented that they regret that it took a cancer diagnosis to wake them up and capture their attention, but they feel that many positive and overdue changes in themselves and their life have resulted from it. In making these changes, these patients have found some positive meaning in their illness.

Why Me? Cancer confronts us with the question of why, as one person among many, we have been afflicted with this disease. Many patients have asked, in open protest or in private anguish, "Why did this have to happen to me?" Of course, the answer is that it did not *have* to happen, it just did. But there is often an emotional poignancy to this issue that cannot easily be dismissed.

One reason for this is religious: those who believe in the God of the Judeo-Christian Bible do not understand how such a God could allow cancer to happen to a good person. There must be some reason for it. It is not uncommon for patients to wonder whether the illness is a punishment for certain wrongs or failings of character. The Bible teaches that disease and death are the result of sin. Of course, many religiously oriented patients do not feel that they are being punished, but they do feel that their illness is somehow part of God's plan for them, and they struggle and pray to discern the higher purpose for which it is intended.

Even those who are not particularly religious can feel a sense of self-blame about their cancer because of the influence of the Judeo-Christian tradition in our culture. (*See* Chapter 11.) Many patients feel that if they can fix whatever is wrong in themselves, or adopt the right attitudes and behaviors, then the malignancy will be stopped. It has been argued, for example, that if patients heal themselves, or heal their lives, then physical healing will follow.

Why Do We Suffer? There are many dimensions to the suffering caused by cancer; physical, mental, emotional and spiritual. The suffering can involve all aspects of the person, including his or her relationships, roles, identity, hopes and plans, and the meaning of his or her life.

A person with cancer is challenged to respond to suffering in some way. Most patients, of course, strive to gain as much relief of their suffering as possible. Beyond that, some patients feel their only option is to endure it, either philosophically or stoically. Others seek to deny or downplay it, while some try to rise above it. Some regard it as an opportunity or challenge to demonstrate certain strengths of character or to bear witness to their faith. Some patients rail against it as an outrage, and others are able to find some personal meaning in their suffering, especially in bringing about changes in themselves that they feel are important (such as acceptance or humility).

The religions of the world all contain, in one way or another, a philosophy or perspective on the meaning of suffering. Perhaps the perspective most widely known in our culture is the Judeo-Christian one, according to which suffering serves the positive purpose of deepening one's spirituality. Religious faith can bring a perspective to suffering that offers consolation or strength to those living through cancer.

RELIGIOUS AND SPIRITUAL PERSPECTIVES ON MEANING

When we talk about the meaning of an experience, we are talking about its relationship or connection to something larger or beyond the experience itself. For example, the meaning of a serious illness can be found in how it is related to the person's life as a whole. The meaning of one's life as a whole can be found in its connection to some larger reality, cause or purpose. Many people feel that their lives are meaningful because of the contribution they make to the lives of others.

To understand the roles of religion and spirituality in defining meaning for us, we must ask about the larger meaning of the lives of these other people. We might argue that the success of a human life contributes to the human adventure as a whole. We then might ask, however, whether the success of human evolution (physical, mental and moral) really matters, since humankind will not survive the eventual demise of our solar system. Suppose there is some realm or cause within or beyond evolution. Fine. But, in order to have any meaning, what is it connected to? Thus, an infinite series of questions is launched here, wherein we can always ask about the larger reality to which something is meaningfully connected. Is there some ultimate reality that finally provides meaning to everything else?

These are the kinds of questions that lie at the heart of religion, faith and spirituality. These systems of belief all acknowledge a transcendent source of meaning and value beyond ourselves as human beings. At times of serious illness or crisis, it is to one of these systems that we may turn for solace, comfort and meaning; for the inner strength to endure the physical and emotional challenges of illness, and for guidance in our personal response to it.

Religion describes both the formal area of study of these belief systems and, more specifically, the organized understanding of beliefs shared by groups of people. The Western religious tradition includes Judaism, Christianity and Islam. The Eastern religious tradition includes Buddhism, Taoism and Hinduism. Each religious system is based on a core of beliefs, often articulated through a set of ancient texts that are considered authoritative and sacred. These bodies of literature incorporate that religion's values and teachings, providing the source of answers to many profound human questions.

Faith often refers to the beliefs held by an individual who is an adherent of one of the formal systems of religion. Each of us, whether we know it or not, holds some kind of faith. We may believe in a personal God or in a Divine Clockmaker (that is, a God who created the world, set it in motion and then left it alone). This faith may be spelled out by a formal systematic theology or comprise pieces of many different religious teachings. This personal faith is frequently deep and forms a foundation of emotional and spiritual strength when we face crisis, cancer and, especially, death.

Spirituality is the connection that many people feel to God or to something beyond us, but not in accordance to the formal teachings of traditional religion. Thus, many people speak about being spiritual but not necessarily religious. While some people seek their answers in religious literature and traditional teachings, others search beyond traditional models to find answers that will bring them emotional and existential meaning.

Religion, Coping and Healing A person's faith or spirituality provides a means for coping with illness and reaching a deeper kind of inner healing. Coping means different things to different people: it can involve finding answers to the questions that illness raises, it can mean seeking comfort for the fears and pain that illness brings and it can mean learning how to find a sense of direction at the time of illness. Religious teachings can help a person cope in all of these dimensions.

Religious teachings can also point the way toward healing, which can be something very different from curing. Modern medicine has been able to recognize that a medical cure is not always possible; nor is it the only appropriate goal for treatment. Sometimes, when treatment is futile, the healing of soul or spirit can provide a deep and sustaining comfort; religion has long focused upon this as its central purpose. Healing of the soul or spirit means recognizing the values in one's life and striving to bring these in line with the teachings of one's religion or the fundamentals of one's faith.

The Quest for Meaning The meaning of life and death, humanity's purpose or direction and the struggle with suffering and pain have long been central themes in religious literature.

Within the context of many traditional belief systems, the ultimate answer to meaning, suffering and death resides with God alone. One conservative religious answer is that God's ways are beyond human understanding, but we must trust in God's goodness and purpose. Many people feel a great sense of confidence and assurance in the belief that an all-powerful, all-knowing deity controls the world. The idea that the reward for a life well lived is eternal rest in heaven is usually associated with this conservative belief.

Liberal theologies offer other explanations about God's place in human experience. Some hold that God has created an imperfect world and that it is our task and responsibility as humans to work toward the world's repair or perfection. This means that we share an obligation to help one another face the struggles of human existence, including illness and death.

Some humanistic religious traditions assert that God has no direct influence on contemporary human events. They assert that when we suffer, all that God can do is to be present with us. The comfort in this belief system comes from the conviction that God feels our pain and knows what we are going through when we suffer.

Religion and "Why Me?" For many patients, the "why me?" issues are essentially religious in nature. Religious people sometimes are concerned that illness relates to some sin that they have committed. Most religions today reject the idea that God punishes us through illness. Many people hold to an alternative view—that illnesses, such as cancer, demonstrate the presence of evil in the world. Religion gives us the opportunity to help others and thereby overcome evil or imperfection by creating good.

Most theologians and religious leaders today acknowledge that there are no simple answers to these questions. They also recognize that the question "Why me?" is really not so much a question requiring an answer as a cry of emotional and spiritual pain. Rather than try to address this question with theological formulas that bring little consolation, they strive instead to honor the emotional anguish behind these questions and to point to the comfort, reassurance and broader perspective offered in religious teachings.

Emotional Comfort In the face of a serious illness, we are often challenged by a range of emotional reactions that can be unfamiliar and more intense than anything we have ever encountered. We feel ourselves vulnerable and in need of a stable and solid support. Religion steps in with comfort and reassurance.

One of the great sources of emotional support in times of illness is the Book of Psalms. For those of us familiar with the Western religious canon, no voice speaks more compassionately and with greater understanding of the emotional upheaval of crisis than the Psalmist. From the 23rd Psalm (King James Version), we read: "Yea, though I walk through the valley of the shadow of death, I will fear no evil: for thou art with me; thy rod and thy staff they comfort me."

When we are confronted by cancer or other serious illness, our sensory experience is often heightened, both in regard to the beauty of life and its more fearful, ugly and painful side. Our emotional connection to the world can become more intense. Religious tradition places this experience in an ancient perspective. We recall the stories of great sages and saints who also faced hardship and death. They instruct us about the intensity and how our path has been traveled before by so many others. Our feelings direct us to a new connection to the world and God's presence in it.

RELIGIOUS GUIDANCE

Another dilemma confronting us when we are faced with cancer relates to what we are to do. We wonder how to act, how to function at this time. It seems that the ordinary ways of living and functioning are inappropriate or trite. Religion again assists us with models of behavior to lift up the values we hold as important. Spiritual disciplines and teachings of various kinds can instruct us in structured exercises.

Asceticism is an example well known through religious history. Simpler examples of responses supported by religion include giving to charity and helping others. Religion teaches us that we can find order and direction by doing things that foster our spiritual well-being and energy. These can include some of the practices that follow.

Religious Resources and Practices Many conventional religious resources and practices help us cope with cancer by offering comfort, support and direction.

Rituals and prayer are the central and best-known religious techniques. Prayer extends comfort in many ways. It offers us consolation, encouragement, connection and solace. We experience a sense of divine presence and divine love as we pray. Prayer and ritual touch deep feelings within us. They allow us to give voice to our pain, joy, grief, loss, isolation, alienation and loneliness. Prayer evokes mem-

ories of our youth and of our family and long-standing relationships. It also brings a sense of power and awesome mystery. Prayer reveals a side of ourselves that may be needy, that we may not want to reveal, that struggles with certainty and in which our "inner child" resides.

Prayer techniques such as centering, traditional prayer, meditation, guided meditation and anointing have long been recognized as effective tools in dealing with illness. Recent scientific studies reported in books such as Dr. Larry Dossey's *Healing Words* prove beyond doubt that prayer makes a difference.

Four nondenominational prayers for healing, selected by the pastoral care staff at the UCSF/Mount Zion Medical Center, are found at the end of this chapter.

The *religious community* is a powerful ally in dealing with crises in our lives. People who know us and care about us from within a community of faith are important partners in the healing process. Apart from the effectiveness of their love and prayers, the religious communicants can often provide practical support for the tasks of daily life that need to be done.

We should not underestimate the value of clergy visits for helping us to cope with cancer. In many ways, the presence of clergy powerfully conveys the message of God's care to those who are ill. Clergy tangibly represent God's caring presence, both through their being there and through the words they speak.

Healing practices associated with religion and focused upon cancer and other illnesses have become much more common today than ever before. Some of these practices come from fringe groups and charlatans seeking to prey upon frightened people. Yet mainstream religion has also recognized the value of healing prayer services and rituals as an adjunct to more typical prayers and rituals. Some rituals of this kind are ancient. Some are contemporary. Many people have sought and found healing and comfort through religious tradition and practice.

NONDENOMINATIONAL PRAYERS FOR HEALING

These four prayers for healing have been composed or selected by the pastoral care staff at the UCSF/Mount Zion Medical Center.

My God and God of all generations, in my great need I pour out my heart to you. Long days and weeks of suffering are hard to endure. In my struggle, I reach out for the help that only you can give. Let me feel that you are near, and that your care enfolds me. Rouse me with the strength to overcome my weakness, and brighten my spirit with the assurance of your love. Help me to sustain the hopes of my loved ones as they strive to strengthen and encourage me. May the healing power you have placed within me give me the strength to recover so I may fulfill my journey in the Divine Plan.

In sickness I turn to you, O God, as a child turns to a parent for comfort and help. Strengthen within me the wondrous power of healing that you have implanted in your children. Guide my doctors and nurses, that they may speed my recovery. Let the knowledge of your love comfort my loved ones, lighten their burdens and renew their faith. May my sickness not weaken my faith in you, nor diminish my love for other human beings. From my illness may I gain a truer appreciation of life's gifts, a deeper awareness of life's blessings, and a fuller sympathy for all who are in pain.

Send me, O God, your healing, so that I may quickly recover from the illness that has come upon me. Sustain my spirit, relieve my pain and restore me to perfect health, happiness and strength. Grant unto my body your healing power so I may continue to be able to bear testimony to your everlasting mercy and love, for you, O Lord, art a faithful and merciful healer.

Be at Peace
Do not fear the changes of life—
Rather look to them with full
    hope as they arise.
God, whose very own you are,
Will deliver you from out of
    them.
He has kept you hitherto,
And He will lead you safely
    through all things;
And when you cannot stand it,
God will bury you in His arms.
Do not be afraid of what may
    happen tomorrow;
The same everlasting Father who
    cares for you today
Will take care of you then and
    every day.
He will either shield you from
    suffering,
Or He will give you unfailing
    strength to bear it.
Be at Peace—
And put aside all anxious
    thoughts and imaginations.
                    —*St. Francis de Sales*

14
VISUALIZATION: THE POWER OF IMAGERY AND MENTAL PARTICIPATION

Andrew W. Kneier, PhD, with Janet Amber Damon, MSW

---◇---

If you have ever made up a story, you know about the creative power of your imagination. Images or scenes just pop into your mind, seemingly from nowhere. Sometimes the image is so right for the story that you are both delighted and taken aback, wondering, "Where did that come from?" or "How did I come up with that?" It often seems that the image was given to you, not created by you, or that you somehow found the image in your mind. Writers of fiction and artists of all types owe their craft and livelihood to the resourcefulness of their imagination, as they draw upon this wondrous source of creativity that resides within all of us.

Cancer patients have also discovered the power of their imagination in dealing with the many challenges posed by their illness. In the most general sense, they do this by mentally visualizing what they hope to achieve, whether it be the destruction of their tumor, relief from pain or overall inner peace. In their mind's eye, they visualize an image of what they are striving for and how they might achieve it. They have found that the imagination is not only a wellspring of ideas and images but also a powerful tool for promoting emotional, spiritual and physical well-being.

In *Healing Yourself*, which has helped countless patients to employ this versatile inner resource, Martin Rossman, MD, described imagery this way:

An image is an inner representation of your experience or your fantasies—a way your mind codes, stores, and expresses information. Imagery is the currency of dreams and daydreams; memories and reminiscence; plans, projections and possibilities. It is the language of the arts, the emotions and, most important, the deep inner self.

Imagery is a window on your inner world; a way of viewing your own ideas, feelings, and interpretations. But it is more than a mere window—it is a means of transformation and liberation from distortions in this realm that may unconsciously direct your life and shape your health.

This chapter discusses the many uses of imagery by cancer patients and offers a first-hand account by a psychotherapist who used imagery in coping with her own cancer.

THE SIMONTON APPROACH TO FIGHTING CANCER

In 1978, O. Carl Simonton, MD, and Stephanie Matthews Simonton presented a method of using imagery to combat cancer in *Getting Well Again*. Their approach was to visualize the process of medical treatments and the immune system successfully destroying cancer cells. After guiding patients into a state of deep relaxation, they offer the following instructions:

Mentally picture the cancer in either realistic or symbolic terms. Think of the cancer as consisting of very weak, confused cells. Remember that our bodies destroy cancerous cells thousands of times during a normal lifetime. As you picture your cancer, realize that your recovery requires that your body's own defenses return to a natural, healthy state.

If you are now receiving treatment, picture your treatment coming into your body in a way that you understand. If you are receiving radiation therapy, picture it as a beam of millions of bullets of energy hitting any cell in its path. The normal cells are able to repair the damage that is done, but the cancer cells cannot because they are weak. (This is one of the basic facts upon which radiation therapy is built.) If you are receiving chemotherapy, picture that drug acting like a poison. The normal cells are intelligent and strong and don't take up the poison so readily. But the cancer cell is a weak cell so it takes very little time to kill it. It absorbs the poison, dies, and is flushed out of your body.

Picture your body's own white cells coming into the area where the cancer is, recognizing the abnormal cells, and destroying them. There is a vast army of white blood cells. They are very strong and aggressive. They are also very smart. There is no contest between them and the cancer cells; they will win the battle.

Picture the cancer shrinking. See the dead cells being carried away by the white blood cells and being flushed from your body through the liver and kidneys and being eliminated in the urine and stool.

Continue to see the cancer shrinking, until it is all gone.

According to the Simontons, a key aspect of successful visualization is the *type* of imagery used, not just the process of using it. They believe the cancer cells should be visualized as weak, confused and extremely vulnerable, and that the medical treatments and immune response should be visualized as powerful, aggressive and invincible. This makes good intu-

itive sense in that the response of immune cells against the cancer can certainly be characterized as an attack. Images of combat and victory can also help a patient feel less vulnerable and helpless against the cancer.

However, some clinicians in this field argue that aggressive imagery is not the best for everyone. Depending on a person's temperament, a more gentle imagery may feel more comfortable and appropriate—for example, the imagery of the cancer melting away or being quietly put to sleep. Some patients feel more protected and healed by soothing images or memories of being held, rocked or comforted than they do by images of a relentless military attack.

The Simontons' work also raises the question (they acknowledge that the answer to this is unknown) of whether imagery that is anatomical in nature is any more or less powerful than symbolic representations. Is it better to picture in your mind what the cancer and immune cells actually look like (photographs of a cancer cell surrounded by immune cells can be found in medical books), or is it better to imagine a shark devouring terrified little sand crabs as a symbol of this process? Again, it is important for each person to find the imagery that feels right.

In their book, the Simontons touched on an important issue that has been further developed by other clinicians who use imagery in working with cancer patients. This is the fact that we can learn from the images that come to us. Just as we can interpret the meaning behind images in our dreams, we can also find meaning in the images that present themselves when we visualize cancer and the healing process. As Dr. Rossman noted, often the images that arise spontaneously come from our unconscious. If we picture the cancer as dark and foreboding, it suggests the ominous nature of cancer that we hold in our minds. If we imagine chemotherapy as a corrosive acid, it could indicate our fear of the treatment rather than our perception of its healing power. Picturing cancer cells as cockroaches, and the treatment as total house fumigation, may betray the person's pessimism about ever completely eradicating the cancer. The image of cancer being stoned to death by an angry mob of immune cells—which implies that the cancer is being punished—may be a reaction to a person's feeling punished or victimized by cancer.

When the images that spontaneously come to us have negative connotations—about ourselves, the future, the nature of cancer, the effects of treatment and so forth—the opportunity arises to grapple with these underlying assumptions and to develop imagery that is more positive and optimistic. You can do this on your own, or by being guided in your imagery by a therapist or using guided-imagery tapes. For more information about negative versus positive imagery, consult the thoughtful *Imagery in Healing* by Jeanne Achterberg and Frank Lawlis.

DOES VISUALIZATION WORK, AND IF SO, HOW?

Whether visualization can impede or reverse the course of cancer has not been proven definitively one way or the other. The scientific evidence on this issue is reviewed in Chapter 10; the conclusion there was that a patient's active participation in combating cancer—and the feelings of hope, optimism and a strong will to live that underlie this effort—appear to make a positive difference to the medical outcome in some cases. Many studies have documented this effect. However, there are also many studies that have failed to do so. On balance, the evidence to date makes a solid case that visualization could have beneficial medical effects and should at least be tried.

There is no controversy, however, about whether visualization is emotionally and psychologically beneficial. The scientific studies on this issue have consistently documented a positive effect on a patient's emotional state and psychological adjustment. The main reason is that visualization offers an active and potentially effective means for self-help in the healing process and thereby diminishes the feelings of vulnerability, helplessness and lack of control that so often accompany the experience of cancer.

How visualization sometimes works in assisting recovery from cancer is one of the many mysteries having to do with mind-body communication. Some people can lower their heart rate by imagining themselves in a peaceful, natural setting. Others have lowered their body temperature by imagining that they are in a tub of ice water. Under hypnosis, people have caused warts to go away by directing and imagining their dissolution. Countless studies on the placebo effect have demonstrated the physical changes caused by a person's belief in the healing effects of what they thought was a real medicine. In classical conditioning studies, a stimulus (such as sugar water) is given along with an immunosuppressive drug; later, the stimulus alone leads to a decrease in certain immune measures. People afflicted with multiple personalities sometimes exhibit certain physical conditions in one personality state that are not present in another state. There have been cases where cancer has regressed spontaneously, sometimes in association with a strong emotional catharsis. We do not know the mind-body mechanisms by which these wonders occur.

It is also unknown why these mechanisms sometimes appear to result in marvelous outcomes while in other cases they seem to have no effect. Often, for example, a person's belief in a placebo counts for nothing; only the real medicine works, independent of expectation. Some highly suggestible subjects, under hypnosis, will develop a blister when they are told (and imagine) that the ice cube they are touching is really a hot coal; others will just feel the ice.

Although we do not understand the why and how of the mechanisms involved, the powerful effect of mental images on bodily processes has become an added source of hope for cancer patients and provides an additional means for their active participation in the recovery effort. To many, it makes good sense that mentally participating in the healing processes at work within their bodies (such as the immune response to a tumor, or the poisoning of cancer cells by chemotherapy), through visualizing those processes, will assist these processes. This is the major application to cancer that has grown out of the mind-body interactions that have been documented in recent years.

The improved emotional state of patients who practice visualization may also help explain why these patients sometimes enjoy better-than-expected medical outcomes. Research in the growing field of psychoneuroimmunology has consistently demonstrated the connections between emotions and the immune response.

APPLICATIONS OF IMAGERY

Cancer patients have used their own visualization and the guided imagery offered by others in a variety of ways and for a variety of purposes. Here are some of the many applications that may help you in your own struggle with cancer.

◆ *To Maintain Hope.* You can imagine yourself completely healthy, and hold this image in your mind several times a day. Let this be the image that inspires and sustains you. In their tapes and their book, the Simontons advise: "Imagine yourself well, free of disease, full of energy. Picture yourself reaching your goals in life. See your purpose in life being fulfilled [and]

… your relationships with people becoming more meaningful. Remember that having strong reasons for getting well will help you get well, so use this time to focus clearly on your priorities in life."

◆ *To Promote an Effective Immune Response.* Without any mental participation on your part, your body's own defense against cancer is working away at destroying it. As we have mentioned, you may be able to assist this process by mentally participating in it, through imagery. Try to find images that feel right for you, whether they are biological pictures in your mind or powerful symbols of the body's defense processes at work.

◆ *To Prepare for and Heal from Surgery.* Surgery for cancer can create intense anxiety because of the vulnerability involved and the uncertainty about the outcome. Before surgery, you might imagine the operation and the active presence of your will or soul in preventing the cancer cells from evading the scalpel. You might imagine yourself at peace in the caring and competent hands of your surgeon. To promote your healing from surgery, you can visualize the opening of blood vessels and the increased flow of blood (and infection-fighting white blood cells) to the surgical site.

◆ *To Participate Mentally in Chemotherapy.* It is not uncommon for patients to dread chemotherapy and to feel that something awful is being done to them. Through imagery, you can embrace the process and participate in it. Try to welcome these medicines into your body and visualize how they expel the cancer and restore you to health. You can use the images suggested by the Simontons or develop your own. Invite your imagination to help you: it is often best to let the images come to you, as a gift from an inner source of wisdom, rather than to force an image that you intellectually think is right.

◆ *To Reduce Side Effects.* The nausea and vomiting caused by chemotherapy are partly due to the anticipation and dread of these side effects. Patients have successfully reduced these effects by visualizing, during chemotherapy, the healthy cells in their gastrointestinal tract being protected from the drugs or bouncing back rapidly from the toxic effects. Positive imagery can be used to reduce the nausea that often comes in anticipation of receiving chemotherapy. The smell of the rubbing alcohol to cleanse the skin before infusion often elicits the nausea; patients who attach a more positive image to this smell have been able to offset this effect.

◆ *To Cope with Pain.* You can use imagery to reduce pain by distracting yourself from it and by altering the meaning behind the pain. Pain often creates anxiety, which can make the pain worse. Try to find an image for your pain that has a blunting effect on it, or an image that soothes and heals the source of the pain.

To quote the Simontons again: "If you are experiencing pain anywhere in your body, picture the army of white blood cells flowing into that area and soothing the pain. Whatever the problem, give your body the command to heal itself. Visualize your body becoming well."

◆ *To Offset Stress and Anxiety.* Like many cancer patients, you may often feel extremely weary and distraught, and feel like you need a respite from all that you are going through and dealing with. In your mind, you can retreat to a place for peace and restoration. Many guided-imagery and relaxation exercises can take you to such a place. You can learn to take a deep breath, close your eyes and imagine yourself in this special scene. Symptoms of anxiety may subside when you do this. Dr. Rossman's book contains a lovely exercise that escorts you to a serene imaginary location of your own creation.

A FIRST-HAND ACCOUNT

Janet Amber Damon, MSW

My cancer diagnosis came totally out of the blue. I was 48 years old, had been working as a psychotherapist for over 15 years, and was about to leave for Paris to study art. Two weeks before leaving, I had my annual gynecological exam. I learned I had cancer, an ovarian sarcoma, Stage 4. It had already metastasized to other organs.

Before this moment I had always been a fighter. I always found a way to cope with the tragedies, stresses and struggles of life. Now—completely unexpectedly— attack came from within my own body. I had no knowledge of cancer or what I was facing. It all felt overwhelming!

I had a hysterectomy and four tumors removed, and then began chemotherapy. The reality was that I was a basket case. I withdrew, I isolated myself, I was immobilized, fragile, I had no energy for anything. I was undone. I had used up my bag of hope; the blackboard was erased and I had run out of chalk.

My journey through cancer then turned toward greater hope and strength. I met a doctor at UCLA, Bernard Towers, doing research on the body-mind connection. I began weekly visits to learn visualization techniques. It was a process that helped me connect with my internal world. My strength began to return despite the massive doses of chemotherapy.

By experiencing the effects of the visualization on my healing and recovery, and later, from reading and hearing about others who had similar experiences, and through teaching patients and seeing the benefits of their use of visualization, I am convinced that it is a valid, effective path for releasing tensions and stresses and for increasing the body's ability to fight disease.

For me, visualization became a means of focusing my mind in order to release the healing forces of my body and to encourage the healthy parts of my body to maintain and protect themselves while chemotherapy worked at killing the cancer. It was also a way to take control. I felt empowered. At the very least, it improved the quality of my life. I also believe that visualization can release enough of the healing forces in the body to effect a cure.

When I first learned of visualization techniques, I was surprised to realize that I had been visualizing all the time. It's something we all do without being aware of it. We think in images, but we usually don't focus and concentrate on these images or change them in order to reach certain goals.

Something that I learned from the research on imagery was the idea that images in the mind are perceived as real events to the body. For example, athletes who practice their toning and muscle-strengthening exercises in their imagination often receive similar benefits to those received by the athletes who physically do the exercises.

In a state of deep relaxation with images coursing through the mind, the body moves into a state of heightened alertness and heightened ability to achieve whatever it is attempting to achieve. There are phrases that describe this phenomenon: athletes refer to it as being "in the zone," and religious people refer to it as ecstasy.

HOW I GOT STARTED

I was introduced to visualization by listening to guided-imagery cassette tapes. I found this to be a simple and effective way of getting started. These tapes are available in bookstores and some health food stores and through catalogs.

I also used guided-imagery scripts from books such as those suggested by the Simontons and Martin Rossman. I later developed my own visualization script, which I offer for your consideration. I created my own tape of this script to help me through the process.

I also took advantage of biofeedback in order to reduce stress and obtain inner calmness. I found that biofeedback can be easily learned from written or spoken instructions. The process employs an electronic device to measure your body's reaction to stress. There are small, inexpensive models available. A light or a tone emanates from these devices, and the intensity of the signal reflects many of the body's reactions to stress, such as brain wave activity and skin temperature. I found it invaluable to learn from the device I used when a state of total relaxation was attained, how to create that state mentally and what factors would raise or lower the relaxation response in my body.

I also sought professional help from a therapist who helped people learn visualization techniques. For a referral to someone in your community who specializes in this work, call your local American Cancer Society office. I found it essential to work with a therapist who helped me develop the type of imagery that was right for me, that fit my temperament and interests.

You might want to keep this in mind in creating your own imagery. Think of your hobbies and of activities that interest you and that you know something about, and try to develop a visualization exercise that builds on these. For example, if you are a gardener, you might want to visualize weeds growing, the bugs and poisons that destroy them, and the fertilizers and sunlight that enrich healthy plant life.

A SAMPLE VISUALIZATION

This is a visualization exercise that I developed and found to be a powerful tool in dealing with my cancer. I recorded it onto a tape and listened to it every day. You could also have someone quietly read the steps to you. It is good to follow the steps carefully the first couple of times.

Before you start, think of something that you consider a healing liquid. This could be a particular medicine, a tonic your parent used to fix you when you were sick, the honey from flowers, a magician's potion, a particular hue of spray paint that stops rust or whatever has a certain poignancy for you.

1. Find a comfortable, quiet, darkened place to sit or lie down in, and relax completely. If this is difficult, get earplugs and a dark material to put over your eyes. Do whatever is necessary to get about 20 minutes of uninterrupted time. Turn the phone's ringer off, and put a sign on the front door. Ask your family to help with this.
2. Breathe gently and slowly five times, drawing your breath down into your lungs and stomach, feeling your ribs moving and expanding with each breath.
3. Keep breathing gently and regularly. Focus all your attention and imagine that you are bringing that warm breath into any place of tightness or tension in your body.
4. Release the tension with each exhalation as though the warm air was gradually being released from a balloon. Let it drain away.
5. Imagine (or see in your mind's eye) the healing liquid in a container. This is your healing force.
6. Imagine the container is at the location where cancer cells exist.
7. Pour or spray the liquid over the cancer so it covers or coats it.
8. Picture the cells beginning to melt

away as the healing force coats and covers them.

9. Then allow that coating to remain in place as you slowly open your eyes and become aware once again of the room around you.

10. During the coming hours, take a moment to close your eyes and imagine the coating on the cells as you left it. The cells are being smothered and are dying.

11. Repeat the visualization at least three times a day. Return to the site of the cancer, using the same method, and add more of the healing force to the now dissipating and dissolving cancer cells.

12. Do this visualization at bedtime, but when you are done do not open your eyes. Let yourself drift off into sleep with the image of the dying cancer cells in your mind.

I believe not only that visualization helped me to recover from my cancer but that it also provided a direct means of encouraging the healthy parts of my body to maintain and protect themselves while drugs and radiation did their job.

Our medical doctors work at destroying the cancer, and each day they are discovering better techniques and drugs to carry out their work. We have tools to help them. Visualization gave me a way of participating in what my doctors were doing, a way of using the power of imagery to fight cancer. Although I placed myself in the hands of the medical team, I also found a way of doing my part to see to it that the best results were achieved.

Our body wants to be well. There is great wisdom in the way the systems of the body work each day for our benefit. Our job is to encourage and help those systems to become strong. If we take charge of our body, if we become part of the team of medical people who are working to return us to health, then I believe our chances for survival are heightened. In my case, there is no doubt in my mind that the combination of the medical care I received and the visualization skills I learned (and have continued to practice for 10 years) are the two major reasons for my regaining and maintaining my health.

15
CREATIVE EXPRESSION TO IMPROVE YOUR QUALITY OF LIFE

Ernest H. Rosenbaum, MD, and Isadora R. Rosenbaum, MA

A merry heart doeth good like a medicine.

—Proverbs 17:22

———◇———

Courage, hope, faith, sympathy and love promote health and prolong life. A contented mind, a cheerful spirit is health to the body and strength to the soul. How you live has a major effect on your health and your life. Not only your attitude but also your activities can promote better health. Enhancing and enriching your quality of life heightens your emotional experiences and reduces depression. Your attitude depends in part on what you expect from life and how good you think your life has been. Health depends on the interaction between mind and body, joys and sadnesses, as well as the sense of security and being loved and appreciated.

To achieve a better quality of life, you need to involve yourself in a positive living program for the promotion of a healthy mind. The quality of life can be enhanced by the spiritual uplift and relaxation provided by interests and hobbies such as art, music, writing and humor. These can enrich your life through positive experiences. We achieve a special satisfaction through things that we create ourselves. This improves feelings of self worth, decreases depression and promotes a sense of well-being.

THE ROLE OF THE MIND IN HEALTH
Good health is one of the greatest assets we have in life, for without it your future

is uncertain. The mind plays a key role in promoting good health. If your health is impaired, through an accident or illness, life may become compromised by subsequent debilitation. Some of the new problems you may face are economic, social, emotional or psychological.

Recently there has been a shift in the philosophy of health care to a more "holistic" way of medical care as suggested by Plato a few thousand years ago. We can't separate the mental from the physical, since they are related as part of the whole body. Being a health care provider is like being a juggler trying to balance many balls—the medical, physical, environmental, psychological and nutritional in an attempt to keep the heart, brain and body healthy. Many authorities feel that 50 to 80 percent of illnesses are stress related, including high blood pressure, colds, depression and certain skin diseases.

Research at the University of Utah evaluated the role of stress during a recent economic depression. There were more fatal strokes and heart attacks than were predicted. Continuing studies are looking at how stress relates to a decrease in the function of the immune system. If a direct link is found, an immune defect could precede many diseases. There is a relationship between anger, stress and disease. One of the secrets of good health and longevity is knowing how to control stress. (*See* Chapters 8 and 9 on stress.)

How one accepts and deals with adversity, or controls stress and anger, determines one's coping skills. Norman Cousins found a means to cope with his incapacitating arthritis and used his inner strength to not only fight his way back to good health but also to increase his longevity through humor.

Attitude Attitude has a major influence on your life and has become one of the important ingredients in living well and longer. It is in part shaped by our experiences and education, failures and successes. A positive attitude can help increase our ability to cope with life's problems or with a disease. We have a chance each day when we get up to make this a great day and achieve what we wish, or to merely accept events that occur and not try to improve your lot or set new goals. Some things in life are more difficult to change than others. Thus, how we live is in part controlled by our attitude toward life.

The Will to Live The will to live is nurtured by a positive attitude. A negative attitude can diminish or undermine the mind by fear, anger or loss of self-esteem. These emotions, when unresolved, can lead to hopelessness, futility, resignation and the loss of the will to live. (*See also* Chapter 7.) Here are a few examples:
◆ The phrase "frightened to death" is more than a figure of speech. An early reference to stress and fear is recorded in the Bible, in Acts 5, when Ananias and his wife, Sapphira, suddenly die after being castigated by Peter for withholding from the disciples some of the money paid for the sale of land. This has been attributed to a sudden coronary death from stress.
◆ In primitive societies people have been literally frightened to death by the imposition of a curse or spell, known as bone pointing. Such deaths have not been explained medically, even with an autopsy, but it seems apparent that the paralyzing effect of fear, aided by ignorance and superstition, played an important role. The victim has been encouraged to believe in the power of the curse. Thus, ignorance and superstition play a role in how the mind functions to help or hinder a person in living.

People with a positive attitude are able to be open, to talk about their problems with their family, friends and physicians. They feel good about themselves and generally have been that way all their lives. It is often very hard to change lifelong patterns such as your psychological reaction to daily living.

The will to live is therefore a spiritual, emotional and ethical commodity. It needs nurturing and development and, if controlled, can strengthen a person's resolve to survive. We soon discover that the mind plays an important role in trying to control life, that there is a direct correlation between a person's mental and emotional states.

We measure successes and failures in life by our standards and ideals as we strive for goals in work, relationships and health. Just to survive makes for a shallow life. Victory is for those who have the courage and stamina to fight and endure each of life's many struggles and who always have goals and the satisfaction of aspiring to reach them whether they succeed or fail. This is the "challenge of life."

The answer lies in your attitude toward life. We can help ourselves and others live better if we:
◆ Live in the present and in the future, not in the past.
◆ Set reasonable goals as to what can be accomplished.
◆ Accept new problems and attempt to solve them through understanding and increased awareness.
◆ Try to resolve depression and negative emotions.
◆ Actively do things to help ourself and others.
◆ Learn techniques to relax and practice mind control by using simple methods to calm down, such as yoga or tai chi, or practice biofeedback or visualization.

THE ROLE OF CREATING ART IN HEALTH

Cynthia D. Perlis, BS, Ernest H. Rosenbaum, MD, and Isadora R. Rosenbaum, MA

A hundred years ago, it was commonly believed that people could not be creative past middle age. Now, reports Lydia Bronte in *The Longevity Factor*, most Americans can expect a "second middle age"—a stage of adulthood between 50 and 75 that has not existed before. Today, people in middle age and beyond sometimes feel that life is just beginning. A new sense of identity is discovered and defined along with an enhanced sense of self. During these years, art can be a healing force.

Artistic expression is an important psychosocial activity. We can create art by ourselves, alone in a studio, or we can attend classes ranging from beginning drawing to advanced printmaking. Sometimes we can express ourselves visually when we are unable to express ourselves verbally. Art can help us express what we are feeling in the present, yet it can also help us to express a memory, a moment that has happened that we do not want to forget. Music, drawing, painting and creating sculpture provide a means of communication and self-expression—and a way to alleviate stress.

Art also helps us to change our moods, come out of depression or simply relax.

Art can be richly therapeutic for people, including the elderly, with a serious illness such as cancer. Suzanne, a woman approaching 80 who is living a full and energetic life in spite of her advanced cancer, has continued to teach art classes, take printmaking classes and work in her home studio. Her recent works have included drawings and watercolors that express what it feels like to cope with life-threatening illness. She has created drawings that tell the story of her disease. One watercolor, *The Cell of Positive Thinking*, was created when she began a course of chemotherapy.

Creating art, says Suzanne, improves her self-worth and leaves a permanent gift to be enjoyed by all. She has received constant encouragement and support from her friends and family. They drive her to art classes and create along with her. Together they are participating in a shared experience, a shared community of meaning; the essence of what it means to be human.

You do not have to have artistic ability to be creative. Sometimes just doodling or experimenting with art materials can open up a wide range of ideas. People often become too critical of their work—or are afraid others will judge their ability. It is important to express yourself for yourself and not for everyone else's approval. There really is no right or wrong in expressing who you are. For instance, if you feel you cannot draw, try making collages of pictures cut from magazines.

Creating art at any age gives people an opportunity to express what they are feeling. Creating art provides the ability to make decisions for oneself. With the opportunity to make decisions, to exercise control over choice, people enhance their quality of life, improve self-esteem and create ways to relate to others in a meaningful way.

A whole life or one experience can be shared in a work of art. One artist writes, "No, I will never say my work is finished. I must live forever—on and on. The reason we artists enjoy such longevity is that we are always looking ahead to the 'masterpiece' to come."

Here are some recommended creative art activities:

◆ Draw a self-portrait. Include words to describe who you are.

◆ Create a family tree—ask everyone to draw their own portrait on the tree.

◆ Take painting, drawing or sculpture classes at your local community college. If you feel you're not good enough, take a beginners' class—everyone will be in the same boat.

◆ Draw your dreams.

◆ Make a collage with pictures cut out of magazines. Decide on a theme before you start or let the theme evolve.

◆ Do a drawing with a friend, child, grandchild or spouse.

◆ Take photographs.

◆ Learn needlepoint or knitting.

◆ Buy fabric paint and paint on T-shirts.

◆ Don't be judgmental—there is no right or wrong, no rules, no grades.

◆ Smile as you create.

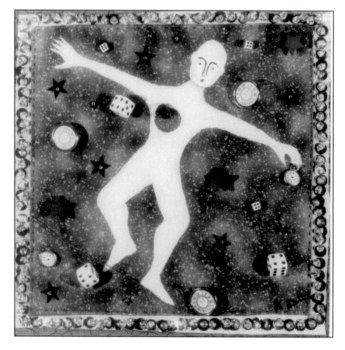

Art for Recovery Breast Cancer Quilts Project

BREAST CANCER QUILTS

Cynthia D. Perlis, BS, Ernest H. Rosenbaum, MD, and Isadora R. Rosenbaum, MA

Inspired by the AIDS quilt, in the summer of 1996, Dr. Rosenbaum suggested to the Susan G. Komen Foundation a project designed to give women with breast cancer a creative voice. The tradition of quilt-making has been nurturing and creative for countless women throughout history and, as it had for people with AIDS, could serve to bring the terrible epidemic of breast cancer before the public in a moving and beautiful way.

Cynthia Perlis, who directed the project, remembered the touching stories and drawings that women with breast cancer had shared with her. It was time to give these women a voice in the larger community, to let them speak through their creative spirits and to share their pain, their hopes and their dreams. Women recovering from and coping with breast cancer would be able to express visually their feelings about this illness.

Soon, fabric squares began to arrive at the UCSF/Mount Zion Art for Recovery office and, collectively, these squares began to represent the entire scope of this devastating illness. One square read: "I WON THE LOTTERY NO ONE CARED TO ENTER." On another piece of fabric, written in ballpoint pen, was the entire story of one woman's breast cancer experience. Another woman embroidered "THE GIFT OF A LIFETIME" and dedicated the square to her doctor. The quilt-maker then sewed the fabric squares into a beautiful quilt.

One year later, there were five quilts, each measuring eight feet by eight feet, and each including images by 25 women with breast cancer or in memory of a loved one. More quilts are in progress.

The quilts have been on display across the country. One of the most poignant parts of this project are the stories that women have written about their own squares that tell the painful reality of breast cancer. Here is one example:

I wanted to make this square as a thank you to my three daughters who have been so loving and supportive these past ten months. The design idea came from a beautiful Christmas tree ornament given to me by my second daughter. I was extremely touched by this gift and displayed it prominently on our tree.

I didn't really understand why it made such an impact on me and I'm not sure I know the answer yet. However, I suspect one of the reasons was that it was possible to have something beautiful represent a difficult and challenging time in my life. It also served as a daily reminder to be ever-vigilant and to never forget. I wear a pink ribbon of some kind every day now to continue to remind myself, my thirtyish daughters and the world that the ENEMY is still out there ready to strike 180,000 more women this year alone.

—Elisa Bambi Schwartz

The Breast Cancer Quilts Project continues to invite women from around the country to create images for the quilts. In May, 1998, the eleven quilts were exhibited at the National Institutes of Health as part of the National Cancer Institute's Breast Cancer Think Tank to support other women battling cancer and increase public awareness of the disease. As a result of this prestigious exhibition, calls have been coming to Art for Recovery from all over the United States wanting information about participating in this significant project.

THE ROLE OF POETRY AND PROSE IN HEALTH

Ernest H. Rosenbaum, MD, *and Isadora R. Rosenbaum,* MA

The Veil of Illusion

The night time is brutal,
  there is no "snuggling in."
All of the aches and pains and horrors
  come to haunt me.
In the deep dark stillness of the night
I am left with myself,
A loneliness I can't describe
Nothing seems real.
Even the light of a beautiful day
  can't diminish the darkness.
The hustle, bustle of Saturday morn-
  ing sounds
Can't break the silence, the stillness.
But once in a while
  in a blissful moment of distraction
I can almost remember the other side
  when I still wore the veil.
                —*Elisa Bambi Schwartz*

Since the development of written language, humans have tried to capture their
lives and history through writing. The
ancients used pictures and signs to record
their lives and thoughts. Over the centuries this has evolved into written history as well as literature. Like art and music,
literature, whether prose or poetry, is
another way to support and enhance
patient care and well-being. Like art and
music, literature can be "the best medicine" and, through the benefits of self-
expression, can have healing powers.

Reading or writing poetry or prose can
reduce boredom and help relieve depression. It can divert your mind from your
medical situation, providing creative stimulation and helping you to communicate
your feelings with your family, friends
and medical team. Enjoying the use of
your creative spirit and intelligence can

provide a vital force to improve your state
of wellness, daily living and quality of life.

You may feel unsure about your ability to create literature, but do not be too
critical of your early efforts, since it takes
time to learn techniques and to discover
your unique "voice." Your talent will
develop if you give yourself a chance.
Many people find that taking a creative
writing class or joining a poetry or fiction
writers group provides guidance and
reduces their initial frustrations.

When people are seriously ill or
depressed, they often feel hopeless. Such
feelings can be heightened by receiving
bad news about their disease or treatment.
Even during the recovery process, people
may feel sadness and a heaviness of heart.
Reading great literature, whether prose
or poetry, as well as attempting to express
your own feelings of sorrow and loss
through writing can raise your spirits,
provide relaxation and give creative satisfaction. Working with others in a class or
group can also help to prevent isolation.

A patient who is a poet described the
deep effect that reading Pushkin,
Lermontov and Pasternak has on her
heart and spirit. She also said, "Sometimes
when I have had a sad or hard day, I create poetry myself. Poetry makes my heart
'burn bright' through its magical strength.
It also pleases me with an unusual inner
feeling when people read my poetry,
which for me is a 'lyric confession.' They
appreciate my lyric confession when they
understand my point of view and this creates an impulse to create more and more
poetry."

This poet is also a journalist and writes
articles and reviews on art, dance and
music. She says, "I have also enjoyed the

recognition I have received. It has led to important moments in my life during the past two and a half years, such as when a small four-page newspaper *Odessky Listok* told stories [I had written] of people from other cities and countries. Readers appreciated the stories about people's adventures and life which is not only a personal declaration of their importance on earth but for mankind as well."

> "I want to live—to think and suffer"
> The poet said, and I agree.
> I want to live to sing in poems
> The taste of life, its smell, its joy, its
>   dreams.
> I want to share my deepest feelings
> How free and happy—I am blessed to
>   live
> In Golden State—unique and gorgeous
> In the mysterious Bay waves.
> I want to suffer, but not from pain
> Not from the evil—my inevitable fate
> I want to cry from love, to love again,
> Be loved, forget my age, be able to create.
> —*Tamara Belorusets,* translation by
>   *Yelena Nechay*

Alexander Morrison, also a poet, said, "I also have written poetry for many years. I find it interesting to observe how, in different ways, I expressed the same philosophy at 18 as I do now. I was amazed then as I am now at how the human being, screwed by circumstances beyond all belief, can manage to stand up despite the unmitigating bullshit that presses down on him. I'm talking about mankind and people like myself—the survivors and the contributors, the people I think have become successful human beings."

> Trace the affinity
> Of the will to be
> with the ability
> To Be no longer.
> Ah … such a narrow way divides.
> And yet, in the precarious clime

> Of this most eccentric inch
> A world of men lived
> Triumphant!
> —*Alexander Morrison*

"I'm looking for the same answers I looked for at 18. I haven't changed, but I do know that even with the odds tremendously against you, most of us manage somehow to make it."

> The vulgar splendor of a noise
> Contents the appetite of ears
> Insensitive to subtleties
> The really loud occurrence falls
> without the benefit of sound
> How silently are these:
> The awakening to love,
> The audacity to dream,
> The will to live.
> —*Alexander Morrison*

The Recovery

> No longer can I bear
> To dwell in this misbegotten state
> Of involuntary confinement
> The sorrow is too deep
> The truth of it too great
> For human comprehension
> And so, with anxious hands I break
>   away
> The larval crust and shake myself free!
> Outside carillon bells
> Sing of my resurrection and celebrate
> My reawakening with soft murmurs
> Bird songs and forgotten lullabies
> They call to me, beckon me
> Into the blazing light of day
> And direct me toward the path
> Of undisturbed freedom!
> With grateful tears
> I squint into the blinding sun
> And with an innocence of childhood
>   born
> I join the living once again
> All is forgotten
> —*Diane Behar*

ART FOR RECOVERY/BRANDEIS PEN PAL PROJECT

Cynthia D. Perlis, BS

In 1992, I developed the Art for Recovery/Brandeis Pen Pal Project for patients to enjoy the art of writing letters to pen pals. The idea developed from my hospital visits at the bedsides of patients for the Art for Recovery program, where I noted that although these people in many cases were quite frail, weak and in pain, their spirits were very much alive. I felt that they had much to offer in the way of personal experiences, insight and wisdom. Seriously ill patients could become, in effect, teachers. I matched 12 patients, half with cancer and half with AIDS, with 24 grade seven and eight students (aged 12, 13 and 14). The teens would write letters to the patients, including drawings if they chose. They could ask absolutely any question, such as, "Are you afraid to die?" "How did you ever tell your parents that you had cancer?" One 12-year-old girl wrote to a 32-year-old woman with leukemia, "I could never tell that to my parents." In their letters back, the patients would write about their jobs, their families, their illnesses. They would answer the teens' questions about their conditions and difficulties.

Originally the letters went back and forth for nine months, but the program was later extended to five years. Over 60 students and as many patients have built bridges and have created their own community. At the end of each school year, there is a healing service, where the students and the patients meet face-to-face for the first time. The students read aloud blessings that they have written and the patients bring the students symbols of healing. This experience defines the true meaning of the word *mitzvah* (a Jewish word for a good deed).

The following letters are excerpted from the correspondence.

Dear Katherine,
How did you know you had cancer? My sister has a muscular disease, so I know about muscular problems, but I don't really know anyone with a serious disease. Was it really scary when you found out you were ill? How long have you had cancer?
    I'm really looking forward to writing to you.
        Love,

Lily
P.S. Please send a picture

Dear Lily,
It was really nice to get your letter.
    I have breast cancer and I found a lump in my breast that felt big and hard. I could also feel swollen lymph nodes under my arm. It was very scary when I first found out.
    I had to go through a lot of treatment and make decisions about the treatment that was hard. I seem to be doing well so far and hope it continues this way.
    Because I am a physician I see a lot of children with serious diseases and also a lot of children who are healthy. I'm sorry to hear that your sister has a muscular disease. How has it been for you to deal with this and help her?
    Thank you for your very nice picture — Write soon.

Katherine

Dear Emily:

I got some bad news recently. My leukemia is back. The doctors are very surprised, it is unusual for someone who has done well for two years to get their cancer back now. I always knew there would be a chance for it to come back, but I was hoping it would be longer (or not at all).

I had thought there was nothing more the doctors could do. But they want to try a procedure on me where they get some cells from the man who donated some of his bone marrow to me before. These cells are white blood cells and they fight off infections. The doctors hope by giving me these cells, it will help boost my immune system to fight off and maybe destroy the leukemia.

It is a hard decision for me to make. It might be hard to understand why I might just decide to just let the leukemia kill me. The procedure will make me pretty sick again. And the doctors are not too sure it will work anyway. I was not very happy last time I was in the hospital and I am not looking forward to being sick again. But my friends and family seem to really want me to try this procedure because it is my only chance to live.

It is hard to realize that I have to make these kinds of decisions. I am just a regular, normal person. These kinds of things happen in the movies or TV.

Whatever happens, I would like to keep writing you. We can write about all sorts of things still. And you can ask me questions about what is happening to me if you want. The leukemia is part of my life, but not all of it.

My knees are better, I almost walk normal. But I am still pretty weak. Only my left leg can go up the stairs. It is like someone is holding me back if I try with my right leg.

Carol

Dear Carol,

I am very sad right now because you have got leukemia again. I had no idea this could happen again and I am very sorry. But I have a lot of hope that you will get better and I know you will too.

When did the leukemia come back? Is it as bad as it was before? How does your family feel about this? Are you afraid? How do you feel about coming back to the hospital after you've been out of it for so long? I have so many questions about this.

I heard from Cindy that you feel okay right now and I'm really glad about that. I hope that the new procedure the doctors are going to try will work.

It really is going to be a hard decision for you to make, but I think that if I were in this same situation, I would just try whatever the doctors think might work. I don't know why, but I hope whatever they do works and I hope you'll feel better soon.

I would like to keep writing to you too. Thanks for saying I can ask questions about what is happening. … I'm glad your knees are better.

Bye,

Emily

THE ROLE OF HUMOR IN HEALTH

Ernest H. Rosenbaum, MD, Malin Dollinger, MD, and Stu Silverstein, MD

Humor and laughter have been found to have a positive effect on the body's physiology as well as inducing relaxation. They help people cope and produce improved relations among family members and friends. A light-hearted attitude can reduce the chance of illness, reduce depression and thereby promote longevity.

Humor reduces stress almost immediately. It also helps alleviate pain. Laughter has even been used as an aide in treating disease. As Norman Cousins stated, "I made the joyous discovery that 10 minutes of genuine belly laughter had an anesthetic effect and would give me at least two hours of pain-free sleep." He discovered that watching funny movies with the Marx Brothers or the Three Stooges was therapeutic. Cousins wrote in *Anatomy of an Illness* that he deliberately tried to increase his laughter to help improve his health.

There is an old joke that a man was wondering what the meaning of life was, and he became morbidly depressed over this question. He even tried to shoot himself in the head, but missed. Finally, in desperation, he wandered randomly into a movie theater, where a Marx Brothers movie was showing. There he realized that as long as there is laughter there is meaning to life.

Thus humor can do wonders to help lift the spirits. Some studies have shown that if you just smile, the body's response is a positive one. Try it and see what happens.

THE PHYSIOLOGY OF HUMOR AND LAUGHTER

Humor usually results in laughter, which arouses the emotions, resulting in physical changes. These include short-term increases in blood pressure, heart and respiratory rate and reduction of stress.

Laughter stimulates the brain to produce endorphins (morphinelike relaxants that have a euphoric—uplifting—or analgesic—pain-relieving—effect). The result is muscle relaxation with a resolution of stress and anxiety, an improvement in mental and spiritual well-being and, often, a decrease in hostility and anger. Laughter also confers several long-lasting benefits on your body; in the long run it lowers blood pressure, and it also serves as a mini aerobic workout without the expense of joining a health club.

Scientific studies are looking at exactly how laughter, mirth and a humorous perspective can have a positive effect on health and improve quality of life.

Laughter from jokes, speeches, comedies, plays, movies, operas or other humorous events is a socially accepted way of getting a message across. It is sometimes a means of getting through personal tragedy or crisis (for those creating the humor as well as those responding to it). Some people find that telling jokes about themselves removes some of the heaviness they may feel about their lives.

Humor can be spontaneous or specifically created, but no matter how it evolves, it can make a difference to your life. It is a healing power for both body and soul as well as a help in sustaining oneself through some of the depressing episodes of life.

There are many benefits of humor. Here are some of them.

1. Humor can help us expand our per-

spective on life and enhance creativity.

2. The more we laugh, the better our chance of decreasing depression and promoting the healing process. Promoting the laughter factor injects more happiness into daily life.

3. Humor can improve family relations and smooth communications.

4. Humor provides physical and mental energy and rejuvenation through emotional relaxation.

5. Humor helps people cooperate and communicate, as well as decreasing anger and fear.

6. Humor can promote a will to live, promote energy, improve self-esteem and increase self-worth.

7. Humor is considered by many one of the great medicines of all time.

8. Humor can reduce anxiety and thereby improve the enjoyment of social experiences such as dining.

There is an old Dutch saying that humor often comes from telling a tragic story after enough time has passed. In this way you can laugh at many hard times in your life. It wasn't funny at the time, but after you triumph over the tribulations of life the stories can later be uproariously funny.

HOW TO MAKE HUMOR WORK FOR YOU

1. Collect or write down humorous anecdotes, mementos, cartoons and jokes. Refer to them often to improve your emotional energy and revive sag-ging spirits.

2. Create humorous cards and cartoons to make you laugh every day. Often telling personal or family stories about life is a way of sharing humor and funny events.

3. Take a class on writing or telling jokes.

4. Keep humorous books, articles or cartoons nearby. Refer to them frequently to make yourself smile and laugh.

5. Try to avoid frequent contact with depressing people who drain your emotional energy. Associate with positive people who use humor.

6. Promote parties and fun social events, such as birthdays. You need to make them happen.

7. Arrange a get-together with friends or relatives to tell jokes, recall happy and funny events or share a funny video or movie.

8. Regularly visit a local comedy club.

9. Maintain a compendium of humor and philosophy to help you reduce isolation, anger, despair or loneliness.

By using vignettes, jokes or philosophical or practical sayings or words, you can improve your coping skills and reduce despair. A bit of humor, when appropriate, can make a sad event a little lighter and more positive. For grave or serious situations, a little humor can decrease your level of unhappiness. Apply the techniques of Norman Cousins.

Don't leave it to chance. Actively seek humor in your life. Those who laugh last laugh best!

THE ROLE OF MUSIC IN HEALTH

Isadora R. Rosenbaum, MA, *Ernest H. Rosenbaum,* MD, *Jim Murdock, and*
Malin Dollinger, MD

Music has healing powers. It has been said that "music soothes the savage beast." It is said that Plato believed that health in body and mind is obtained through music. Florence Nightingale used the healing powers of music as part of nursing the ill. Music affects the physiologic and psychological aspects of an illness or disability. In the Bible, David the shepherd boy played his harp to help the psychologically anxious, insomniac King Saul relax and sleep. And music was used to calm shell-shocked soldiers in World War II.

Music has a personal meaning to each of us, often recalling or eliciting a positive emotional response. It has a universal appeal, it is inexpensive and it crosses cultural barriers. It is available by radio, TV, tape player, CD player, vinyl records and live. It can be listened to quietly, through earphones or out aloud for all to enjoy.

There is always a place for music in our daily life. It gives a special pleasure and enjoyment and improves our mood. It affords us a way of expressing ourselves in a nonverbal way that can give us joy, calm us down or lead to great excitement. It can provide us an escape or reach down into our deeper soul and elicit emotions that are pent up. For some people and their relatives and friends, music offers a special way to pass time that may sometimes seem endless.

It can provide a way to decrease stress, promote emotional recovery and provide relaxation. It can also afford a means of communication without the need to use a common spoken language.

PHYSIOLOGIC AND PSYCHOLOGICAL EFFECTS

Music can increase or decrease heart rate and blood pressure, depending on the tempo and type of music. It can relax and reduce anxiety or stimulate and heighten awareness. The intense emotions evoked by music can affect the nervous system and induce production of endorphins. Music can help relax muscles to decrease nervous tension. It can also reduce alienation and feelings of isolation, and improve self-control and confidence.

Both age and illness and its therapies can affect a person's psychological equilibrium, causing depression as well as negatively affecting spiritual and emotional feelings and social interactions.

Music offers a bridge in helping to support a person through many of the crises in life. It reduces stress and thus reduces stress-related illnesses.

EMOTIONAL ENHANCEMENT

There is a type of music to fit any emotion or mood. John Philip Sousa playing "The Stars and Stripes Forever" brings cheers and elicits patriotism. The Verdi *Requiem* or Rossini's *William Tell* may elevate the mood and give waves of relaxation to reduce stress or help alleviate grief. Listening to Mendelssohn's *A Midsummer Night's Dream*, or a Count Basie or a Turk Murphy jazz program, can provide an emotional lift. Listening to the soft sentimental music of Nat King Cole, Glenn Miller or Tommy Dorsey is relaxing; it can also provide fun and exercise if you get up and dance.

Music offers immediate gratification. You can sit and tap your feet to the rhythm, play simple instruments or stand up and march. You can hum a tune to yourself or sing it out, but you can also sing songs, clap your hands or even sing in the shower. Pretend for a moment that no one else is around. Think of your favorite song, the one that brings back pleasant memories—especially of someone close to you. How do you feel now? Do you understand how powerful music can be in helping us gain emotional peace and happiness? Music is a form of communication that can be enjoyed with others. It requires no active participation, unless you wish it to.

A music program
◆ reduces boredom and disillusionment
◆ creates and enhances a happy mood
◆ recalls pleasant experiences, bringing pleasure
◆ offers immediate gratification

◆ creates distraction from problems of daily living
◆ may improve bonding among family and friends
◆ leads to an opening up of communication as people reminisce after enjoying music together.

In the hospital or treatment setting, music
◆ helps improve coordination, when music is used with physical therapy rehabilitation
◆ gives psychological, social, physical rehabilitation and emotional and supportive benefits
◆ enhances the effectiveness of speech training in persons who have had brain damage
◆ helps reduce anxiety commonly seen during medical therapy, thereby making therapy more acceptable.

Music is truly a vital part of our lives—when we are well and especially when we are ill.

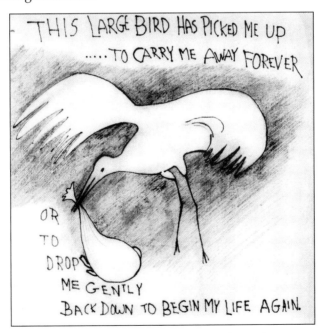

Art for Recovery Breast Cancer Quilts Project

PART III:
THE BODY

16
NUTRITION FOR THE CANCER PATIENT

Ernest H. Rosenbaum, MD, Isadora R. Rosenbaum, MA, and Julie Matel, MS, RD

———————◇———————

Good nutrition is needed for general good health and is particularly crucial when you are ill. During this time, it is important to give your body the protein, fat, carbohydrate, vitamins and minerals it needs for energy, repair of normal tissue, and to keep your immune system strong to fight disease. Food is not only something to delight the taste buds—it is an essential ingredient in the fight against disease. It is as important as your medicine or medical therapy. Because of your illness or treatments you may not be able to eat in the same way and might find that your pleasurable experiences around eating are affected.

When you are ill, you will be more attuned to the smell, taste and texture of foods. As your senses will be acute, it is important to savor and enjoy foods now more than ever. However, you may find that your tastes have changed and you are turned off by foods that you once enjoyed. This is called food aversion. Allow your memory of the enjoyment to encourage you to eat these foods as well as to develop a taste for new foods.

Think of yourself as an explorer. Sample small portions of foods you used to eat, try new tastes and note the reaction your body and spirit have to them. Even an explorer needs a map to chart unknown territory. With the help of a registered dietitian you can learn to explore alternative tastes and foods.

In the following chapters, we
◆ discuss the basics of good nutrition—what foods you need to eat, and how much you need to eat;

◆ describe the various side effects of therapy that may interfere with adequate nutrition;
◆ recommend ways for you to deal with these problems through diet and medication, and
◆ provide a variety of special diets that will make it easier for you to eat if you are unable to eat a regular diet.

You will not be asked to follow difficult and unpleasant diets. Rather, it is our intent that you can use the information here, within the guidelines given you by your health care experts, to plan a nutritious diet around your own food preferences. In Chapter 20 you will find a large selection of recipes.

Always consult your health care team experts if you are having problems or plan to change your diet.

The dietary principles discussed in this chapter apply to most cancer patients, but if you have special dietary needs because of other problems, such as diabetes, heart disease, liver disease, kidney disease, etc., it is especially important for you to consult your medical team before changing your diet in any way.

The goal of these chapters is to provide current information that will help you maintain or improve your nutritional status and help you better fight your illness.

How to Use Chapters 16 to 20
◆ Learn the basics of good nutrition from Chapter 16.
◆ In the section "What Foods Should You Eat?" (*see* page 159) you will learn why you must be particularly concerned about getting adequate protein and calories, in contrast to the American public in general, which gets more than enough of both.

◆ Determine the amounts of the various nutrients and calories you need for good health from page 161, "How Much Should You Eat?"

◆ Plan your daily menus to include the proper balance of foods from the food guide pyramid, paying particular attention to the proper amounts of protein and calories (*see* page 162).

◆ Keep a daily record of what you eat. Enter the amounts in the Food and Weight Summary chart (*see* page 163).

◆ If you are losing weight, refer to "Helpful Hints for Better Nutrition" (page 164) for suggestions on how to increase your protein and calorie intake. Add appropriate supplements to your menu as described in "Nutritional Supplements" (page 213). Experiment with the recipes given in Chapter 20.

◆ If you are not feeling well enough to eat your regular diet, *see* Chapter 19, "Modified Diets," for diets starting with simple foods that are easy to tolerate and gradually progressing back to normal foods.

◆ If you are experiencing a specific problem, such as nausea, diarrhea, a sore mouth or lack of appetite, *see* Chapter 17, "Nutrition Problems: Causes and Solutions," for helpful recommendations. Suggested diets are described in Chapter 19. These diets list foods you will find easy to tolerate and foods you should avoid. Sample menus are given to help you plan your own diet.

◆ If you are not feeling well enough to do much cooking, "Cooking with Convenience Foods" in Chapter 20 will give you suggestions on cooking with canned, packaged and frozen foods, with emphasis on your need for adequate protein and calories.

NUTRITIONAL NEEDS OF CANCER PATIENTS

To help your body function at its best, it is vital to choose a variety of nutritious foods each day. Good nutrition is even more important for people with cancer for the following reasons.

◆ Well-nourished patients are better able to cope with the side effects of treatment and may even be able to handle higher doses of certain treatments.

◆ A well-balanced diet can prevent breakdown of body tissue and help rebuild tissues that cancer treatment may harm.

◆ A healthy diet can maintain the body's immune system, which will help prevent and treat infections.

The following nutrients are essential when you are starting cancer treatment.

Calories A calorie is a unit of energy derived from food that is required to keep our bodies functioning. The body has the ability to store excess calories as fat, and when needed, convert this fat to energy. During illness, the body may require more calories for healing after surgery, radiation treatment or chemotherapy and for recovering from the side effects of treatment.

It is important to maximize calorie intake by selecting calorie-dense foods. You may find that you are uncomfortable with eating more fat, since diets to prevent cancer often emphasize lower amounts of fat. However, during this period, foods higher in fat make it a lot easier to provide the calories you need when you are dealing with problems such as nausea, loss of appetite and unwanted weight loss.

Proteins Protein is made up of individual units called amino acids. The body uses amino acids to build and repair tissues, to manufacture antibodies to fight infection and to assist in many other body functions. Your body requires more protein for healing if you have lost weight, had surgery or been through radiation or chemotherapy. Keep in mind that in order for the body to use protein efficiently, adequate calories must first be supplied in the diet.

Good sources of protein include meat, fish, poultry, eggs, milk and milk products, soy and soy products, beans, nuts and dried peas. Nutritional supplements such as Ensure Plus, Sustacal and Carnation Instant Breakfast or homemade shakes can supply extra protein when you are unable to eat enough high-protein foods. According to the food guide pyramid, the suggested number of servings from the food groups high in protein are two servings of lean meat, fish, chicken and meat substitutes (6 to 8 ounces each) and two or three servings of milk or milk products. However, your protein needs may be increased at this time. Consult with a registered dietitian about recommendations for your age, sex, weight and medical condition.

A good example of a low-cost high-calorie/high-protein nutritional supplement is Carnation Instant Breakfast, fortified milk, High-Protein Smoothies, or milkshakes (*see* Chapter 20). For high-calorie/high-protein snack ideas, *see* page 165.

Fat Requirements A high-fat diet may be necessary for those who have lost weight or are underweight.

Vitamins and Minerals Vitamins and minerals are essential nutrients that help to activate, regulate and control many of our body's metabolic processes. The National Academy of Sciences has established recommended dietary allowances (RDAs) for 13 essential nutrients. Most people can get all of these vitamins and minerals from eating a balanced diet. A multiple vitamin may be required, however, if you are unable to eat properly. Make sure that the vitamin and mineral supplement that you choose supplies all of the needed nutrients at about 100 percent of the RDA.

Although megavitamin therapy (vitamin dosages far in excess of recommended levels) has been suggested as a treatment for cancer and other diseases, no reliable scientific evidence proves that it is effective. In fact, some vitamins taken in excess can be harmful. For example, while the body has the ability to excrete excess amounts of the water-soluble vitamins (B and C) in the urine, the fat-soluble vitamins (A, D, E and K) are stored in the tissues and can accumulate to toxic levels if consumed in excess. If a vitamin is to be taken in therapeutic amounts (many times greater than the recommended amount), it should be prescribed by a physician.

Antioxidants Human studies show that antioxidants, including beta-carotene and vitamins A, C, E and selenium, may reduce the risk of cancer. Antioxidants act by destroying harmful molecules called free radicals that form in the body naturally. Free radicals can damage DNA, RNA and fat and protein molecules, and may be involved in the development of cancerous cells. Antioxidants decrease DNA damage, and it is possibly through this route that they help prevent the transformation of normal cells into malignant cells, thus acting as protective substances. However, there is no conclusive evidence that a diet rich in these antioxidants is able to reduce the incidence of, or to cure, cancer.

Fluids and Hydration
It is important to maintain adequate hydration by drinking enough fluids daily. Drink at least eight glasses of water a day, unless your physician has told you to monitor your fluid intake. Avoid too many caffeinated drinks, as these act as diuretics and can increase water loss. Some chemotherapeutic agents increase your need for water. Therefore, be sure to follow your doctor's, nurse's or pharmacist's instructions concerning your fluid intake.

POTENTIAL TOXIC SIDE EFFECTS OF VITAMINS AND MINERALS

Vitamin/Mineral	Toxic Side Effects
Beta-carotene	unknown
Vitamin A	liver, kidney and bone damage, headaches, irritability, vomiting, hair loss
Vitamin C	nausea, diarrhea
Vitamin E	rare; fatigue, skin reactions and abdominal discomfort may occur
Selenium	hair loss, fingernail changes

ALTERNATIVE DIETS

Vegetarian Many Americans have elected to follow a vegetarian diet, which, when well planned, can be a healthy alternative to the conventional diet. Several terms are used to describe vegetarian diets. Lacto-vegetarians include milk and seafood, and lacto-ovo-vegetarians include eggs as well. Those who consume vegetables only, with the exclusion of all animal foods, dairy products and eggs, are referred to as vegans. There are more details about following a balanced vegetarian diet in Chapter 19.

The vegetarian diets that are less restrictive and include animal products such as milk or eggs or both are hearty, healthful and easier to plan. However, highly restrictive vegan and Zen macrobiotic diets can cause serious malnutrition.

Vegan Diet More careful planning is required when following a vegan diet. It is limited in calcium, iron, riboflavin and vitamin B_{12} and lacks concentrated protein sources. In order to provide an adequate supply of essential amino acids, include whole grains and cereals with each meal. In addition, a complementary protein, which can be provided by legumes, vegetables or a combination of nuts and seeds, should be included each day. Furthermore, the iron from grains is not absorbed by the body as well as the iron from meat. Therefore, to increase iron absorption, include a source of vitamin C (e.g., orange juice, citrus fruits, kiwifruit or strawberries). Be sure to include nuts and dark green vegetables for calcium, and cereal for riboflavin. Since vitamin B_{12} is found almost exclusively in animal products, vegans may need to use vitamin B_{12}–fortified soy milk or breakfast cereals.

Maintaining an adequate vitamin intake is a concern for people with cancer and can be a challenge when following a strict vegan diet. Therefore, include plenty of nuts and seeds, an additional one to four servings of fruits and vegetables, and three to five servings of grains and cereals, using the Food Guide Pyramid for Vegetarians on page 211.

Macrobiotic Diets Another vegetarian diet is the Zen macrobiotic diet. Macrobiotic diets are not recommended for people with cancer.

This diet is based on the Zen Buddhist belief that one's health and happiness depend upon a proper balance between the "yin" and the "yang" foods. This balance is achieved by progressing through 10 steps, which range from the lowest-level diet, made up of 30 percent vegetables, 30 percent animal products, 15 percent salad and fruit, 10 percent soups, 10 percent cereals and 5 percent desserts, to the highest-level, which contains 100 percent cereals. The highest and most extreme level, where people consume only brown rice and tea, has resulted in vitamin deficiencies and several deaths.

WHAT FOODS SHOULD YOU EAT?

Basic Nutrition—The Food Guide Pyramid

One of the most important ways you can help yourself to get well is to eat the right amount of essential food nutrients needed by your body to repair tissue and maintain your weight. These essential food nutrients—proteins, fats, carbohydrates, vitamins and minerals—are also vital for normal body functioning and for maintaining good health.

The food guide pyramid has been developed as an outline to assist you with daily meal plans. Foods are divided into groups according to the nutrients they contain. Each group provides some, but not all, of the nutrients you need each day. Be sure to choose a variety of foods from each group daily.

Bread, Cereal, Rice and Pasta Group The recommended emphasis in the diet is reflected in the base of the pyramid. This group provides primarily the B vitamins and carbohydrates for energy. Include 6 to 11 servings from this group daily.

Examples of 1 serving are: 1 slice bread, ½ cup (125 mL) cooked rice or pasta, ½ cup (125 mL) cooked cereal, 1 oz. (25 g) ready-to-eat cereal.

Vegetable Group Include 3 to 5 servings from this group daily. Choose at least one serving of a dark green or a deep yellow vegetable for beta-carotene (the plant form of vitamin A).

Examples of 1 serving include: ½ cup (125 mL) chopped raw or cooked vegetables, 1 cup (250 mL) leafy raw vegetable.

Fruit Group The recommended amount of fruits is 2 to 4 servings daily. Include at least one serving of a fruit rich in vitamin C, such as orange, kiwifruit, strawberry or grapefruit.

Examples of 1 serving size include: 1 piece fresh fruit or 1 melon wedge, ¾ cup (175 mL) fruit juice, ½ cup (125 mL) canned fruit, ¼ cup (50 mL) dried fruit.

Milk, Yogurt and Cheese Group The 2 to 3 recommended daily servings of this group are a good source of calcium, phosphorus, vitamins A and D, protein and riboflavin.

Examples of 1 serving size are: 1 cup (250 mL) milk or yogurt, 1½ to 2 oz. (40 to 50 g) cheese.

Meat, Poultry, Fish, Dry Beans, Eggs and Nuts Group (includes peanut butter and tofu)

Protein, B vitamins and iron are the important nutrients found in this group. Include 2 to 3 servings per day.

Examples of 1 serving size are: 2 to 3 oz. (50 to 75 g) cooked lean meat, poultry or fish, ½ cup (125 mL) cooked beans, 1 egg, 2 tbsp. (25 mL) peanut butter (equivalent to 1 oz./25 g of meat), 4 oz. (125 g) tofu.

Fats, Oils and Sweets Group This group includes butter, cream, margarine and vegetable oil, along with candies and sweet desserts. Foods from this group contain calories, vitamin E and negligible amounts of other nutrients. Therefore, most people should limit foods from this group daily.

Examples of 1 serving include: 1 tsp. (5 mL) margarine, oil or mayonnaise, 1 tsp. (5 mL) salad dressing.

HOW MANY SERVINGS DO YOU NEED?

A range of servings is shown for each group of the food guide pyramid. The number of servings that is right for you depends on the number of calories you require each day. You will learn how to calculate your estimated calorie needs in the section "How Much Should You Eat?" If your calorie needs are lower (1,600 to 1,800 calories or less), select from the lower number of servings from each food

The Food Guide Pyramid: A Guide to Daily Food Choices

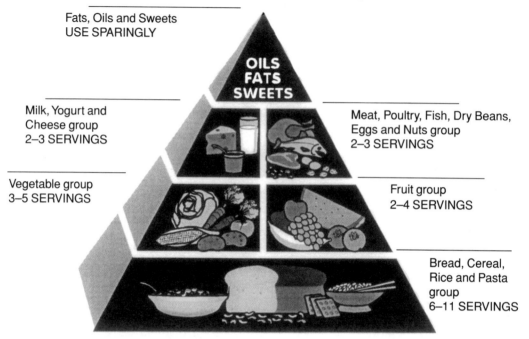

Fats, Oils and Sweets
USE SPARINGLY

**OILS
FATS
SWEETS**

Milk, Yogurt and
Cheese group
2–3 SERVINGS

Meat, Poultry, Fish, Dry Beans,
Eggs and Nuts group
2–3 SERVINGS

Vegetable group
3–5 SERVINGS

Fruit group
2–4 SERVINGS

Bread, Cereal,
Rice and Pasta
group
6–11 SERVINGS

Source: U.S. Department of Health and Human Services

group. If your calorie needs are in the average range (2,000 to 2,400 calories), select from the middle number of servings from each food group. If you have higher calorie needs (2,600 calories or more), select from the higher number of servings from each group.

The chart below is an example of the number of servings from each of the food groups appropriate to various calorie requirements.

Monitor your weight weekly to determine whether you are getting enough calories. If you find that you are losing weight, start including more calorie-dense foods from the fats, oils and sweets group. However, if you cannot tolerate fat, consider increasing your consumption of calorie-dense low-fat foods such as dried fruit and fruit juices. Note the range of the fruit and fat servings listed above. These

ranges are to allow flexibility in your food choices, depending on your fat tolerance. For more ideas on how to increase calories, *see* pages 165 and 167.

HOW MUCH SHOULD YOU EAT?

Protein and Calorie Requirements This section shows you how to determine your desirable weight and the amounts of protein and calories you require to maintain this weight.

The Desirable Weight table shows average desirable weights for healthy adults. You may want to make allowances for the effects of your illness. If you are overweight, maintain your weight, as this is not a good time to lose weight. Try to maintain your weight within your range. Ask your dietitian for advice and determine a realistic desirable weight to maintain during your therapy. Enter this weight on your Food and Weight Summary chart on page 165.

Minimum Daily Protein Requirement
A healthy adult has a daily nutritional requirement of approximately 0.5 grams of protein per pound of desirable body weight. Cancer patients may have increased protein and calorie needs. In addition, if you are already malnourished because of your illness or treatment, you will need an even greater amount of protein (0.7 to 0.9 grams per pound of desirable body weight).

To find your minimum daily requirement of protein in grams, multiply your desirable body weight (in pounds) by 0.5 (or by 0.7 to 0.9 if you have already lost weight). Enter this figure on your Food and Weight Summary chart. When planning your daily menu, try to get at least this amount of protein from the foods you choose.

minimum daily protein requirement
= desirable weight x 0.5

Minimum Daily Calorie Requirement
Your sex, age and activity level affect the amount of calories you need. Men need more calories than women. Children need extra calories for growth, while the elderly need fewer calories. The more active you are, the more calories you need.

To estimate your daily calorie needs, multiply your desirable weight (in pounds) by 18 if you are a man (by 20 if you have already lost weight) or by 16 if you are a woman (by 18 if you have already lost weight). Enter this amount on your Food and Weight Summary chart once a week. Plan your daily menu to get at least this estimated amount of calories.

minimum daily calorie requirement
(women) = desirable weight x 16

minimum daily calorie requirement
(men) = desirable weight x 18

Meeting Your Daily Requirements You can determine whether you are meeting your daily protein and calorie requirements by keeping a list of everything you eat. Add up your total protein and calorie intake each day and enter the amounts on your Food and Weight Summary chart. The protein and calorie content of most foods can be found in *Bowes & Church's Food Values of Portions Commonly Used*, which may be available in the resource center at your hospital, a bookstore or a library. There are also computer programs, such as Nutritionist IV and Foodworks, that can help you to keep track of protein and calories.

Weigh yourself weekly rather than daily, since daily weights reflect your body's fluid content rather than overall changes in body weight. Enter your weight on your Food and Weight Summary chart. If you are losing weight, increase your daily calorie intake. See Chapter 20 for high-calorie/high-protein recipes.

READING FOOD LABELS

Nutrition information on food packages can help you make informed food choices to better suit your specific needs. Food labels will assist you with maximizing

Calories	Milk	Meat	Vegetables	Fruit	Bread	Fat
1,600–1,800	2	2	3	2–4	6	3–5
2,000–2,400	3	2	4	4–5	9	6–7
2,600+	3	3	5	5–6	11	8–9

your calorie and protein intake and developing an awareness of the fat content of various foods.

If you are usually careful about the amount of fat you eat, you can afford to relax a bit while you are undergoing cancer treatment, and possibly losing weight as a result of it. At this time, the calories in fat may be beneficial (unless you are significantly over- or underweight).

When reading food labels, keep in mind that the amounts of calories, protein, fat and so forth are stated per serving. Almost all bagged, wrapped and canned items contain more than one serving.

DESIRABLE WEIGHT

| Height* | Weight (in Pounds and Kilograms)†‡ | |
	Age 19–34	35 and Older
5'0" (152 cm)	97–128 (44–58 kg)	108–138 (49–63 kg)
5'1" (155 cm)	101–132 (46–60 kg)	111–143 (50–65 kg)
5'2" (157 cm)	104–137 (47–62 kg)	115–148 (52–67 kg)
5'3" (160 cm)	107–141 (49–64 kg)	119–152 (54–69 kg)
5'4" (163 cm)	111–146 (50–66 kg)	122–157 (55–71 kg)
5'5" (165 cm)	114–150 (52–68 kg)	126–162 (57–74 kg)
5'6" (168 cm)	118–155 (54–70 kg)	130–167 (59–76 kg)
5'7" (170 cm)	121–160 (55–73 kg)	134–172 (61–78 kg)
5'8" (173 cm)	125–164 (57–74 kg)	138–178 (63–81 kg)
5'9" (175 cm)	129–169 (59–77 kg)	142–183 (64–83 kg)
5'10" (178 cm)	132–174 (60–79 kg)	146–188 (66–85 kg)
5'11" (180 cm)	136–179 (62–81 kg)	151–194 (69–88 kg)
6'0" (183 cm)	140–184 (64–84 kg)	155–199 (70–90 kg)
6'1" (185 cm)	144–189 (65–86 kg)	159–205 (72–93 kg)
6'2" (188 cm)	148–195 (67–89 kg)	164–210 (74–95 kg)
6'3" (191 cm)	152–200 (69–91 kg)	168–216 (76–98 kg)
6'4" (193 cm)	156–205 (71–93 kg)	173–222 (79–101 kg)
6'5" (196 cm)	160–211 (73–96 kg)	177–228 (80–104 kg)
6'6" (198 cm)	164–216 (74–98 kg)	182–234 (83–106 kg)

*Without shoes.
†Without clothes.
‡ The higher weights in the ranges generally apply to men, who tend to have more muscle and bone; the lower weights more often apply to women, who have less muscle and bone.

Source: Adapted from *Nutrition and Your Health: Dietary Guidelines for Americans.* 3d ed. Washington, D.C.: U.S. Government Printing Office, 1990.

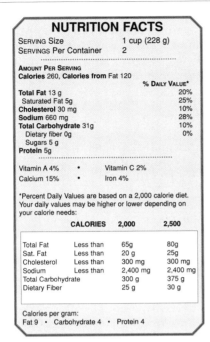

NUTRITION FACTS

Serving Size   1 cup (228 g)
Servings Per Container   2
....
Amount Per Serving
Calories 260, Calories from Fat 120

	% Daily Value*
Total Fat 13 g	20%
Saturated Fat 5g	25%
Cholesterol 30 mg	10%
Sodium 660 mg	28%
Total Carbohydrate 31g	10%
Dietary fiber 0g	0%
Sugars 5 g	
Protein 5g	

Vitamin A 4%	•	Vitamin C 2%
Calcium 15%	•	Iron 4%

*Percent Daily Values are based on a 2,000 calorie diet. Your daily values may be higher or lower depending on your calorie needs:

CALORIES		2,000	2,500
Total Fat	Less than	65g	80g
Sat. Fat	Less than	20 g	25g
Cholesterol	Less than	300 mg	300 mg
Sodium	Less than	2,400 mg	2,400 mg
Total Carbohydrate		300 g	375 g
Dietary Fiber		25 g	30 g

Calories per gram:
Fat 9 • Carbohydrate 4 • Protein 4

SAMPLE MENU FOR GOOD NUTRITION FOR CANCER PATIENTS

The following menu is an example of a well-balanced meal plan that includes the recommended number of servings from each food group. If you have lost weight and need to include extra calories in your diet, add more servings of snacks, appetizers, desserts and drinks from the list of snack ideas below and the recipes in Chapter 20.

Breakfast (265 calories, 5 g protein)
½ cup (125 mL) cooked cereal
½ cup (125 mL) fruit or juice
1 slice toast with 2 tsp. (10 mL) margarine or butter

Midmorning Snack (440 calories, 21 g protein)
1 cup (250 mL) milk
3 crackers
2 tbsp. (25 mL) peanut butter or 1½ oz. (40 g) cheese

Lunch (365 calories, 20 g protein)
Sandwich:
2 slices bread
2 oz. (50 g) meat/fish/poultry or 2 tbsp. (25 mL) peanut butter or 1½ oz. (40 g) cheese slices
1 tsp. (5 mL) mayonnaise
1 slice each lettuce, tomato
1 piece fruit

Midafternoon Snack (160 calories, 12 g protein)
½ sandwich:
1 slice bread
1 oz. (25 g) meat/fish/poultry
½ cup (125 mL) raw vegetables

Dinner (510 calories, 30 g protein)
2 oz. (50 g) meat/fish/poultry
½ cup (125 mL) vegetables
½ cup (125 mL) grain product (rice, pasta, etc.)
1 slice bread
1 tsp. (5 mL) margarine or butter
1 cup (250 mL) milk

This is a guideline. You may find that your day-to-day intake varies. For example, some days nausea and taste changes may prevent you from eating adequate amounts of food in all food groups. On these days, high-calorie/high-protein shakes or supplements that contain added vitamins and minerals may be helpful.

FOOD AND WEIGHT SUMMARY

Personal Daily Requirements	**Amount Required**	**Number of Grams/Calories of Required Eaten Daily**
Desirable weight (range)		
Protein in grams		
Calories		

HELPFUL HINTS FOR BETTER NUTRITION

Whether you are at home or in the hospital, you can make good use of a planned approach to your eating. You may have to work hard to overcome the obstacle of a poor appetite, but there are techniques to help you.

In the Hospital

1. Consult with the hospital dietitian. When you are in the hospital, you have the advantage of being able to consult with the hospital dietitian. Have him or her help you plan a balanced daily menu that includes the proper amounts of protein and calories. Ask for advice if you are having any eating problems. The hospital dietitian can also help you plan a home nutrition program.

2. Consider adding a high-protein or high-calorie diet supplement to your menu. Ask the dietitian to discuss various diet supplements with you. He or she may be able to let you taste-test brands of supplements and can advise you about the pros and cons of the various brands.

3. Snack between meals. The dietitian will arrange for you to have snacks such as high-protein diet supplements, milk-shakes, eggnogs, puddings or sandwiches. If you must interrupt or miss a meal for a test, therapy or an examination, ask that your food be saved or ask to order another meal when you return to your room.

4. Fill out your daily menu when you are feeling well enough to plan your meals imaginatively. Have someone help you if necessary. Order food that you like. Find out if the hospital has any menu choices not listed on the printed menu. Consider the protein and calorie values of the food you order, but give thought to its eye appeal and aroma so that it will be as appetizing as possible. Giving variety to your menus will improve your appetite. You may want to save some of your menus to use as examples when you are planning your meals at home.

5. Have your family and friends bring your favorite foods. Favorite foods from home will often help your appetite. In some hospitals, families are allowed to use the ward kitchen to prepare special food or to warm up food brought from home.

6. Make your mealtimes pleasant. Your mealtime atmosphere is important to make you feel like eating. Your family and friends can bring flowers and pictures to your hospital room. Ask for candles or wine, if permitted. Whenever possible, eat with family, friends or other patients. If you are alone, turn on the radio, television or music for company. Try to make mealtime a social time.

7. Avoid stress at mealtimes. Relaxation exercises before meals may help reduce tension and may improve your appetite.

Have an aperitif before meals. If your doctor gives you permission, you may find a glass of beer or wine before meals relaxes you as well as stimulates your appetite.

8. Exercise before meals. Light exercise for 5 to 10 minutes approximately a half-hour before meals may stimulate your appetite. The nurse or physical therapist can show you simple range-of-motion exercises you can do in bed; or if you can get out of bed, take a walk up and down the hospital corridors.

At Home In addition to the above suggestions, which apply as well to meals at home (frequent small meals, snacks, high-protein supplements, attractive surroundings, exercise, etc.), there are some techniques to use when you no longer have the hospital facilities and staff avail-

HIGH-CALORIE/HIGH-PROTEIN SMALL MEAL AND SNACK IDEAS

	Calories	Protein (grams)
Apple slices and cheese*	175	7
Apple slices and peanut butter	250	8
Baked potato and cheese	340	10
Buttered popcorn with parmesan cheese	60	3
Carnation Instant Breakfast Drink	130	7
Cheese nachos	345	10
Cinnamon toast and milk	270	10
Cold or cooked cereals and milk	240	11
Commercial supplements: Ensure, Sustacal, Resource	250	8
Cornbread and buttermilk	200	10
Cottage cheese (½ cup/125 mL) with fruit	245	28
Crackers or pretzels and dip	175	10
Crackers with smooth peanut butter or cheese	370	10
Dried fruit, nuts, granola	245	5
Egg custard and graham crackers	250	7
Eggnog and cookies	480	12
English muffins with butter and preserves	220	3
Fruited yogurt (regular) (½ cup/125 mL)	225	9
Gelatin and fruit	80	3
Granola bar	100	2
Hard-boiled or deviled egg	75	6
Hot chocolate (cocoa) and cookies	350	10
Milkshake and graham crackers	450	14
Muffins or bagels with cream cheese	350	10
Pop-Tarts and milk	315	10
Popsicles (pudding or regular)	80	2
Sandwich with protein: meat, egg, poultry, tuna, cheese, peanut butter	400	2
Sherbet or ice cream and topping	300	6
Soup, cream	200	6
Soup, with meat and vegetables	150	14
Tomato or V-8 juice and crackers	130	3
Tomato stuffed with egg, tuna or chicken salad	200	16
Waffles with syrup and butter	350	6
Yogurt (regular or frozen) (½ cup/125 mL)	115	3

*Where no specific serving sizes are given, refer to *Bowes & Church's Food Values of Portions Commonly Used.*

able. Here are some suggestions to help you at home.

1. Plan your daily menu in advance. Include the proper number of servings from the food guide pyramid and your required amounts of protein and calories. As well as planning your menu, plan the time you will eat. If you have no appetite, you will need to rely on specified times to eat rather than on your hunger mechanism.

2. Get help in preparing your meals. If you are not feeling well, you may not feel like making the effort to prepare a nutritious meal. A friend or relative may be able to help you by preparing foods for several days in advance. Home aid in preparing meals or delivered meals are available in many communities. Some grocery stores have shopping services that may be accessed through your computer. Or order take-out from your favorite restaurant.

3. Fix small portions of favorite foods and store them. Prepare several portions at the same time and freeze them. Then you won't have to think about what to fix. It lessens the problem of figuring out what to eat when your appetite may be poor or you do not feel like cooking. Remember to protect against bacterial contamination that can cause food poisoning: Do not leave food at room temperature for long periods, and refrigerate or freeze foods immediately.

4. Add extra protein to your diet. Use fortified milk for drinking and in all recipes calling for milk. Use peanut butter, cheese, cottage cheese and hard-boiled eggs as snacks, and devise ways to add them to recipes. See the recipe suggestions in Chapter 20.

5. Add extra calories to your diet. Add cream or butter to soups, cooked cereals and vegetables. Use gravies, sauces and sour cream with vegetables, meat, poultry and fish. Add a high-calorie diet supplement to your normal recipes. The chart below provides some suggestions.

6. Make food visually appealing. The eye appeal of food can stimulate your appetite. Choose foods with attractive colors. Garnish your meal with parsley, lemon wedges, olives, cherry tomatoes, shredded raw vegetables and so on. Use a small plate if you cannot take normal portions of food, so that your meal will not look too small.

7. Appeal to your sense of smell. Cook dishes with tantalizing aromas and special sauces. Gravies and sauces are aromatic and enhance the taste of food; they also add calories and make swallowing easier. The smell of bread baking can stimulate hunger and contribute to a sense of well-being. Avoid foods with odors that trigger queasiness.

8. Be creative with dessert. Desserts are an appealing part of the meal. Take advantage of this for a caloric boost.

9. Follow your own preferences in eating. Even if you have dietary restrictions, there is still room to improvise and to choose foods that you like and mealtimes that suit your appetite.

ADDING EXTRA CALORIES

	Calories	Protein (grams)
Butter (1 tbsp./15 mL)	100	0
Cheese (1 oz./25 g)	112	7
Cottage cheese (½ cup/125 mL)	120	16
Cream, heavy (¼ cup/50 mL)	202	1
Gravy (¼ cup/50 mL)	50	2
Hard-boiled eggs (2)	162	12
Peanut butter (1 tbsp./15 mL)	115	5
Sour cream (2 tbsp./25 mL)	50	1

MYTHS OF NUTRITION THERAPY FOR CANCER

Many people have their own ideas about treating cancer either with special vitamins, foods or chemicals, or by changing their diet. Many of these ideas are myths, unsupported by scientific evidence.

Natural and Organic Foods Patients are often curious about the superiority of "natural" or "organic" foods over regularly grown and processed foods in the dietary management of cancer. "Natural" is a general term covering all foods that are processed without artificial coloring, preservatives or any kind of synthetic additives. "Organic" is a more specific term that refers to foods grown without chemical fertilizers, pesticides or herbicides. There is no scientific evidence that either natural or organic foods offer any nutritional advantage over regular foods, and frequently their greater cost makes them less financially desirable as nutritional sources.

Concerns about the relationship between additives and cancer are based for the most part on speculation, and there is no good evidence that a person eating regular foods from the supermarket is at any greater risk than a person who eats natural foods. Cancer existed long before food additives were invented.

Natural and organic diets are often tried by desperate patients who choose to listen to family or friends and who do not want to follow one of the standard medical therapies. Thus far there is no clinical or research support for the effectiveness of such diets in curing, palliating or containing disease.

Starving the Tumor Probably the most commonly held myth is that you can starve the tumor by starving yourself. Many patients have expressed the fear that by eating proper diets they will be feeding the tumor more than they will be feeding their normal body tissue. There is no scientific evidence to support this theory. Some careful experimental studies with animals with cancerous tumors found no improvement in those put on a starvation diet. On the other hand, we know for certain that patients who are malnourished have more toxic and nutritional side effects from therapy, do poorer medically, lose their strength earlier, heal more slowly, have reduced immunity and become an invalid or bedridden more quickly.

Megavitamin Therapy Much attention has recently been focused on megavitamin therapy for certain diseases, including cancer. In some animal studies, certain vitamin A or E compounds have been shown to be related mainly to the prevention of tumors rather than to treatment of them. These results have yet to be confirmed in humans, and the experts have generally agreed that there is no benefit to any form of megavitamin therapy for cancer.

Vitamins and minerals should come from the food you eat. A properly planned diet makes vitamin and mineral supplements unnecessary, although at times vitamin and mineral preparations may be prescribed for patients unable to eat a balanced diet. A trained professional should prescribe such supplements, and only on the basis of a dietary analysis and assessment of individual need as determined by your medical team.

Much has recently been written about the role of minerals such as zinc, copper, selenium and magnesium in human nutrition. These metals are present in the human body (and in our foods) in minute amounts and are therefore termed "trace minerals." They are important for nutritional health, but their precise functions in the body are just beginning to be understood. The effects on cancer of ingesting increased amounts of minerals have not been well studied. Animal experiments have shown that some metals can actually cause cancer, but we do not know the implications for human cancer treatment.

It has been shown that zinc deficiency in humans may result in loss of appetite, sometimes a loss of sense of taste and smell, and slower wound healing. However, it is not clear whether some of the loss of appetite and taste distortion experienced by cancer patients is due to zinc deficiency, rather than to the cancer itself.

One fact is clear: a well-balanced diet supplies adequate amounts of the trace minerals for known human requirements. The first and best nutritional goal is to maintain an adequate, well-balanced diet.

GENERAL DIETARY GUIDELINES FOR THE CANCER PATIENT

◆ Eat foods at room temperature.
◆ Drink 10 to 12 cups (8 oz./250 mL) of fluid each day. Stir carbonated drinks until the bubbles have disappeared before you drink them.
◆ Nutmeg added to food and sauces will help reduce motility (the movement of food through the gastrointestinal tract).
◆ Start a high-fiber, low-residue diet (*see* Chapter 19) on the day you begin radiation therapy.

Food That May Cause the Nutrition Problems Discussed in Chapter 17.
◆ Alcohol and tobacco
◆ Chocolate, coffee, tea and soft drinks with caffeine
◆ Fried, greasy and fatty foods
◆ Milk and milk products, because of potential lactose intolerance. Exceptions are buttermilk, yogurt and processed cheese because the lactose has been altered or removed. Milkshake supplements such as Ensure are lactose-free and may be used. (*See* "Milk (Lactose) Intolerance" on page 185.)
◆ Nuts and seeds
◆ Popcorn, potato chips and pretzels
◆ Raw vegetables
◆ Rich pastries
◆ Strong spices and herbs
◆ White bread and toast

Foods to Encourage
◆ Baked, boiled or mashed potatoes
◆ Bananas, applesauce, peeled apples, apple and grape juices
◆ Cooked vegetables that are mild, such as asparagus tips, green and waxed beans, carrots, spinach and squash
◆ Fish, poultry and meat that is cooked, broiled or roasted
◆ Fresh and dried fruit and some fruit juices such as prune juice
◆ Macaroni and other noodles
◆ Whole-bran bread and cereal
◆ Yogurt, processed cheese, eggs, smooth peanut butter and buttermilk

17
NUTRITION PROBLEMS: CAUSES AND SOLUTIONS

Ernest H. Rosenbaum, MD, Isadora R. Rosenbaum, MA, and Julie Matel, MS, RD

———————◇———————

Maintaining adequate nutrition can be exceptionally difficult for patients with cancer. Many problems—most commonly loss of appetite—occur as side effects of cancer therapy. The foods you eat can affect these problems—they can make them worse or they can relieve them.

Physical problems may interfere with food intake and proper nutrition. Patients with head and neck tumors may have mouth or throat pain or difficulty swallowing. People who have had part of the stomach or gastrointestinal tract surgically removed may have problems of early filling, diarrhea, cramps and decreased absorption. Removal of parts of the intestine or blockage of the intestine can also inhibit absorption. Those with ileostomies or colostomies may have difficulties with salt and water balance because of diarrhea. Diarrhea commonly causes poor absorption of calories and nutrients, because food moves so rapidly through the gastrointestinal tract.

Radiation therapy to the head and neck area frequently results in a loss of taste perception and decreased production of saliva, along with inflammation, pain and difficulty swallowing. Radiation to the abdomen may cause some damage to the bowel, resulting in cramps, diarrhea, malabsorption or obstruction.

Chemotherapy can inhibit appetite and affect the mouth and esophagus. Decreased food intake is common for a short period around the time of treatment. It is important to try to compensate for weight loss during this time by making a conscious effort to eat more. When you experience any of these problems, first consult your physician or the dietitian on your health care team. With their help and with the suggestions in these chapters, you should be able to plan a diet designed to minimize these problems. Prescription medications may be required. Your dentist and pharmacist may also be of assistance.

In this chapter, we discuss the problems you may encounter and offer suggestions—what foods to eat, what foods to avoid, medication that can help and other tips.

SURGERY TO THE HEAD AND NECK AREA

Surgery to the head and neck area often affects the ability to eat. Proper planning before surgery should include a visit to a dentist to maximize the use of the remaining teeth and minimize problems immediately after surgery. Often a dental appliance can be constructed that will help you control saliva while eating.

Your diet may have to be modified because of a change in your ability to chew some foods. Adapting to surgery involving the tongue or other oral structures often takes time, and may require swallowing rehabilitation with a speech pathologist or occupational therapist specifically trained in head and neck swallowing disorders.

COLOSTOMY AND ILEOSTOMY DIETARY GUIDELINES

A colostomy is formed when part of the colon is surgically moved to open on the surface of the abdomen, usually below the waist. This forms a stoma, or artificial anus, through which stools are excreted. An ileostomy is an opening leading to the small bowel. The person with an ostomy wears a bag attached to this stoma to catch the excretions. He or she can lead a normal life in most respects, including choosing what to eat.

Some of the following foods cause problems for those with colostomies and ileostomies. Experiment to find out whether they cause you gas, discomfort, diarrhea, constipation or pain.

Foods That May Irritate
◆ Foods with seeds, such as strawberries, raspberries, tomatoes
◆ Nuts; popcorn; skin on fruits and vegetables such as apples and corn; coconut
◆ Some fresh vegetables such as coleslaw and salads

Foods That May Produce Gas
◆ Carbonated drinks and beer
◆ Dried beans or peas, broccoli, brussels sprouts, cabbage, cauliflower, corn, cucumber, green pepper, onions, sauerkraut, turnips and winter squash

Foods That May Produce Odor
◆ Onions, eggs, fish

What You Can Do Keep a record of what you eat and when so that you can identify (and avoid) any food that causes symptoms. The general rules for avoiding digestive problems can be helpful, such as eating in a pleasant, relaxed atmosphere and chewing your food slowly and thoroughly. Avoid swallowing air, which can lead to gas formation. Yogurt, buttermilk and cranberry juice have proven effective in helping to control odor.

Be sure to drink plenty of fluids to prevent dehydration. Contact your physician if you are experiencing severe diarrhea or severe constipation.

RADIATION THERAPY TO THE HEAD AND NECK AREA

Irradiation in the mouth and throat may result in painful mucositis, altered or lost taste, dry mouth or dental problems. Radiation to the head and neck can also affect the gums, teeth, production of saliva and type of saliva and the mouth's ability to respond to infection.

A dentist should examine your teeth before radiation therapy and determine which teeth, if any, have problems that should be treated before radiation therapy, when your ability to heal is at its best. If it is necessary to remove teeth, the extraction site must be completely healed before the radiotherapy to avoid irreversible bone damage. Radiation treatment generally should not start until about 14 days after the extraction.

Radiation will make your teeth susceptible to decay. You will want to avoid foods and drinks that leave sugar on your teeth (sugar-free gum, candy and drinks may be helpful). Daily mouth care should include brushing at least twice a day followed by a fluoride treatment as instructed by your dentist.

A sore or dry mouth may also occur as a side effect of radiation therapy. Radiation mucositis frequently occurs with radiation to the head and neck. You may need a nourishing, soft diet.

If mucositis causes you to cut down on eating, you may need a protein supplement. A dietitian can help you plan an adequate diet. Occasionally, when swallowing becomes too painful, temporary tube feeding may be necessary.

A common problem of radiation to the oral cavity and pharynx is xerostomia, or dry mouth, which is caused by a reduction in saliva after irradiation of the salivary glands. You should increase your fluid intake, particularly while eating, to ease swallowing and help moisten your mouth. Avoid dry, hard food, and use creams, gravies and sauces to moisten food.

Loss of taste can result from radiation to the oral cavity. Taste will usually return within two months after therapy is completed. Adding spices and sauces and emphasizing foods with distinctive flavors and aromas may help combat the problem.

RADIATION THERAPY TO THE CHEST AND ESOPHAGUS

Radiation is frequently delivered to the chest and esophagus to treat lung cancer, esophageal cancer and lymphoma. Doses in excess of 3,000 cGy may, within three weeks, result in esophagitis (esophageal inflammation), with symptoms of painful swallowing. Reducing the daily dose or a short interruption in the treatment will usually allow rapid healing.

RADIATION THERAPY TO THE ABDOMEN AND PELVIS

Radiation to the upper abdomen or pelvis may cause radiation enteritis (inflammation of the bowel). However, only a very small percentage of patients treated with radiation to the abdomen will develop chronic problems.

Because of their rapidly dividing cells, the mucosa of both the large and small bowel, including the rectum, are sensitive to even modest doses of radiation. The severity of symptoms depends on the extent of the irradiated area, the daily dose, the total dose required and the pos-

sible simultaneous use of chemotherapy. In addition, patients with a history of abdominal surgery, pelvic inflammatory disease, atherosclerosis, diabetes or hypertension are predisposed to radiation-induced nausea and vomiting.

Treatment to the upper abdomen is more likely to lead to nausea and vomiting, while pelvic irradiation is more likely to result in rectal irritation, frequent bowel movements or diarrhea, resulting in malabsorption of fat, bile salts and the B vitamins.

Your physician will evaluate the extent of the enteritis by assessing the frequency of diarrhea, the character of the stools and the presence of rectal bleeding or abdominal distension, as well as possible dehydration or electrolyte imbalance resulting from diarrhea or malabsorption.

What You Can Do Treatment of radiation enteritis includes adjusting the diet, medication and, in severe cases, interrupting radiation treatment. Patients receiving abdominal or pelvic radiation should follow a low-fat, low-fiber/residue diet, beginning with the first radiation treatments. "Residue" refers to indigestible material in food, sometimes called fiber. They should limit their intake of milk products, except for buttermilk, yogurt and acidophilus or lactose-free milk.

◆ Greasy, fried or fatty foods tend to be difficult to digest.
◆ Vegetables should be cooked.
◆ Whole-grain and high-bran products, such as whole wheat bread, and nuts, popcorn, potato chips and beans should be avoided.
◆ Patients can drink fruit juices (except prune juice), but they should not eat raw fruits. They should also reduce alcohol consumption.

Medication If radiation enteritis persists despite diet changes, medications will be needed. A 250 mg 5-ASA suppository every night has helped reduce or control symptoms during and after radiation therapy.

Relief from abdominal pain may be obtained with narcotics. If proctitis is present, a steroid foam given rectally may offer relief. Finally, if patients with pancreatic cancer are experiencing diarrhea during radiation therapy, their doctor may recommend oral pancreatic enzymes (pancreatin) to be taken with meals to assist with digestion and absorption of food.

CHEMOTHERAPY

Detailed information on nutrition and chemotherapy is often not easily available. The specific dietary recommendations in this book show that many drug side effects can be reduced or controlled. Ideally a qualified dietitian should be working with the oncologist and the patient. When no dietitian is available, nutritional counselling and diet planning may be done by a nurse or the physician.

LOSS OF APPETITE (ANOREXIA)

Cancer therapy or the cancer itself may cause changes in your body chemistry that result in a loss of appetite. Pain, nausea, vomiting, diarrhea or a sore or dry mouth may make eating difficult and cause you to lose interest in food. You can also lose your appetite because of anxiety or depression about your disease. Often patients who have been informed of the possible diagnosis of cancer lose 5 to 10 pounds (2.2 to 4.5 kg) while waiting for test results.

The brain produces chemicals (cytokines and serotonin) that can cause loss of appetite. A study by the Eastern Cooperative Oncology Group showed that as little as 6 percent loss of body mass was related to a decreased length of survival. The reduction of calorie intake can lead to a loss of muscle mass and strength

and other complications by causing
◆ interruptions of medical therapy, impeding effective cancer therapy
◆ poor tolerance of surgery
◆ impaired efficacy of chemotherapy and radiotherapy
◆ decrease in quality of life
◆ decrease in immunity

A totally different approach to eating is required when you no longer have enough appetite to make you want to eat. You will need to learn to eat even when you do not feel like eating and to approach eating as an important part of your therapy. Talk to a dietitian, nurse or your doctor about ways to improve your appetite. It is important both for your general sense of well-being and your ability to fight the disease that you eat a nutritious diet and try to maintain your weight.

As appetite may no longer motivate you to eat well, now you will need a planned approach. You may improve your appetite by experimenting with different ways of preparing and serving food. Choose foods high in calories and proteins, so you can get maximum energy and avoid losing weight (which will cause weakness).

If you don't seem to be making progress, you might ask your doctor about medications that can stimulate your appetite, such as
◆ Megace
◆ Marinol, a legally available synthetic form of THC (the active ingredient in marijuana) in capsule form. It is usually used as an antinausea drug, but it also stimulates the appetite. Some states legally allow marijuana to be used to reduce nausea symptoms for patients receiving chemotherapy under the supervision of their physician.

Tips for reducing loss of appetite are found under "Helpful Hints for Better Nutrition" in Chapter 16. Also, choose from the high-calorie/high-protein small meal or snack ideas in that chapter.

ABNORMALITIES IN SMELL AND TASTE PERCEPTION

Abnormalities in smell and taste perception are common, especially for those who have received radiation therapy to the neck and mouth area. "Taste blindness," or an altered sense of taste and smell, is a temporary condition that occurs when the tongue's lining and taste buds, or taste receptors, are altered by surgery, radiation therapy (especially of the head and neck) or chemotherapy or because of the cancer itself. The most common complaints are of food tasting too sweet or too bitter or of a continuous metallic taste or smell.

A loss of taste perception makes it more difficult to eat, which leads to weight loss. Taste loss tends to increase in proportion to the extent of tumor. With time and healing the sense of taste returns.

Often a strong aversion to certain tastes or foods follows an illness. Taste aversions may also be associated with chemotherapy, so avoid eating your favorite foods on the day you receive chemotherapy.

What You Can Do If Foods Taste Too Bitter
◆ Add sweet fruits to meals.
◆ Add honey or sweetener to foods and drinks.
◆ If meat tastes too bitter, eat it cold or at room temperature.
◆ In place of meat, eat blandly prepared chicken and fish, mild cheeses, eggs, dairy products or tofu. All of these foods may taste better when prepared in casseroles or stews.
◆ Marinating foods may make them taste better. Marinate meats or fish in pineapple juice, wine, Italian dressing, lemon juice, soy sauce or sweet-and-sour sauces.
◆ Mouth care can help. Brush your teeth several times a day, and use mouth rinses (water mixed with salt, hydrogen peroxide or baking soda, or diluted Cepacol or Chloraseptic).

What You Can Do If Foods Taste Too Sweet
◆ Gymnema Sylvestra, a herbal tea that is often used by professional wine tasters, will deaden the taste buds to sweet tastes for about 20 minutes if it is held in the mouth for about five minutes before eating.
◆ Dilute fruit juice or other sweet drinks with half water or ice.
◆ Avoid sweet fruits; vegetables may be more appealing.

What You Can Do If Foods Taste "Off"
◆ Drinking water, tea, ginger ale or fruit juices mixed with club soda may remove some of the strange tastes in your mouth. It might also help to munch on hard candies, such as sugar-free mints or Tic Tacs. Sugar-free gum or hard candies often reduce after-tastes.
◆ Add wine, beer, mayonnaise, sour cream or yogurt to soups and sauces to disguise the off tastes of other foods.
◆ Eat starchy foods such as bread, potatoes, rice and plain pasta. Do not add butter, margarine or other fatty substances to these foods.
◆ Choose bland foods. Eggs, cheeses (including cottage cheese), hot cereals, puddings, custards, tapioca, cream soups, toast, potatoes, rice and peanut butter are less likely to taste strange than foods with more distinctive flavors.

What You Can Do in General
◆ Eating in relaxed and pleasant surroundings can help reduce problems of taste blindness.
◆ You may have cravings for spicy and salty foods. Spicy, highly seasoned foods are irritating to many people. However, if your doctor does not advise against such foods, and if you can tolerate them, by all means satisfy such urges.
◆ Often flavorings such as herbs, spices or food seasonings may help. Also, acidic foods such as grapefruit may stimulate taste buds (but avoid them if they irritate your mouth).

◆ High-protein foods and supplements are particularly important when taste blindness prevents you from eating properly.

NAUSEA AND VOMITING

Nausea and vomiting are a frequent side effect of cancer therapy. They can also be brought on by an obstruction in the intestine, irritation of the gastrointestinal tract (gastritis) or brain tumors. (*See also* Chapter 18.)

Constant vomiting naturally makes it impossible for you to eat or take fluids, so whatever can be done to reduce nausea should be done before vomiting starts. Paying attention to psychological causes and using antinausea drugs and antianxiety and relaxing medications will help control symptoms.

Nausea and vomiting may begin one to three hours after treatment or even as long as two to four days later. You may start to fear therapy, a fear that can gnaw at you and make you want to avoid treatment. Nausea and vomiting may also make pain control and maintaining an overall good quality of life much harder to deal with. A wide variety of antinausea drugs are available to minimize or prevent the problem.

Anticipatory Nausea and Vomiting It is estimated that up to half of all people receiving chemotherapy experience some nausea or vomiting not after they receive the drugs but before their treatment. This is known as anticipatory nausea and vomiting (ANV) and it usually makes the nausea and vomiting even more severe when the chemotherapy is actually given. ANV can become such a set psychological pattern that the amount of chemotherapy that can be given must be reduced. And once the psychological pattern of ANV is established, it is much harder to control nausea and vomiting before and after treatment. (This behavior pattern was described 90 years ago by the Russian physiologist Pavlov and is referred to today as Pavlov's syndrome.)

The aim in chemotherapy is to deliver a therapeutic amount of drugs with the least side effects. But each chemotherapy agent and each drug combination has a potential for causing nausea and vomiting. Getting three or four drugs at a time, which is often the case, can make the reaction even more severe. The dosage and the number of cycles to be given also contribute to the reaction.

You, your family and even your friends should talk with your doctor about the type of chemotherapy you will be getting. For each drug or drug combination, a program should be established that allows you some control over the situation. With psychological factors playing such a big part, it is very important that you be a participant in preventing nausea and vomiting.

Your anxiety state, how you feel about yourself and your cancer and how you respond to stress and disease are all important factors in setting up this psychological pattern. And once the pattern is established, all kinds of stimuli can trigger feelings of nausea: the colors or smells in the room where the chemotherapy is given, the smell of rubbing alcohol used to prepare you for the IV needle, the sight of the nurse entering the room or even the sight of the hospital.

What You Can Do To deal with this problem, you will have to take steps both to relax before your chemotherapy and to not inadvertently set up situations that become associated with nausea. Some patients benefit from meditation, psychological support and aversion training (through media such as audiotapes to help prevent fear and nausea). Here are some other suggestions.

◆ Try to relax in a quiet, darkened room before your treatment sessions.

Negative Talk	Positive and Supportive Talk
◆ I'm too tired or weak to eat	◆ I'll feel stronger after my frozen dinner. It will take only 3 minutes to microwave.
◆ I'm already nauseated, I don't want to eat.	◆ Having light foods in my stomach (crackers, jello, apple juice) may help me to feel better.
◆ I'm eating as much as I can and haven't gained a pound.	◆ Have patience, it takes time to gain weight. Just keep on eating high-calorie foods every few hours.
◆ I'm sick. I can always eat more tomorrow.	◆ Do the best I can do today. I'm in control of this aspect of my life.
◆ My medication has caused me to gain a lot of weight. I'm not going to eat today.	◆ Eating low-fat food will prevent weight gain and eating the right foods will help me to fight my illness.

◆ Use behavioral techniques to help you relax and control any triggering stimuli: hypnosis, relaxation therapy, imagery or listening to a tape of your favorite music or a relaxation tape.

◆ Perhaps try acupuncture or acupressure, which have been effective in controlling nausea and vomiting in some cases.

◆ The time of day when you get treatment can sometimes make a difference. If you usually get nauseated in either the morning or the afternoon, try to change your appointment schedule.

◆ Avoid eating hot, spicy foods or other dishes that might upset your stomach or gastrointestinal tract. Replace fluids and electrolytes. Drink extra fluids before a chemotherapy treatment to help your body get rid of chemotherapy byproducts.

◆ Avoid eating for at least two hours before your treatment. Eat foods that are easily digested (high-carbohydrate, low-fat). Take a snack with you to treatment. If you experience "dry heaves," you may be able to get relief by eating something light, such as crackers or dry toast, before your therapy. Pregnancy antinausea programs can provide helpful suggestions.

◆ Eat and drink slowly. Do not force foods past the point of tolerance. Eat smaller, more frequent meals. Take clear, cool foods and chilled drinks at first, especially apple and cranberry juices, fruit drinks such as Kool-Aid and Gatorade, ginger ale and 7-Up, Jell-O, tea or iced tea.

◆ Popsicles, salty foods, soda crackers and toast are often well tolerated. Avoid overly sweet, greasy, hot or spicy foods and foods with strong aromas, as they often aggravate nausea. Food served chilled or at room temperature may be more appealing.

◆ Avoid cooking odors that may bring on nausea by having friends or family prepare your meals at their own homes and bring them over to you, or order in from a restaurant. To reduce the smell of beverages, drink them through a straw.

◆ Always avoid your favorite foods when you are getting chemotherapy. You might start to associate these foods with treatment, nausea and vomiting and develop a strong aversion to them.

Medications Two areas in the brain have been identified as being responsible for nausea and vomiting, and certain drugs and other methods can selectively block these areas. Your doctor can work out a program to combat your nausea, although if one drug or drug combination doesn't work as well as you would both like, you may have to experiment with various programs.

Generally, antivomiting drugs (antiemetics) should be taken 30 minutes before chemotherapy so that they have time to take effect.

◆ If vomiting has already started and you cannot keep a pill down, antinausea suppositories such as Compazine or Tigan may help.

◆ Long-acting capsules such as Compazine Spansules can be very helpful, since they work for 6 to 12 hours.

◆ Ativan (lorazepam) and Decadron (dexamethasone), both sedatives, may help block the brain's vomiting center. This is also a powerful combination for blocking anticipatory nausea and vomiting. Ativan can be taken under the tongue for rapid absorption during severe nausea. Xanax (alprazolam), another sedative, may also help to reduce anxiety.

◆ Ativan is an antidepressant, antianxiety and sleeping tablet that can cause amnesia, which might take the edge off any memory of vomiting once the episode is over.

◆ Some forms of marijuana—the natural tetrahydrocannabinol (THC) and the synthetic Marinol—may control nausea and vomiting. However, they can also cause drowsiness, dry mouth, dizziness, a rapid heartbeat and sweating. The use of marijuana to alleviate cancer therapy side effects is legal in some states.

◆ Granisetron (Kytril), ondansetron (Zofran) and dolasetron mesylate (Anzemet) are the most significant new drugs used to control nausea and vomiting caused by intensive chemotherapy and radiotherapy. They may be needed when you are receiving highest-potential chemotherapy drugs or when you cannot get relief with other antinausea agents. They are often given with Decadron IV. They suppress vomiting in 60 to 80 percent of patients and are even more effective in combination with other antinausea drugs. Kytril lasts longer, often for one day.

SORE MOUTH AND THROAT

A sore or ulcerated mouth or throat is a frequent side effect of chemotherapy or radiation therapy to the head and neck area. This condition will clear up in a few days, unless your recovery is slowed by malnutrition. (If symptoms persist, consult your physician; you may have an infection such as monilia, also known as thrush.)

The lining, or mucosa, of the gastrointestinal tract, which includes the inside of the mouth and throat, is one of the most sensitive areas of the body. Many chemotherapy drugs can inflame the lining, a condition called mucositis. Many drugs can also cause small ulcerations or sores to develop. Radiation delivered to the head and neck can irritate the lining and cause sores, and so can mouth or throat infections, especially fungus infections like monilia (thrush). All these can be very painful or at least uncomfortable.

Oral Hygiene Mouth care is very important when you have mucositis. You will have to make sure your mouth stays clean and moist and that you eat the proper foods and get medication for any infection that develops.

A good oral hygiene program includes dental cleaning and scaling, followed by daily brushing and flossing to reduce plaque.

Any scaling, cleaning, tooth extractions or repair of cavities should be done before your cancer therapy begins. Extractions especially should be completed at least two weeks before therapy to give your mouth a chance to heal. Ill-fitting dentures should be fixed or replaced. Any periodontal or dental work has to be coordinated with your oncologist.

Before any dental work is to be performed, your blood counts should be checked to be sure that your body can take care of any infection or bleeding (low white cell counts can lead to infections, and a low platelet count may lead to bleeding). If you have any mouth injury because of a dental procedure, antibiotics are recommended.

The following daily steps will help your mouth stay in good shape:

◆ Use a soft-bristle toothbrush and soften it more by soaking it in warm water. You may find that brushing with a paste of baking soda and water is less irritating than commercial toothpaste.

◆ If brushing your teeth is painful, use either a cotton swab or Toothettes, a sponge-tip stick impregnated with a dentifrice.

◆ Avoid commercial mouthwashes. Some of these have ingredients (especially alcohol) that can irritate your mouth even more. Lemon glycerin swabs may make your mouth feel clean but they are *not recommended*, because glycerin can dehydrate and will make your mouth drier.

◆ A Water-Pik to cleanse your mouth is helpful.

◆ Peridex (oral rinse) will help gum inflammation and bleeding.

What You Can Do If You Have Mucositis
If the soreness in your mouth becomes severe, there are quite a few anesthetic agents you can use on a short-term basis. If your symptoms persist, you should have a complete dental hygienic evaluation. There is an increased risk of mucositis for those who wear dentures or tooth devices, who have a history of oral lesions (herpes, canker sores, monilia or gum infections) or who smoke.

◆ Benadryl elixir, lozenges and analgesics may help reduce mouth pain.

◆ Swishing and swallowing the anesthetic jelly viscous Xylocaine or Hurricane (benzocaine) can help you eat if you have pain in your mouth, pharynx or esophagus. Gargle with 1 tbsp. (15 mL) viscous lidocaine before meals. Also available are a spray and a liquid to put directly on sore spots.

◆ Frequent use of a gentle mouthwash may help reduce the discomfort or pain. A solution of baking soda and salt dissolved in warm water should be used instead of commercial mouthwashes, which may be irritating to the oral mucosa.

◆ Swish diluted milk of magnesia, Carafate slurry or Mylanta around your mouth.

◆ Orabase, with or without Kenalog, is a dental salve that covers mouth sores while they are healing. You may have to apply it several times a day.

◆ GI Cocktail

1 tbsp. (15 mL)	Cherry Maalox
1 tsp. (5 mL)	Nystatin
½ tsp. (2 mL)	Hurricane Liquid original flavor

Mix ingredients thoroughly. Swish and gargle for one minute, and then swallow, immediately before each meal.

Infections Mouth infections can be dangerous. Examine your mouth every day for any irritation or early fungus growth (white spots inside your mouth that don't wash off). Look under your tongue and at the sides of your mouth and report any changes to your doctor. If you do get an infection, it should be treated promptly.

◆ If you have a herpes virus—acute or recurrent—your doctor may prescribe oral acyclovir tablets or cream.

◆ Monilia requires antifungal agents, such as Mycostatin (nystatin) oral suspension, Mycelex Troches, Mycostat Pastilles, Nizoral (ketoconazole) tablets, Diflucan (fluconazole) capsules, fluconazole oral solution, Fungizone (amphotericin) or Sporanox (itraconazole) oral solution.

◆ You can freeze nystatin liquid in medicine cups or ice cube trays and let it melt in your mouth.

Nutrition A normal high-protein, high-calorie diet with supplements as needed will help your sore mouth or tongue heal faster. Drinking lots of fluids will also help with healing as well as help make your mouth sores more comfortable.

A high-calorie, high-protein diet includes scrambled eggs, custards, milk-shakes, malts, gelatins, creamy hot cereals, macaroni and cheese and blenderized or pureed foods. Commercial supplements such as Ensure, Sustacal and Carnation Instant Breakfast Drink can be helpful.

Until your mouth sores heal, you should avoid
◆ very hot or very cold foods
◆ tomatoes and citrus fruits such as grapefruit, lemons and oranges, which can burn your mouth
◆ salty foods, which can cause a burning sensation
◆ hot, spicy, coarse or rough foods, including toast, dry crackers and potato chips
◆ alcoholic beverages and tobacco, which irritate the lining of the mouth
◆ any medications that contain alcohol, such as mouthwashes or cough syrups

Your diet should consist of soft, bland foods. Solid foods should be soft or cooked until tender. A liquid diet or a pureed diet may be needed if you find solid food too irritating. Frequent small meals served warm or at room temperature will be more tolerable.

Foods especially well tolerated are: applesauce, cool or room temperature drinks, cooked cereal, strained cream soup, custard and puddings, soft-cooked eggs, plain ice cream, sherbet, Jell-O, milk-shakes, mashed potatoes and popsicles.

Dry Mouth (Xerostomia) Saliva serves many functions. It initiates the digestion of starch. It mixes with food to form a bolus that can be swallowed. And it is the first line of defense to protect the teeth from oral bacteria. Radiation therapy to the head and neck area affects the salivary glands. Saliva production is decreased, and saliva becomes thicker, resulting in a dry mouth, a condition called xerostomia. This can interfere with chewing and swallowing or simply be an uncomfortable sensation. This may be temporary, but if doses exceed 4,000 cGy, you may be left with some degree of permanent dryness.

What You Can Do If You Have Dry Mouth Choose foods with a high liquid content, such as
◆ applesauce
◆ custard, puddings
◆ hard candies, especially sugar-free lemon drops
◆ ice cream, sorbet
◆ most fruits
◆ water (add lemon juice)
◆ yogurt, cottage cheese

Tips for Moistening Foods
◆ Add gravies, sauces, melted butter or margarine, broth or salad dressing.
◆ Dunk breads or other baked goods in your beverage.
◆ Drink generous amounts of nutritious liquids with meals. You may find that you eat less because you fill up on the liquid. Add lemon juice to water.
◆ Suck on sugar-free hard candy (such as Tic Tacs) or chew sugar-free gum. This may help to stimulate saliva production. Avoid sweet products, since your teeth have lost the natural protection that saliva provides. You can also suck on popsicles or flavored or plain ice cubes.
◆ Artificial saliva products may be help-

ful. Ask your physician, dentist or speech therapist about these.

◆ Salagan (pilocarpine) is a medication in pill form that increases saliva production.

◆ Commercial preparations such as Moi-Stir and MouthKot, an oral saliva substitute, or Oral Balance, a moisturizing gel, may help.

◆ Use a special dry-mouth toothpaste such as Biotene.

◆ Make your own mouthwash with liquid lidocaine (Xylocaine), baking soda and salt dissolved in 1 quart (1 L) of water, or mix 1 quart water and 1 tsp. (5 mL) salt and 1 tbsp. (15 mL) baking soda.

◆ Use lip balms, chapsticks or lipstick if your lips are dry.

SWALLOWING DIFFICULTIES

Bernadette Festa Bell, MS, RD, CNSD, *and Jillian Chelson*, MSCCC, SLP

Difficulty swallowing may be a result of surgery to the mouth and throat, radiation therapy or generalized weakness. The severity of your swallowing problem will vary depending on the type of surgery you have had and whether you have undergone radiation therapy. You may experience only temporary discomfort due to pain and swelling or more severe problems requiring supplementation by tube feeding until your ability to swallow is restored. If your swallowing difficulties are minor and you feel you can manage them without a swallowing therapist, the following suggestions might help.

WHAT YOU CAN DO

If swallowing difficulties prevent you from eating your normal meals, eat frequent small meals and snacks to ensure that you get enough calories. Choose soft foods or foods that can be cooked until tender. This will make chewing and swallowing easier. Many people find liquid nutritional supplements in addition to their meals an easy way to get all the protein and calories they need.

Cut the foods into bite-sized pieces or grind them so that less chewing is required. If you are having trouble using your tongue to move the food from the front to the back of your mouth, or to move food around inside your mouth, moisten foods with gravies, sauces or yogurt.

If you continue to have trouble swallowing (coughing, choking, changes in breathing, frustration with eating) or experience weight loss, ask your doctor for a referral to a swallowing therapist.

SWALLOWING TRAINING PROGRAM

If your swallowing difficulties are more severe, you may need a swallowing training program to relearn how to swallow safely and comfortably. The basic components of this program are (1) proper food consistency, (2) proper positioning of body and head, (3) specific, prescribed swallowing techniques, and (4) appropriate feeding methods.

Food Consistency The consistency of your food will be critical to your success. Ideally, a team that includes a dietitian, a swallowing therapist and your physician will choose the type of food and consistency most appropriate for you. Their evaluation will take into account your ability to move and feel the structures of your mouth, to cough, to clear your throat and to handle secretions.

While relearning how to swallow, you will need to progress from those foods that are easier to swallow to those that are most difficult. For many people, thin liquids are the most difficult because of the highly complex coordinated movements and sensory perception required to swallow them. The following list gives some examples of food consistencies that may be prescribed for you.

Foods That Tend Not to Fall Apart in the Mouth applesauce, avocados, banana, custard, egg dishes, ground foods with sauces or gravies, hot cereal, mashed potatoes, puddings, most pureed foods, quiches, soft vegetables with sauces, soufflés, tapioca

Foods That Fall Apart in the Mouth crackers, dry breads, dry cereals, meats, nuts and seeds, rice, raw vegetables

Liquids

Thin alcohol, broth, coffee or tea, Ensure or Sustacal, hot chocolate, ice cream, juices, Jell-O, milk, popsicles, sherbet, soda, water

Semithick blenderized or cream soups, buttermilk, Ensure or Sustacal (or equivalent supplement with 2 tbsp./25 mL thickening agent such as Thicken-up), milkshakes, nectars, tomato juice, V-8 juice

Thick Ensure or Sustacal (or equivalent supplement with 3 tbsp./50 mL thickening agent such as Thicken-up), pureed fruit, thickened shakes, thickened thin liquids

Solid Diets for Swallowing Difficulties Solid food diets vary in consistency; there are four levels. Your swallowing therapist or dietitian will help you choose the right level for your needs. In most cases, the principle is to eat foods that do not fall apart when placed on the tongue. Other people may need to eat food that is smooth and nonfibrous. Still others may only be able to drink their nutrition. It will all depend on your specific type of swallowing problem.

Level 1—Pureed baby foods; blenderized cottage cheese; cream of wheat or rice; custard; mashed potatoes; puddings; pureed fruits and vegetables; pureed meats, fish and beans; pureed soft-cooked egg; thinned plain yogurt

Level 2—Ground custards; finely chopped pasta; ground meats; junior baby foods; macaroni and cheese; moist cakes; pancakes in bite-sized pieces; soft canned fruits in bite-sized pieces; soft moist scrambled eggs; soups without chunks; vegetables in bite-sized pieces

Avoid nuts, seeds, skins and connective tissue on fruits and in meats.

Level 3—Chopped beans; boiled eggs; breads without crust, seeds or nuts; casseroles; chopped tender cuts of meat, poultry and fish; cooked cereals; corn flakes and puffed rice; french toast; fresh peeled fruits in bite-sized pieces; omelets; pasta dishes; peanut butter; potatoes without skin; puddings; soft-cooked vegetables in bite-sized pieces; waffles

Level 4—Soft-textured breads without seeds, nuts or dried fruit; all cheeses; all cooked cereals; dry cereal without nuts or dried fruit; cooked fruits and vegetables; cream soups; eggs; raw fruits and vegetables without skins or seeds; whole moist tender meats, fish and poultry

Amount and Pacing In most cases, foods should be eaten in small bites (1/2 tsp/2 mL/). Sometimes a larger amount (say, 1–2 tsp/5–10 mL) will provide the sensation required to swallow. Be careful when you experiment with sizes. Until you are once again proficient at swallowing, eat with someone nearby.

Completely swallow each bite before taking another bite. "Feel" or look to see if the food has cleared the mouth. "Sense" whether food has cleared the throat.

Do you feel or see any food in the mouth? Do you feel food stuck in your throat? If you answer yes to either of these questions, attempt dry swallows until no food pieces can be seen or felt.

Hydrating the Mouth A dry mouth can make it difficult and even impossible to swallow. There are a few tricks for hydrating, or moistening, the mouth and increasing saliva. Use popsicles, hard sugarless candy or crushed ice or take frequent sips of water throughout the day. You can buy artificial saliva products such as Salivart at a drugstore. When saliva production is a problem, choose sour foods, which increase saliva, and avoid sweet foods, which decrease saliva production. Always be sure that you are capable of swallowing your own saliva and thin liquids.

Positioning of Body and Head The proper position can often markedly reduce swallowing difficulties. In the beginning, eat without the distraction of conversation or noise so that you can concentrate on the swallowing process. The standard position for swallowing is sitting as upright as possible with the hips at a right angle to the body. Sit in a firm chair, preferably one with a high back so you can place a pillow behind your head. Place your feet on the floor or another firm surface.

After you swallow, tilt your chin down toward the chest to close off the trachea (windpipe) and help prevent food moving into the lungs, which can cause pneumonia.

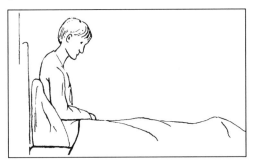

If you have to eat in bed, sit up and use a wedge-shaped cushion behind your back to achieve as upright a position as possible. If you are in a hospital bed, put the head of the bed in a full upright position. Never eat lying down or in a reclining position unless your swallowing therapist has suggested these positions.

The position of your head is also important to effective and safe swallowing. Your swallowing therapist will prescribe the best head position for your particular swallowing problem.

FEEDING METHODS

The following feeding methods may be helpful while you are relearning to swallow and to manipulate foods of different consistencies. Be patient with yourself during all stages of your swallowing rehabilitation.

◆ Never rush feeding. Time and patience are needed on your part and on the part of your caregiver.

◆ Always make sure your mouth, tongue and teeth are brushed and clean before you start to eat.

◆ After eating, sit upright for at least 20 minutes.

◆ Do the exercises for lips, tongue, jaw and swallow response that may be prescribed by your swallowing therapist. Do these four to eight times a day. The more frequently you do them, the faster you will recover.

You may wish to keep a record of your progress. The goal of your training program is to be able to swallow safely and enjoy your normal diet. By achieving this goal, you will help achieve another vital goal, a highly nutritious diet, which is crucial to your healing.

See also Swallowing Training Program recipes, page 222 to 226.

HEARTBURN, REFLUX AND INDIGESTION

Over one million people experience heartburn, which commonly is caused by acid reflux (the movement of acid from the stomach into the esophagus). Heartburn is a sensation of burning or pressure in the upper stomach and the esophagus. It can cause an inflammation of the esophagus called esophagitis.

Indigestion, an uncomfortable feeling in the abdomen after eating, is usually caused by eating too much or by eating foods that are too spicy or too fatty. Indigestion may also accompany stress, constipation, bloating or eating when you have no appetite.

What You Can Do about Heartburn

◆ Avoid spicy, acidic, tomato-based or fatty foods such as citrus fruits, fruit juices and chocolate.
◆ Limit your intake of tea, alcohol, colas and coffee, including decaffeinated versions of these.
◆ Stop or at least reduce smoking.
◆ Watch your weight. Obesity causes an increase in intra-abdominal pressure, which can aggravate reflux.
◆ Eat small, frequent meals.
◆ Avoid strenuous exercising too soon after eating.
◆ Walk around after meals rather than sitting down.
◆ Avoid bedtime snacks. Eat meals at least three or four hours before lying down.
◆ Elevate the head of your bed with 4 to 6 in. (10 to 15 cm) of blocks to help gravity drain stomach and gastric acids. Or use several pillows to elevate your head when you are lying down or sleeping.

Medication for Heartburn An antacid taken one or two hours after meals and at bedtime may provide relief. If heartburn is excessive or recurrent, consult your doctor about stomach-acid blocking medicines such as Tagamet, Zantac, Pepcid, Axid, Prilosec, Prevacid and Propulsid. Over-the-counter antacids include Maalox, Mylanta, Gaviscon, Tums and Gelucil.

What You Can Do about Indigestion

Again, frequent small meals and a bland diet can be helpful. In general, avoid overeating and avoid foods you have found cause you indigestion.

Medication for Indigestion An antacid taken one or two hours after meals may help relieve discomfort. Antispasmodic drugs such as Donnatal block acid production in the stomach.

ESOPHAGITIS

Esophagitis—inflammation of the lining of the esophagus, the tube leading from the throat to the stomach—may be a side effect of chemotherapy or radiation therapy to the head and neck area, or may occasionally occur because of infection.

What You Can Do The recommended dietary approach is similar to that used with a sore or ulcerated mouth or throat (*see* above). In general, eat slowly and only small amounts at a time.

Medication Any medications should be prescribed by your physician. You might ask your doctor about gargling with and swallowing an analgesic solution such as liquid or viscous Xylocaine before meals to lessen irritation. A similar solution may be made by dissolving 1 tbsp. (15 mL) baking soda and 1 tsp. (5 mL) salt in 1 quart (1 L) warm water. Use 2 to 4 tbsp. (25 to 50 mL) before each meal. Systemic analgesics such as Tylenol or codeine may be needed to relieve pain. Carafate (sucralfate) Suspension may reduce symptoms and discomfort and help healing by coating the esophagus.

If symptoms persist, a candida (monilial-fungal) infection may be present, which can be effectively treated with ketoconazole (Nizoral), nystatin (Mycostatin), fluconazole (Diflucan), amphotericin (Fungizone), itraconazole (Sporanox) or Mycelex.

EARLY FILLING AND BLOATING

A common problem during radiation therapy or chemotherapy is early filling—a feeling of being full after having taken only a few bites of food.

Bloating may be defined as an over-full feeling occurring after eating, often after just a few bites. Bloating is due to the inability of the stomach and intestines to properly digest the food you eat. It may also occur because of a slowdown of the passage of food from one part of the intestines to another, which may be caused by nervousness and tension; anticancer drugs, narcotics, strong pain-relieving and other medications; lack of adequate exercise, or constipation. Bloating may also be related to the type of food you eat. Fatty, fried and greasy foods tend to remain in the stomach longer and may cause you to feel full. Carbonated drinks, gas-producing foods and milk may also cause bloating.

What You Can Do Eat frequent small meals instead of three large meals a day and emphasize sweet or starchy foods and low-fat protein foods. Sit up or walk around after meals.

Avoid fatty, fried and greasy foods, gas-producing vegetables (such as dried beans and peas, broccoli, brussels sprouts, cabbage, cauliflower, corn, cucumber, green peppers, sauerkraut, turnips and winter squash), carbonated drinks, chewing gum and milk. Stir carbonated drinks to remove gas bubbles.

Medications Mylanta Gas Tablets (simethicone) help relieve and reduce symptoms of excess gas.

DIARRHEA

Diarrhea is a condition marked by abnormally frequent bowel movements that are more fluid than usual. It is sometimes accompanied by cramps. You may get diarrhea because of chemotherapy, radiation therapy to the lower abdomen, malabsorption because of surgery to the bowel or sometimes a bowel inflammation or infection. Some antibiotics, especially broad-spectrum antibiotics, can cause diarrhea. Diarrhea may also develop because of an intolerance to milk (*see* "Milk (Lactose) Intolerance" below), difficulty in absorbing fats, sensitivity to a specific food or group of foods, food allergy or emotional or psychological problems.

Treatment Effective treatment depends on finding the cause. A general approach is to limit your diet solely to fluids to allow the bowel to rest. Drink plenty of mild liquids, such as fruit drinks (Kool-Aid and Gatorade), ginger ale, peach or apricot nectar, water and weak tea. Hot and cold liquids and foods tend to increase intestinal muscle contractions and make the diarrhea worse, so they should be warm or at room temperature. Allow carbonated beverages to lose their fizz or stir them before you drink them. Inform your physician, nutritionist or health care team if you are on this diet longer than one day.

When you are feeling better, gradually add foods low in roughage and bulk. Examples include steamed rice, cream of rice, bananas, applesauce, mashed potatoes and dry toast and crackers. These foods should be eaten warm or at room temperature.

As your diarrhea decreases, you may move on to a low-residue diet (*see* Chapter 19). Frequent small meals will be easier on your digestive tract.

Foods to Avoid Many types of foods are likely to aggravate your diarrhea and should be avoided. These include

- fatty, greasy and spicy foods
- coffee, regular (not herbal) teas and carbonated drinks containing caffeine
- citrus fruits such as oranges and grapefruit
- popcorn, nuts and raw vegetables and fruits (except apples)
- drinks and foods that are served too hot or too cold

What You Can Do

- Talk to your physician and other health team members to determine the cause of the problem. It may be due to a variety of causes as mentioned above, including an intestinal blockage, antibiotics or the cancer.
- Diarrhea can cause dehydration, so you will have to drink plenty of fluids. (*See* "Clear Liquid Diet" in Chapter 19.) When you have diarrhea, food passes through the gut more quickly, so many nutrients are not absorbed. You also lose electrolytes, which are vital to the fluid balance of your body. To replace the fluid, sugar and salt you will lose, a good general formula is: 1 quart (1 L) boiled water, 1 tsp. (5 mL) salt, 1 tsp. (5 mL) baking soda, 4 tsp. (20 mL) sugar and flavor to your taste. As with any specially prepared concoction, however, check with your dietitian or doctor to make sure you can tolerate the ingredients.
- Potassium is lost in diarrhea. It is a necessary mineral and must be replaced. Foods high in potassium include bananas, apricot and peach nectars, tomatoes, potatoes, broccoli, asparagus, citrus juices and milk. A potassium supplement may be needed if diarrhea persists.
- Gatorade may be useful for replacing fluid, potassium and electrolytes.

- Try the BRAT diet: bananas, rice, applesauce, tea and toast.
- Eat foods that are high in protein and calories.
- Reduce your intake of foods that are high in roughage and residue.
- Talk with your dietitian about ways to improve your diet.
- Ileostomy and colostomy diarrhea may be severe enough to require specific medical and dietary treatment and foods.
- An antidiarrhea medication such as Kaopectate, Imodium or Lomotil may be prescribed.

Diarrhea Medications for Radiation Therapy

- Kaopectate (30 cc to 60 cc after each loose bowel movement)
- Lomotil (one or two tablets every two to six hours as needed to a maximum of eight tablets a day; most patients require only two or three tablets per day after the diarrhea has been controlled.
- Imodium (two tablets initially followed by one tablet after each loose stool, not to exceed 16 tablets per day); Imodium is also available in liquid or tablet form without a prescription.
- Donnatal (one or two tablets every four hours for abdominal cramping).
- Paregoric (1 tsp./5 mL every four hours) (requires a physician's triplicate prescription.)
- Tincture of opium is very successful for severe uncontrollable diarrhea (requires a physician's triplicate prescription)
- For severe diarrhea, octreotide (Sandostatin) injections can be helpful.

Milk (Lactose) Intolerance Lactose intolerance can sometimes develop after intestinal surgery, radiation therapy to the lower abdomen or chemotherapy. Some people are also born with lactose intolerance or develop it later. The intolerance results from a deficiency of lactase, an enzyme that digests milk sugar (lactose) in the intestine, and is marked by bloating, cramping and diarrhea.

◆ If your diarrhea is caused by lactose intolerance, avoid milk and milk products such as ice cream, cottage cheese and cheese. Depending on how sensitive you are to milk, you may also have to avoid butter, cream and sour cream.

◆ If you are very sensitive, use lactose-free, nonfat milk solids or soy milk.

◆ You can make your own lactose-free milk by adding Lactaid—a tablet containing lactase—to your milk and keeping it in the refrigerator for 24 hours before drinking it.

◆ You can use buttermilk and yogurt because the lactose in them has already been processed and is easily digested.

◆ You might tolerate some processed cheeses.

◆ Try Mocha-mix, Dairy Rich and other soy products, or some lactose substitutes like Imo (an imitation sour cream), Cool Whip and Party Whip.

◆ *See* the "Lactose-Free/Lactose-Restricted Diet" in Chapter 19.

CONSTIPATION

Constipation may be defined as infrequent bowel movements, compared with your normal pattern. It is often accompanied by decreased appetite and a bloated feeling. It commonly results from inadequate fiber or bulk-forming foods in the diet, not drinking enough fluid, emotional stress or lack of exercise.

Constipation may be caused by some chemotherapy neurotoxic drugs such as vincristine, vinblastine and vinorelbine. Other drugs that are constipating include pain-relieving narcotics such as morphine and codeine, gastrointestinal antispasmodics, antidepressants, diuretics, tranquilizers, sleeping pills and calcium- and aluminum-based antacids.

When prescribing these drugs, your doctor should anticipate the need for a stool softener or a laxative. Enemas or suppositories might also be needed.

What You Can Do Add foods to your diet that are high in fiber and bulk, such as fresh fruit and vegetables, dried fruit, dried beans, whole-grain breads, cereals and bran. If you are not used to eating these foods, proceed slowly. A product such as Beano may help eliminate the bloating sometimes associated with eating these foods.

◆ Drink plenty of liquids.

◆ A glass of prune juice or hot lemon water taken in the morning may help.

◆ Eat fresh fruits and vegetables, leaving on the peel. (Raw fruits and vegetables must be avoided when the white blood cell count is lower than 1,500 and absolute neutrophil count is less than 1,000.)

◆ Eat cooked dried beans and peas such as lentils, split peas and kidney, garbanzo and lima beans.

◆ Eat whole-grain products–cereals such as bran cereals or shredded wheat, foods made with whole-grain flours, other whole grains such as bulgur and wheat berries.

◆ Add unprocessed wheat bran to homemade breads, cereals, pancakes, casseroles and baked goods.

◆ Add bran to your diet. Start with 2 tsp. (10 mL) per day. Increase your fluid intake when you eat bran, as bran works by absorbing fluid, increasing stools and promoting a bowel movement.

◆ Exercise routinely. Your doctor or physical therapist can help design a program for you (*see* Chapter 21).

◆ Check with your doctor before taking any medications.

Medication Laxatives and enemas are sometimes needed in addition to these other measures, but should be used only under the direction of your physician. Many types of laxatives are available; your physician and other health care team members will help you find the best one to fit your specific situation.

Patients requiring narcotics should not take bulk-forming laxatives because the combination causes constipation; stool softeners may be used instead. Certain other laxatives, when used continually, irritate the digestive tract and often make it difficult to regain normal bowel habits once they are discontinued. Increasing doses may also make your colon and rectum insensitive to the normal reflexes that stimulate a bowel movement.

Don't try to diagnose and treat yourself, since there may be more to the situation than you realize. For example, diarrhea can occasionally develop at the same time as a stool impaction, with the liquid stools moving around the impaction. If you take antidiarrheal drugs, you can make their situation much worse.

◆ Stool softeners help the stool retain water and so keep it soft. Stool softeners such as Colace (docusate) should be used early, before the stools become hard, especially as it can be days before any effect is noticeable.

◆ Mild laxatives help promote bowel activity. Examples are milk of magnesia, Doxidan, cascara sagrada and mineral oil (a lubricant).

◆ Stronger laxatives include Phospho-soda (Fleet's), magnesium citrate and sennoside (Senokot).

◆ Contact laxatives, such as castor oil, glycerin suppositories and Dulcolax suppositories or tablets, cause increased bowel activity. (Dulcolax may cause cramping.)

◆ Bulk laxatives include dietary fiber, bran, methyl cellulose (Cellothyl) and psyllium (Metamucil).

◆ Laxatives with magnesium should be avoided if you have kidney disease. (Laxatives that contain magnesium can also cause diarrhea.) Laxatives with sodium should be avoided if you have a heart problem.

◆ If you are taking narcotics, use stool softeners and mild or strong laxatives rather than bulk-forming laxatives, because the combination can cause high colon constipation. A good prescription is Colace and Senokot.

◆ Nonstimulating bulk softeners such as Colace help to soften the stool, and mineral oil or olive oil can be used to loosen the stool.

◆ Bowel stimulants such as Reglan may be useful.

◆ Lactulose (Chronulac) has an osmotic effect, drawing water into the gut to soften the stools and stimulate an increase in the number of bowel movements. This is usually effective and well tolerated.

Treating Stool Impaction A stool impaction develops when all of a stool doesn't pass through the colon or rectum. The stool gradually gets harder as the bowel absorbs water, and then it gets larger. If you cannot pass it, it may partly obstruct the bowel or irritate the rectum or anus. If you do pass it, it may cause small tears or fissures in the anus. You may need to see a proctologist (rectal specialist).

The primary treatment is to get fluids into the bowel to soften the stool so it can be passed or removed. Using enemas—oil-based, tap or saline water, or phosphate (Fleet's)—may help accomplish this goal. Sometimes it might be necessary for a health professional to use a gloved finger in the rectum to break up and extract a large stool or to give you a high warm saline colonic enema.

MALABSORPTION
Cancer sometimes results in food not being absorbed normally from the intestines into the bloodstream. For example, a decrease in the digestive juices that regulate absorption may be caused by cancer of the pancreas, the organ that produces many of these juices.

If you decrease your normal food intake, the intestines become unable to absorb nutrients as they did before. A healthy gastrointestinal tract requires food to stimulate it and maintain it in a healthy state. When you resume eating, bloating or diarrhea occur, and your ability to correct this cycle by eating lessens as your nutrition becomes poorer. So to keep your gastrointestinal tract healthy, you must eat, even though you don't feel like it.

DEHYDRATION

Dehydration is a lack of fluid in the body. It may occur after surgery, radiation or chemotherapy, or as a result of diarrhea, sweating, fever, nausea or an inability to drink fluids.

What You Can Do Try different drinks, or foods that become liquid in the stomach: juice, fruit drinks such as Kool-Aid and Gatorade, punch, soft drinks, decaffeinated tea, milk, milkshakes, eggnogs, soup, low-salt broth, fruits with a high fluid content such as grapes or watermelon, jelly desserts, ice cream, sherbet, fruit ices and popsicles. (*See* Chapter 20 for high-protein, high-calorie beverages.)

WATER RETENTION

The body may retain excess salt and water in the arms or legs because of removal of or radiation of the lymph glands, which filter excess fluid from body tissues. Water retention may also occur in the abdomen, chest, head or neck because of cancer therapy or the cancer itself. Hormonal drugs, such as cortisone, prednisone, testosterone and estrogens, also cause the body to retain excess salt and water.

What You Can Do Decrease your intake of salt, because salt causes you to retain fluids. There are two levels of salt-restricted diets, one allowing a small amount of salt, the other restricting salt severely.

Low-Salt Diet This diet restricts sodium to about 2 to 3 grams a day, the equivalent of 1 to 1½ tsp. (5 to 7 mL) salt. Do not add any salt to food while it is being cooked, and (depending on your diet) add only a very small amount to food at the table. Foods vary in their natural salt content. Ask your dietitian for guidance.

Salt substitutes such as Co-Salt, Morton's Salt Substitute and Adolph's Salt Substitute will help satisfy your need for a salty taste without adding to fluid-retention problems. Some salt substitutes taste better than others, and you may need to try several before finding the one that suits you best. Also, some contain sodium (which you are trying to avoid), so read the label carefully before you buy.

You must also read the labels on all foods you eat to avoid foods with naturally high salt content, such as
◆ bouillon and canned soups
◆ canned, cured and dry meat and fish, such as bacon, cold cuts, corned beef, canned herring and sardines
◆ salted crackers, nuts, potato chips, corn chips and other snack foods
◆ soy sauce, catsup and barbecue sauce
◆ cheeses (you may need to limit total dairy consumption)

Restricted-Salt Diet This diet restricts salt to about ½ gram a day, equivalent to ¼ tsp. (1 mL) salt. It requires the use of special milk, bread and other food products low in salt. Your physician will prescribe a special diet for you.

Medications Your physician may prescribe a diuretic, a drug that will cause you to lose excess fluid and salt through the urine.

Diuretics may cause you to lose too much potassium, a mineral important to body functioning. If you are taking diuretics, you may need to eat foods high in potassium such as apricots, bananas, cantaloupe, dates, dried figs, milk, orange juice, potatoes, prunes, raisins, tangerine juice and tomato juice. Your physician may suggest a potassium supplement.

KIDNEY STONES

Some drugs can cause patients to form

kidney stones. There may be no symptoms, or patients may have an ashen pallor combined with very severe back pain. The degree of pain depends on the amount of urine backed up behind the obstruction caused by the kidney stone.

If a stone is small enough to pass through the urinary tract, collect it and give it to your doctor. It is important that your doctor determine the type of kidney stone you have (uric acid or calcium oxalate) before a special diet is prescribed.

What You Can Do If You Have Calcium Oxalate Kidney Stones Take these steps to acidify the urine:
◆ Reduce intake of foods high in calcium, such as milk, cheese and other dairy products.
◆ Reduce intake of foods high in phosphate, such as dairy products, eggs, organ meats and whole grains.
◆ Reduce intake of foods high in oxalic acid, such as asparagus, spinach, cranberries, plums, tea, cocoa and coffee.
◆ Drink at least 10 to 12 glasses of water a day, unless the local water is "hard." Hard water contains more calcium and magnesium; substitute distilled water.
◆ Consider taking vitamin B_6 and magnesium supplements.
◆ See your dietitian to determine other diet changes.

What You Can Do If You Have Uric Acid Kidney Stones These are the most common type of kidney stone among those caused by chemotherapy. Take these steps to alkalinize the urine:
◆ Increase intake of alkaline-forming foods such as dairy products, fruits (especially dried fruits), vegetables (especially green beans and peas) and breads prepared with baking soda or baking powder.
◆ Reduce intake of meat, eggs, fish, poultry, cereals, breads, pasta, rice, cranberry juice, prune juice and plums.
◆ Your physician may prescribe al-lopurinol (Zyloprim) to prevent uric acid precipitates.

What You Can Do for All Types of Stones
◆ Drink large amounts of water—except "hard" (high-mineral-content) water—and fluids throughout the day and night. Aim for 12 glasses every 24 hours.
◆ Drink plenty of fluids with meals and snacks.
◆ Choose foods with a high water content.

WEIGHT LOSS

When you are being treated for cancer, it is important to try to maintain your desirable weight as closely as possible. (*See* Chapter 16 and the specific directions in this chapter for dealing with loss of appetite and various intestinal problems.) The key is to maintain adequate calorie and protein intake.

Cancer patients (like patients being treated for burns, stress or infections) may need up to 25 percent more calories than their body normally requires. Keep a daily record of your calorie and protein intake. If you are losing weight, increase your calorie intake until you are no longer losing weight. (*See* "High-Calorie/High-Protein Small Meal and Snack Ideas" in Chapter 16. It can be particularly helpful to develop a regular pattern of nibbling on high-calorie snacks.)

Here are some ideas you can use at home to add extra calories and proteins to your everyday cooking:
◆ Add cream, evaporated milk or fortified milk (*see* the recipe in Chapter 20) to cooked cereals, cream sauces, puddings and soups.
◆ Use sour cream on baked potatoes and in cream soups.
◆ Use gravies and sauces on meats and vegetables.
◆ Add extra butter or margarine to cooked cereals, noodles, rice, sauces, soups and vegetables.

◆ Add cheese or hard-cooked eggs to casseroles, noodles, rice or sauces.

◆ Spread peanut butter on apple wedges or celery, and in cookies, frostings and sandwich fillings.

See "Cooking with Nutritional Supplements" in Chapter 20 for ideas on adding high-protein and high-calorie supplements to your cooking.

WEIGHT GAIN

Weight gain can result from chemotherapy, prescribed steroids, abnormal fluid retention, and eating because of anxiety or frustration about your cancer.

Steroids (e.g., prednisone, dexamethasone) may change your metabolism or the way your body uses calories when these drugs are taken over an extended period. Steroids may also increase your appetite and cause fluid retention.

Keep track of how much weight you have gained and where you have gained it. When you are being treated for cancer is not a time to go on a strict weight-loss program, as your body requires nourishing food. However, there are things you can do to reduce weight gain. If you are gaining weight because of chemotherapy or steroids, switch to a low-fat diet (*see* "Fat-Restricted Diet" in Chapter 19). If you are retaining fluid, a low-sodium diet or diuretics may be needed. Your dietitian can suggest appropriate food choices.

PAIN

Pain is a problem for many cancer patients. Its effects can be mild or totally disabling. Pain can result in nutritional problems because pain can cause loss of appetite and seriously limit your ability to eat.

What You Can Do Your physician's guidance in taking pain medications is important for effective pain control. Your physician can also help you learn special pain-control techniques. Mental relaxation and reduction of stress and anxiety will also work to reduce pain.

One point of great importance should be stressed: Be sure your doctor is aware of all the medications you are taking. You may be treated by more than one doctor or dentist, and anyone prescribing medication must know of all medications you are receiving. (*See* "Pain" in Chapter 5.)

DEPRESSION, ANXIETY AND FEAR

Most people eat less when they are depressed. Seeing their bodies waste away may further convince depressed patients of the hopelessness of their situation—an often unfounded fear. Anxiety and fear can also take away appetite. The best treatment here is a positive approach toward your cancer therapy at all stages. (*See* Chapters 10, 11 and 12.)

18
SIDE EFFECTS OF CHEMOTHERAPY

Robert Ignoffo, PharmD, Ernest H. Rosenbaum, MD, and Isadora R. Rosenbaum, MA

———————◇———————

To reduce the side effects that may affect nutrition, *see* Chapter 17.

Adrenocorticosteroids (prednisone, cortisone, dexamethasone [Decadron])
　Toxic Side Effects Could lead to mood changes, hypertension (high blood pressure), edema (fluid and salt retention), headaches, sleeplessness, vertigo, psychiatric problems, muscle weakness (low potassium), osteoporosis, increased hair growth, cataracts, malaise and increased infections.
　Side Effects That May Affect Nutrition nausea and vomiting, altered taste and smell, loss of appetite, stomach or esophageal inflammation or ulcers, ulcerated mouth and throat (mucositis), diabetes, pancreatitis, dehydration, electrolyte imbalance, increased appetite, protein breakdown (catabolism)
　Food-Drug Interactions Give in morning to help imitate the body's normal hormone production time. Give one hour before or two hours after breakfast or when fasting. Antacids and antiulcer drugs (Tagamet, Zantac, Pepcid, Prilosec) can help reduce heartburn, upset stomach or ulcers.

Anastrozole (Arimidex)
　Toxic Side Effects include hot flushes in about 12% of patients. Edema occurs in about 7% of patients. Dry scaling rash occurs in about 5% of patients. Thromboembolic disease has been reported in about 3% of patients. Weight gain occurred in about 1% of patients.
　Side Effects That May Affect Nutrition nausea, vomiting, anorexia, mucositis, stomatitis occur infrequently
　Food-Drug Interactions food does not interfere with absorption of Arimidex

Bicalutamide (Casodex)
　Toxic Side Effects hot flashes, breast pain, breast enlargement in men, hepatitis (rare)
　Side Effects That May Affect Nutrition nausea and vomiting, diarrhea, constipation, flatulence
　Food-Drug Interactions none known

Bleomycin (Blenoxane)
　Toxic Side Effects pulmonary dysfunction, faintness, confusion, sweating, wheezing, cough, shortness of breath, skin darkening, rash, fluid retention in fingers
　Side Effects That May Affect Nutrition loss of appetite, nausea and vomiting, sore mouth or throat (mucositis), weight loss
　Food-Drug Interactions none known. Avoid excess doses of vitamin C.

Busulfan (Myleran)
　Toxic Side Effects low blood counts, skin pigmentation, male breast enlargement, loss of menstrual periods, cough, fever, bruising, confusion, dizziness, malaise
　Side Effects That May Affect Nutrition loss of appetite, nausea

and vomiting, diarrhea, dry mouth, elevated uric acid (hyperuricemia)
Food-Drug Interactions Full meals may reduce drug absorption. Take one hour before or two or three hours after a meal. Take with a starchy food such as bread or crackers that will help clear the stomach quickly and not interfere with absorption.

Carboplatin (Paraplatin)
Toxic Side Effects low blood counts, hearing loss, neuropathy, numbness and tingling in hands and feet
Side Effects That May Affect Nutrition loss of appetite, nausea and vomiting, diarrhea, constipation, sore mouth or throat (mucositis), altered taste and smell, high uric acid levels (hyperuricemia)
Food-Drug Interactions none known

Chlorambucil (Leukeran)
Toxic Side Effects low blood counts, rash, hair loss, pulmonary fibrosis, low sperm count, secondary leukemia (rare), fever, cough, chills, sore throat, joint pains, shortness of breath, fluid retention in legs, skin bleeding
Side Effects That May Affect Nutrition nausea and vomiting, high uric acid (hyperuricemia)
Food-Drug Interactions Full meals may reduce drug absorption. Take an hour before or two hours after a meal. Take with starchy food such as bread or crackers that will help empty the stomach and will not interfere with drug absorption.

Cisplatin (Platinol)
Toxic Side Effects low blood counts, hearing loss, loss of feeling in hands and tingling of fingers and toes, muscular weakness, facial swelling, fast heartbeat, wheezing, fever, chills, sore throat, joint pains, swelling of feet and legs, blurred vision, bleeding and bruising. Kidney insufficiency may be reduced by drinking more fluids and increasing salt intake.
Side Effects That May Affect Nutrition loss of taste, distorted taste, nausea and vomiting, loss of appetite, sore mouth or throat (mucositis), electrolyte imbalance, high uric acid (hyperuricemia)
Food-Drug Interactions none known

Cyclophosphamide (Cytoxan, Neosar)
Toxic Side Effects low blood counts, bladder scarring and bleeding, loss of menstrual periods, decreased sperm count, lung scarring (fibrosis), respiratory insufficiency, skin pigmentation, hair loss, liver toxicity
Side Effects That May Affect Nutrition lactose intolerance, loss of appetite, nausea and vomiting, sore mouth and throat (mucositis), diarrhea, high uric acid (hyperuricemia), bleeding and ulceration of the gastrointestinal tract, altered taste
Food-Drug Interactions Decreased absorption when taken orally if you have stomach inflammation. Do not take with a full meal. Take one hour before or two to three hours after meals. Take with a starchy snack such as bread or crackers that will help clear the stomach and will not interfere with absorption.

Cytarabine/cytosine arabinoside (ara-C, Cytosar)
Toxic Side Effects low blood counts, bleeding, bruising, confusion, disorientation
Side Effects That May Affect Nutrition lactose intolerance, loss of appetite, nausea and vomiting, sore mouth and throat (mucositis), loss of taste, loss of smell
Food-Drug Interactions none known

Dacarbazine (DTIC, imidazole carbox-amide)

Toxic Side Effects fever, chills, sore throat, mouth sores, bleeding and bruising. Sun exposure one or two days after taking the drug can produce facial flushing and light-headedness.

Side Effects That May Affect Nutrition lactose intolerance, loss of appetite, nausea and vomiting, sore mouth or throat (mucositis), high uric acid (hyperuricemia)

Food-Drug Interactions none known

Docetaxel (Taxotere)

Toxic Side Effects low blood counts, flushing, hypertension, itching, sweating, hair loss, rash, phlebitis, peripheral neuropathy

Side Effects That May Affect Nutrition nausea and vomiting (usually mild to moderate), mouth sores (mucositis), diarrhea

Food-Drug Interactions none known

Doxorubicin (Adriamycin)

Liposomal doxorubicin (Doxil)

Toxic Side Effects low blood counts, potential heart damage and risk of congestive heart failure, hair loss. Urine may be orange or red on first day after chemotherapy. Doxil can cause hand-foot syndrome (red rash, swelling, pain).

Side Effects That May Affect Nutrition nausea and vomiting, loss of appetite, loss of taste, sore throat and mouth (mucositis), diarrhea, iron loss

Food-Drug Interactions Vitamin C may enhance action of Adriamycin.

Etoposide (VP-16, VePesid)

Toxic Side Effects low blood counts, wheezing (rare), fever, chills, sore throat and mouth, bruising, numbness and tingling in toes and fingers, shortness of breath, rapid heart rate, weakness

Side Effects That May Affect Nutrition loss of appetite, altered taste and smell, nausea and vomiting, sore throat and mouth (mucositis), diarrhea, protein loss, loss of fluids and electrolytes

Food-Drug Interactions Full meals may reduce absorption when drug is taken orally. Take one hour before or two to three hours after meals. Take with a starchy snack such as bread or crackers that will help to clear the stomach and will not interfere with absorption.

Fareston (Toremifene)

Toxic Side Effects The major side effects are hot flashes and sweating. vaginal discharge, dizziness and edema occur in 5 to 13% of patients. Vaginal bleeding is reported in about 2% of patients. Thrombo-embolic complications are rare but increased in patients with a history of thrombosis.

Side Effects That May Affect Nutrition nausea in about 14% of patients, vomiting in about 4% of patients

Food-Drug or Drug-Drug Interactions phenobarbital, phenytoin and carbamazepine may decrease the metabolism of toremifene. Ketoconazole and erythromycin may inhibit the metaboism of toremifene

5-Fluorouracil (5-FU, Adrucil)

Floxuridine (FUDR)

Toxic Side Effects low blood counts (rare), hair loss (frequent but usually mild), skin hyperpigmentation, rash, loss of coordination and confusion (rare), headache (rare), cough, shortness of breath, fever, nasal and skin dryness, nose bleeds, bruising, sun sensitivity

Side Effects That May Affect Nutrition loss of appetite, nausea and vomiting, sore throat and mouth (mucositis), bleeding and ulceration of the gastrointestinal tract, bile salt losses, bitter taste, diarrhea, niacin deficiency, thiamine deficiency

Food-Drug Interactions none known

Flutamide (Eulexin)

Toxic Side Effects hot flashes, loss of libido, impotence, male breast enlargement

Side Effects That May Affect Nutrition loss of appetite, nausea and vomiting, diarrhea. About 12 percent of patients taking this drug have diarrhea, often associated with lactose intolerance. Taking flutamide with Lactaid or a lactase supplement may prevent diarrhea.

Food-Drug Interactions none known

Gemcitabine (Gemzar)

Toxic Side Effects low blood counts, skin rashes, flu-like symptoms

Side Effects That May Affect Nutrition loss of appetite, nausea and vomiting, diarrhea, sore mouth (mucositis)

Food-Drug Interactions none known

Goserelin (Zoladex)

Toxic Side Effects Common side effects include hot flashes, breast tenderness and enlargement in men, breast pain. Infrequent side effects include fluid retention, worsening bone pain from tumor flare reaction, vaginal spotting or breakthrough bleeding, hepatitis with increased hepatic enzymes (rare).

Side Effects That May Affect Nutrition (all infrequent) nausea, vomiting, diarrhea, constipation, flatulence

Food-Drug Interactions none known

Hydroxyurea (Hydrea)

Toxic Side Effects low blood

counts, fever, chills, sore throat, bruising, hallucinations, headache, joint pains, swelling of the feet and lower legs

Side Effects That May Affect Nutrition loss of appetite, nausea and vomiting, sore mouth (mucositis), diarrhea, constipation, high uric acid (hyperuricemia)

Food-Drug Interactions Full meals and stomach inflammation may delay absorption. Take one hour before or two to three hours after meals. If taken on an empty stomach, may cause nausea. A starchy snack such as crackers or bread will help clear the stomach and will not interfere with absorption.

Ifosfamide (Ifex)

Toxic Side Effects low blood counts, urotoxicity with bladder/urine bleeding (reduced with a uroprotector such as mesna), hair loss, central nervous system toxicity (dizziness, sleepiness, confusion, depression, hallucinations, disorientation and cranial/head nerve dysfunction), painful urination, cardiotoxicity, allergic reactions

Side Effects That May Affect Nutrition loss of appetite, nausea and vomiting, altered taste

Food-Drug Interactions none known

Interferon-alpha (Intron A, Roferon-A)

Toxic Side Effects flu-like syndrome with fatigue, fever, chills, muscular pain and headache. Also dizziness, rash and dry skin. Decreased mental status, visual and sleep disturbances, hypertension, chest pain, arrhythmia and palpitations. Skin bleeding, night sweats, itching, conjunctivitis and irritation at the site of injection.

Side Effects That May Affect Nutrition flu-like syndrome, loss of appetite, weight loss, nausea and vomiting, diarrhea, dry mouth, altered taste and smell

Food-Drug Interactions none known

Irinotecan (Camptosar, CPT-11)

Toxic Side Effects low blood counts, hair loss, skin rash, liver enzyme elevation

Side Effects That May Affect Nutrition nausea, vomiting, diarrhea, (can be severe, starting about six days after chemotherapy), mouth sores (mucositis)

Food-Drug Interactions none known.

Letrozole (Femara)

Toxic Side Effects the major side effect is musculoskeletal pain that occurs in about 20% of patients. Other adverse effects include dyspnea (7%), rash (5%), fatigue (8%), headache (9%), abdominal pain and constipation (6%), somnolence (3%) and weight gain (2%). Thromboembolic complications have occurred in 2 of 362 patients treated with 0.5 to 2.5 mg daily.

Side Effects That May Affect Nutrition nausea in about 13% of patients, vomiting in about 7% of patients

Food-Drug or Drug-Drug Interactions food does not affect the absorption of letrozole. Cimetidine has no effect on letrozole metabolism. Letrozole has no effect on warfarin activity.

Leucovorin (Leucovorin Calcium, Wellcovorin)

Toxic Side Effects allergic reaction

Side Effects That May Affect Nutrition nausea and vomiting (rare)

Food-Drug Interactions In epileptics, large amounts of folic acid may counteract the antiepileptic effect of phenobarbital, Dilantin and primidone, increasing the frequency of seizures, especially in susceptible children. Leucovorin increases the toxicity of 5-fluorouracil.

Melphalan (Alkeran)

Toxic Side Effects low blood counts, increased risk of secondary leukemia, fever, chills, bruising, joint and stomach pains, swelling of the feet and lower extremities

Side Effects That May Affect Nutrition nausea and vomiting, sore mouth and throat (mucositis), high uric acid (hyperuricemia)

Food-Drug Interactions Full meals and stomach inflammation may delay absorption. Do not take with a full or fatty meal. Take one hour before or two to three hours post meal. Nausea is common when taken on an empty stomach. If nausea is a problem, take with crackers or bread to help clear the stomach.

Methotrexate (Folex, Methotrexate, Mexate)

Toxic Side Effects low blood counts, sunlight sensitivity, elevated liver enzyme. Toxicity can be reversed by the use of folinic acid (leucovorin factor). Do not take vitamin supplements one to two days before taking methotrexate.

Side Effects That May Affect Nutrition loss of appetite, nausea and vomiting, diarrhea, bleeding and ulceration of the gastrointestinal tract, lactose intolerance, loss of taste, protein loss, fat-soluble vitamin loss

Food-Drug Interactions Food containing high amounts of salicylates (plums, gums, mints, jelly beans, root beer, apple, cherry and blueberry turnovers, and breakfast squares) should be avoided one to two days before and after methotrexate. Avoid drugs that can increase methotrexate toxicity: aspirin, sulfa, penicillin and non-steroidal anti-inflammatories (ibuprofen, Naprosyn).

Mitomycin-C (Mutamycin)

Toxic Side Effects low blood counts, hair loss, long-term pulmonary toxicity, kidney failure

Side Effects That May Affect Nutrition loss of appetite, nausea and vomiting, diarrhea, sore mouth and throat (mucositis), loss of protein, fluids and electrolytes

Food-Drug Interactions none known

Mitoxantrone (Novantrone)

Toxic Side Effects low blood counts, cardiac toxicity (congestive heart failure, arrhythmia, chest pain; increased risk in patients who have previously taken doxorubicin or daunomycin), low blood pressure, itching, rash, hair loss (rare), shortness of breath

Side Effects That May Affect Nutrition nausea and vomiting, diarrhea, sore mouth and throat (mucositis), bleeding and ulceration of gastrointestinal tract, high uric acid (hyperuricemia)

Food-Drug Interactions none known

Nilutamide (Nilandron)

Toxic Side Effects interstitial pneumonia (rare), visual disturbances, abnormal light adaptation, hepatitis with increased hepatic enzymes (rare), alcohol intolerance (rare)

Side Effects That May Affect Nutrition nausea, constipation, diarrhea (rare)

Food-Drug Interactions none known

Paclitaxel (Taxol)

Toxic Side Effects low blood counts, numbness in the hands and feet, hypersensitivity reaction

Side Effects That May Affect Nutrition nausea and vomiting, loss of appetite

Food-Drug Interactions None known. Vitamin C may improve action of Taxol.

Procarbazine (Matulane)

Toxic Side Effects low white blood cell and platelet counts, headaches, dizziness, fever, abdominal or back pain, muscle and joint pains, shortness of breath, tiredness, weakness, weight loss (rare)

Side Effects That May Affect Nutrition loss of appetite, nausea and vomiting, diarrhea, constipation, altered taste and smell, dry mouth, swallowing difficulties, iron loss, vitamin B_6 loss, protein loss

Food-Drug Interactions Procarbazine can elevate norepinephrine and serotonin in the nervous system, increasing the risk of reaction with certain food substances such as tyramine, which can cause a "pressor effect" characterized by transient high blood pressure, headache, palpitations, nausea and vomiting and (rarely) cerebral hemorrhage.

Foods high in tyramine include ripened cheese (especially Cheddar), wines (especially Chianti), fermented milk products like yogurt, broad beans and bananas.

High blood pressure can occur when taken with these drugs. Concurrent use of barbiturates, antihistamines, narcotics, hypotensive agents and phenothiazines with procarbazine may cause central nervous system effects. Avoid alcoholic beverages and hidden sources of alcohol such as sauces and desserts.

Tamoxifen (Nolvadex)

Toxic Side Effects hot flashes, menstrual irregularities, vaginal irritation (discharge, dryness, occasionally bleeding), leg cramps

Side Effects That May Affect Nutrition loss of appetite, altered taste and smell, nausea and vomiting, fluid retention in legs, weight gain

Food-Drug Interactions To promote absorption, take pill one hour before or two hours after a meal. If taken on an empty stomach, nausea or upset stomach may occur. Take with starch such as bread or crackers to help empty the stomach.

Thiotepa (Thioplex)

Toxic Side Effects Dizziness, headaches, hives and bronchospasm. Rare side effects are amenorrhea, loss of fertility, irritability and bladder bleeding.

Side Effects That May Affect Nutrition loss of appetite, nausea and vomiting

Food-Drug Interactions none known

Topotecan (Hycamtin)

Toxic Side Effects low blood counts

Side Effects That May Affect Nutrition diarrhea, loss of appetite, nausea and vomiting, mouth sores (mucositis)

Food-Drug Interactions none known

Vinblastine (Velban)

Toxic Side Effects low blood counts (lowest between Days 7 and 10 after therapy), tingling in hands and feet, jaw pain

Side Effects That May Affect Nutrition loss of appetite, nausea and vomiting, mouth sores

(mucositis), abdominal discomfort, constipation

Food-Drug Interactions none known

Vincristine (Oncovin, Vincasar)

Toxic Side Effects Nervous system damage (sensory impairment, loss of deep tendon reflexes and nerve pain), skin irritation, hair loss. Rare side effects include abdominal pain and intestinal obstruction, decreased blood sodium and seizures.

Side Effects That May Affect Nutrition nausea and vomiting, constipation, abdominal discomfort, mouth sores and ulcers (mucositis) (rare), dry mouth, altered taste and smell, high uric acid (hyperuricemia)

Food-Drug Interactions none known

Vinorelbine (Navelbine)

Toxic Side Effects decreased white blood cells, anemia, hair loss, vein irritation, numbness in hands and feet (rare), jaw pain (rare), acute shortness of breath

Side Effects That May Affect Nutrition nausea, vomiting, constipation

Food-Drug Interactions Food decreases the oral absorption of vinorelbine by 20 percent.

19
MODIFIED DIETS

Ernest H. Rosenbaum, MD, *Isadora R. Rosenbaum,* MA, *and Julie Matel,* MS, RD

———◇———

The liquid and special diets described in this chapter are designed for various special needs. Your physician will recommend a diet appropriate for your medical condition, and your dietitian will plan an individualized program based on your personal preferences and your cancer treatment.

LIQUID AND SOFT DIETS FOR ILLNESS

On days when you are not feeling well because of illness or therapy, you may not feel like eating your normal diet. You will find you have to eat lighter foods or even liquid foods. As you start to feel better, you can add more solid foods and gradually progress back to your normal diet.

The following diets progress from simple, clear liquids that require little digestion, through liquids of thicker consistency, to a diet of soft-consistency solid foods. These dietary progressions are:
1. Clear Liquid Diet
2. Full Liquid Diet
3. Soft Diet

CLEAR LIQUID DIET

The Clear Liquid Diet is your first step to getting back to a regular diet when you are unable to eat solid foods because of surgery, a partial gastrointestinal obstruction, diarrhea or your therapy. The diet consists of clear fluids or foods that will become liquid at body temperature. There is no fiber or residue in the diet. The foods in the chart below are allowed.

The Clear Liquid Diet alone—without supplements—does not provide adequate protein, calories, vitamins and minerals and is not intended to be used for more than 48 hours.

FULL LIQUID DIET

The Full Liquid Diet contains foods that are easy to eat. They are your next step in gradually returning to a normal diet (unless you are lactose-intolerant). This diet is also good if you are experiencing a sore or dry mouth in therapy or if you have had oral surgery but it may not provide adequate vitamins and minerals. High-calorie/high-protein supplements should be added if the diet is to be used for longer than two days.

FOODS ALLOWED ON CLEAR LIQUID DIET

	Calories	Protein (grams)
clear broth	5–25	0
coffee or decaffeinated coffee	3	0
fruit-ades (Kool-Aid, Gatorade, etc.)	60	0
mild carbonated beverages (ginger ale, 7-Up)	113	0
plain gelatin dessert (Jell-O)	65	1
tea (regular or herbal)	0	0

In addition to the foods in the Clear Liquid Diet, the foods in the chart below are allowed. Where no specific serving sizes are given, refer to *Bowes & Church's Food Values of Portions Commonly Used.*

MODIFIED CONSISTENCY

Soft, pureed and blenderized diets may be used when there are problems chewing or swallowing. A soft or pureed diet contains whole foods that are tender and easy to chew. Foods containing coarse whole grains, tough connective tissue, raw fruits and vegetables, and seeds and nuts are omitted. A blenderized diet is similar to a Full Liquid Diet except that it allows any foods that can be passed through a straw. It too is used when patients have mouth, jaw or esophageal problems after surgery or during therapy.

A pureed diet provides foods that are soft, smooth and semiliquid.

SOFT DIET

The Soft Diet is used when your digestive ability has improved and you are able to advance from liquids to whole cooked foods. You may find, however, that you are still unable to tolerate some foods you normally eat, such as fried or spicy foods, raw or gas-forming vegetables, or hard foods such as nuts, popcorn and pretzels. You may therefore need a soft diet as a step toward resuming a normal diet.

Frequent small meals may be better tolerated than three large meals a day if you are experiencing a lack of appetite or filling up after eating just a few bites of food. Between-meal snacks of eggnogs, milkshakes and liquid high-protein diet supplements are recommended for extra calories and protein.

In addition to the foods in the Full Liquid Diet, the foods on the next page are allowed. Where no specific serving sizes are given, refer to *Bowes & Church's Food Values of Portions Commonly Used.*

The following foods are difficult to digest and should be avoided:
◆ bread with hard crusts, nuts or seeds
◆ dried fruit
◆ fried foods
◆ horseradish, olives, pickles and relish
◆ nuts, seeds and coconuts
◆ popcorn, potato chips and pretzels
◆ raw fruit
◆ rich pastries

FOODS ALLOWED ON FULL LIQUID DIET

	Calories	Protein (grams)
cooked cereal made with fortified milk	215	9
custard	205	9
eggnogs	342	10
fortified milk	161	8
fruit juice (1 cup/250 mL)	120	0
high-protein supplements (e.g., Ensure)	355	14
ice cream (¾ cup/175 mL)	174	4
milkshakes	500	16
plain yogurt (low-fat, 1 cup/250 mL)	122	8
popsicles	40	1
pudding	219	4
sherbet	130	1
strained cream soup made with fortified milk or cream	145	6
vegetable juice	17	1

FOODS ALLOWED ON MODIFIED CONSISTENCY DIET

	Calories	Protein (grams)
avocado, 1	167	2
banana, 1	185	1
butter and margarine, 1 tsp. (5 mL)	45	0
canned fruit, ½ cup (125 mL)	60	0
cooked mild vegetables such as artichoke hearts, asparagus tips, carrot, eggplant, mushrooms, green peas, green wax beans, spinach and squash, ½ cup (125 mL)	25	2
cottage cheese, 1 cup (250 mL)	240	31
cream cheese, 1 oz. (25 g)	105	2
dry cereals, ¾ cup (175 mL), with cream, milk or fortified milk, ½ cup (125 mL)	235	10
eggs, boiled or poached, 1	81	6
eggs, scrambled, 1	125	6
*fish, 3 oz. (75 g)	164	24
macaroni, 1 cup (250 mL)	151	5
mayonnaise, 1 tbsp. (15 mL)	101	0
*meat, 3 oz. (75 g)	225	21
mild processed cheese, 1 oz. (25 g)	112	7
noodles, 1 cup (250 mL)	200	7
omelet, 3 eggs, with 1 oz. (25 g) cheese	355	25
papaya, 1	115	2
plain soft cakes and cookies, 1 oz. (25 g)	140	3
potato, baked, boiled or mashed, 1 med.	75	2
*poultry, 3 oz. (75 g)	225	21
rice, cooked, 1 cup (250 mL)	164	3
salad dressing	75	0
smooth peanut butter, 1 tbsp. (15 mL)	115	5
soufflés, cheese, ½ cup (125 mL)	210	9
tofu (soybean curd), 4 oz. (125 g)	75	8
white bread or toast, 1 slice, buttered	107	2

*baked, broiled, roasted or stewed until tender

SPECIAL DIETS

Sometimes your cancer or cancer therapy will cause problems that require a special diet. Your physician or dietitian may recommend one of the following diets to help you with these problems.
1. Pureed Diet
2. Lactose-Free/Lactose-Restricted Diet
3. Bland Diet
4. Fat-Restricted Diet
5. Low-Residue Diet
6. Neutropenia Diet
7. Vegetarian Diets
8. Alternative Nutrition
9. Nutritional Supplements

Suggested recipes for foods recommended in these diets are given in Chapter 20.

SAMPLE MENU FOR SOFT DIET

	Calories	Protein (grams)
Breakfast (495 calories, 15 g protein)		
fruit juice, ½ cup (125 mL)	60	0
cooked cereal, ½ cup (125 mL)	67	3
fortified milk* or cream for cereal, ½ cup (125 mL)	80	4
egg, soft-cooked, 1	81	6
toast, 1 slice		
with 1 tsp. (5 mL) butter		
and 1 tsp. (5 mL) jelly	157	2
coffee/tea, 1 cup (250 mL), with 1 tbsp.		
(15 mL) cream and 1 tsp. (5 mL) sugar	50	0
Midmorning Snack (405 calories, 13 g protein)		
milkshake or liquid high-protein		
supplement, 1½ cups (375 mL)		
Lunch (745 calories, 35 g protein)		
meat, poultry or fish (roasted, baked,		
broiled or stewed), 3 oz. (75 g)	225	21
gravy, ¼ cup (50 mL)	20	1
potato (boiled, baked or mashed), ½ cup (125 mL)	70	2
green beans, ½ cup (125 mL)	16	1
bread, 1 slice, with 1 tsp. (5 mL) butter	107	2
canned fruit, ½ cup (125 mL)	100	0
whole milk, 1 cup (250 mL)	160	8
coffee/tea, 1 cup (250 mL), with		
1 tbsp. (15 mL) cream and 1 tsp. (5 mL) sugar	50	0
Midafternoon Snack (200 calories, 6 g protein)		
custard or pudding, ½ cup (125 mL)		
Dinner (630 calories, 28 g protein)		
meat, poultry or fish (roasted, baked,		
broiled or stewed), 3 oz. (75 g)	225	21
rice, boiled, ½ cup (125 mL)	82	2
gravy, ¼ cup (50 mL)	20	1
carrots, cooked, ¼ cup (50 mL)	15	1
bread, 1 slice, with 1 tsp. (5 mL) butter	107	2
sherbet, ½ cup (125 mL)	130	1
coffee/tea, 1 cup (250 mL), with		
1 tbsp. (15 mL) cream and 1 tsp. (5 mL) sugar	50	0
Evening Snack (405 calories, 13 g protein)		
milkshake or liquid high-protein		
supplement, 1½ cups (375 mL)		

1. PUREED DIET

A pureed diet provides foods that are soft, smooth and free from whole, minced or ground chunks of food. It eliminates the need for chewing. It is used for people with chewing and swallowing difficulties.

Pureed foods can be purchased in the form of baby food or you can prepare them at home in a blender.

If you are experiencing a loss of appetite or fill up easily, you may find it better to eat frequent small meals instead of three large meals a day. Adding eggnogs, milkshakes and liquid high-protein supplements as between-meal snacks will increase your protein and calorie intake.

The foods on the next page are tolerated well. Unless otherwise indicated, the amounts are for one serving.

2. LACTOSE-FREE/LACTOSE-RESTRICTED DIET

Milk (lactose) intolerance results from a deficiency of lactase, an enzyme that breaks down milk sugar (lactose) in the intestine. It is marked by bloating, cramping and diarrhea. Sometimes it is caused by chemotherapy, intestinal surgery or radiation therapy to the lower abdomen. If you were not previously lactose-intolerant, you should be able to return to your normal diet once your treatment has ended.

What You Can Do
◆ Read food labels and avoid foods containing lactose. Lactic acid or lactate will probably not be a problem.
◆ Buy Lactaid, a lactase enzyme, at your drugstore or supermarket. This breaks down the milk sugar for proper digestion and absorption in the body.

There are different degrees of lactose intolerance. To determine the degree of your sensitivity, first eliminate all sources of lactose (*see* the "Foods Prohibited" list on page 205). Three days later, add back milk treated with Lactaid. Every two or three days add Lactaid to a previously excluded food and try it again in your diet. If you tolerate that food, keep using it; if you don't, exclude it for now, and try it again later. Follow this regimen as long as symptoms are a problem.

Foods Allowed
Beverages Mocha-Mix; Poly Rich; carbonated drinks; coffee; freeze-dried coffee; fruit drinks; some instant coffees (read the labels); Lidalac and other lactose-free milks or milks treated with lactase enzyme (Lactaid); lactose-free products such as Ensure, Ensure Plus, Resource soy milk and Vita Soy

Breads and Cereals breads and rolls made without milk; bagels; Italian bread; some cooked cereals; prepared cereals (read the labels); macaroni; spaghetti; rice and soda crackers

Meat, Fish, Poultry, etc. plain beef, chicken, turkey, lamb, veal, pork and ham; strained or junior meats or vegetables; meat combinations that do not contain milk or milk products; kosher frankfurters; eggs prepared without milk or prepared with Lactaid-treated milk; tofu

Vegetables fresh, canned and frozen artichokes, asparagus, beets, broccoli, cabbage, carrots, cauliflower, celery, corn, cucumbers, eggplant, green beans, kale, lettuce, lima beans, mustard greens, okra, onions, parsley, parsnips, pumpkin, rutabagas, spinach, squash, tomatoes, white and sweet potatoes, yams. Beware of cream-based sauces.

FOODS ALLOWED ON PUREED DIET

	Calories	Protein (grams)
avocado, 1	167	2
banana, 1	185	1
canned, pureed, stewed fruits, ½ cup (125 mL)	100	1
cooked and dry cereals, ¾ cup (175 mL)		
with cream, milk or fortified milk	235	10
cooked pureed vegetables, ½ cup (125 mL)	25	2
cottage cheese, 1 cup (250 mL)	240	31
cream cheese, 1 oz. (25 g)	105	2
cream soups	145	6
custard, ½ cup (125 mL)	205	9
eggnog, 1 cup (250 mL)	300	10
eggs, boiled or poached, 1	81	6
eggs, scrambled, 1	125	6
fish, meat, poultry (finely ground/		
pureed), 3 oz. (75 g)		
served in broth	250	25
served in cream sauce	285	22
high-protein diet supplements, 1 cup (250 mL)	250	14
malted milk drinks, milkshakes, 1 cup (250 mL)	200	12
mashed potatoes, ½ cup (125 mL)	70	2
papaya, 1	115	2
popsicles	60	1
pudding, ½ cup (125 mL)	175	6
regular ice cream, 1 cup (250 mL)	250	4
sherbet, 1 cup (250 mL)	250	1
soufflés	210	9
tofu (soybean curd), 4 oz. (125 g)	75	8
vegetable juices, ½ cup (125 mL)	20	1
yogurt, low-fat with fruit, 1 cup (250 mL)	200	8
If you are able to chew, you may add:		
graham crackers, 4	120	2
macaroni, with cheese, 1 cup (250 mL)	300	5
plain soft cakes (1) and cookies (3)	140	3
rice, 1 cup (250 mL)	250	3
saltines, 6	155	2
white bread or toast, 1 slice, buttered	107	2

The following foods are generally not tolerated well:
◆ bread with hard crusts
◆ coconut, nuts and raisins
◆ fish, meat and poultry pieces
◆ jams and preserves containing seeds or tough skins
◆ olives, peppers, raw vegetables
◆ raw fruit that is not pureed, except bananas and papayas
◆ smoked, spiced or processed meats such as bacon,
luncheon meats and sausage
◆ tart juices if they irritate the mouth

SAMPLE MENU FOR PUREED DIET

	Calories	Protein (grams)
Breakfast (495 calories, 15 g protein)		
fruit juice, ½ cup (125 mL)	60	0
cooked cereal, ½ cup (125 mL)	67	3
soft-cooked egg, 1	81	6
toast, 1 slice, with 1 tsp. (5 mL) butter and 1 tsp. (5 mL) jelly	157	2
fortified milk or cream (for cereal), ½ cup (125 mL)	80	4
coffee/tea, 1 cup (250 mL), with 1 tbsp. (15 mL) cream and 1 tsp. (5 mL) sugar	50	0
Midmorning Snack (405 calories, 13 g protein)		
milkshake or liquid high-protein supplement, 1½ cups (375 mL)		
Lunch (715 calories, 37 g protein)		
finely ground or pureed meat, poultry or fish, 3 oz. (75 g)	225	21
potato (boiled, baked or mashed), ½ cup (125 mL)	70	2
gravy, ¼ cup (50 mL)	20	1
pureed cooked vegetables, ½ cup (125 mL)	25	2
bread, 1 slice, with 1 tsp. (5 mL) butter	107	2
pureed fruit, ½ cup (125 mL)	60	1
whole milk, 1 cup (250 mL)	160	8
coffee/tea, 1 cup (250 mL), 1 tbsp. (15 mL) cream and 1 tsp. (5 mL) sugar	50	0
Midafternoon Snack (200 calories, 6 g protein)		
custard or pudding, ½ cup (125 mL)		
Dinner (530 calories, 27 g protein)		
finely ground or pureed meat, poultry or fish, 3 oz. (75 g)	225	21
boiled rice, ½ cup (125 mL)	82	2
gravy, ¼ cup (50 mL)	20	1
pureed cooked vegetables, ½ cup (125 mL)	25	2
sherbet, ½ cup (125 mL)	130	1
coffee/tea, 1 cup (250 mL), with 1 tbsp. (15 mL) cream and 1 tsp. (5 mL) sugar	50	0
Evening Snack (405 calories, 13 g protein)		
milkshake or liquid high-protein supplement, 1½ cups (375 mL)		

Fruits all fresh, canned and frozen fruits that are not processed with lactose (read the labels)

Fats margarine and dressings that do not contain milk or milk products; oils; bacon; some whipped toppings; some nondairy creamers (read the labels); nut butters and nuts

Soups clear soups, vegetable soups, consommés, cream soups made with Mocha-Mix or Lactaid or nondairy creamer

Desserts water and fruit ices; frozen fruit bars (read the labels); gelatin; angel food cake; homemade cakes, pies and cookies made from allowed ingredients; puddings made with water or milk treated with lactase enzymes

Miscellaneous carbonated drinks; carob powder; cocoa powder; corn syrup; gravy made with water; instant coffees that do not contain lactose (read the labels); jelly, jam or marmalade; molasses (made from beet sugar); olives; pickles; popcorn; pure seasonings and spices; pure sugar candy; soy sauce; sugar; wine

Foods Prohibited
Beverages all untreated milks of animal origin and all milk-containing products (except lactose-free milk), such as skim, dry, evaporated and condensed milk, yogurt, ice cream, sherbet, malted milk, Ovaltine, hot chocolate, some cocoas and instant coffees (read the labels); powdered soft drinks; milk that has been treated with Lactobacillus acidophilus culture rather than lactase

Bread and Cereals some prepared mixes such as muffins, biscuits, waffles, pancakes; Bisquick mix; cornbread; some dry cereals, such as Total, Special K, Cocoa Krispies (read the labels); Instant Cream of Wheat; commercial breads and rolls to which milk solids have been added; zwieback; french toast made with milk

Dairy, Meat, Fish, Poultry, etc. creamed or breaded meat, fish or fowl; sausage products such as frankfurters; liver sausage; cold cuts containing nonfat milk solids or cheese; egg dishes, omelets and soufflés containing milk or cheese; cheese; cottage cheese; yogurt

Vegetables any to which lactose is added during processing; creamed vegetables; breaded or buttered vegetables; instant potatoes; corn curls; frozen french fries processed with lactose

Fruits any canned or frozen fruits processed with lactose (read the labels)

Fats margarine and dressings containing milk or milk products; butter; cream; cream cheese; sour cream; peanut butter with milk-solid fillers; salad dressings containing lactose (read the labels)

Desserts commercial cakes, cookies and baking mixes; custards; puddings; sherbet and ice cream made with milk; ice milk; frozen yogurt; anything containing chocolate; pie crust made with butter; gelatin made with carrageenan; whipping cream

Miscellaneous chewing gum, peppermints, butterscotch, caramels, chocolate; some cocoas; coffee; some instant coffees; dietetic preparations (read the labels); spice blends that contain milk products; MSG extender; artificial sweeteners containing lactose, such as Equal and Sweet'n Low; some nondairy creamers (read the labels); dips made with milk products; some antibiotics and vitamin and mineral preparations

3. BLAND DIET

The Bland Diet consists of foods that are soft and do not irritate the stomach. It eliminates fried, highly seasoned and raw foods. The Bland Diet is recommended if you are experiencing heartburn or indigestion. All foods recommended on the Soft Diet are included. You may find it easier to tolerate frequent small meals than three larger meals a day.

Between-meal snacks of eggnogs, milk-shakes and liquid diet supplements are recommended for extra protein and calories.

The following foods are highest in protein and calories:

cottage cheese; custard; eggnogs; eggs; fish, meat and poultry (baked, broiled, roasted or stewed); liquid diet supplements; milk and fortified milk; milk-

SAMPLE MENU FOR BLAND DIET

	Calories	Protein (grams)
Breakfast (575 calories, 19 g protein)		
fruit juice, ½ cup (125 mL)	60	0
cooked cereal, ½ cup (125 mL)	67	3
egg, boiled or poached, 1	81	6
toast, 1 slice, with 1 tsp. (5 mL) butter		
and 1 tsp. (5 mL) jelly	157	2
fortified milk or cream (for cereal), 1 cup (250 mL)	160	8
herbal tea or decaffeinated coffee,		
1 cup (250 mL), with 1 tbsp. (15 mL) cream		
and 1 tsp. (5 mL) sugar	50	0
Midmorning Snack (405 calories, 13 g protein)		
milkshake or liquid diet supplement, 1½ cups (375 mL)		
Lunch (575 calories, 26 g protein)		
meat, poultry or fish (roasted, baked,		
boiled or stewed), 3 oz. (75 g)	225	21
potato (boiled, baked or mashed), ½ cup (125 mL)	70	2
green beans, ½ cup (125 mL)	16	1
bread, 1 slice, with 1 tsp. (5 mL) butter	107	2
canned peaches, ½ cup (125 mL)	96	0
Midafternoon Snack (575 calories, 19 g protein)		
custard or pudding, ½ cup (125 mL)		
Dinner (550 calories, 27 g protein)		
meat, poultry or fish (roasted, baked,		
boiled or stewed), 3 oz. (75 g)	225	21
rice, boiled, ½ cup (125 mL)	82	2
carrots, cooked, ½ cup (125 mL)	15	1
bread, 1 slice, with 1 tsp. (5 mL) butter	107	2
sherbet, ½ cup (125 mL)	130	1
Evening Snack (405 calories, 13 g protein)		
milkshake or liquid diet supplement, 1½ cups (375 mL)		

shakes; puddings; smooth peanut butter; tofu (soybean curd); yogurt made with whole milk

The following foods are potentially irritating and should be avoided:

coffee and tea; fried foods; raw and dried fruits (except avocados, bananas and papayas); garlic; highly seasoned foods; horseradish; fresh and dried legumes; smoked, spiced or processed meat, such as bacon, luncheon meats and sausage; nuts, seeds and coconut; olives; pepper; potato chips; relishes; gas-forming vegetables, such as broccoli, brussels sprouts, cabbage, cauliflower, corn, cucumber, green peppers, onions, rutabaga, sauerkraut, turnips; raw vegetables

4. FAT-RESTRICTED DIET

The Fat-Restricted Diet is helpful if you are experiencing a full feeling, or bloating, after eating only a few bites of food. This diet eliminates rich, greasy and fatty foods, which tend to "sit" in the stomach. Frequent small meals may be better tolerated than three large meals a day. Between-meal snacks low in fat will help add calories without ruining your appetite.

Nonfat milk or buttermilk should be substituted for whole milk. Plain cakes

and cookies, fruit ices, Jell-O, puddings made with nonfat milk and sherbet make good low-fat desserts. All nonfatty foods are included in the diet.

The low-fat foods listed below are highest in protein and calories. Unless otherwise specified, servings sizes follow *Bowes & Church's Food Values of Portions Commonly Used.*

Foods Prohibited avocados; bacon; more than 1–2 tsp. (5–10 mL) butter, margarine or mayonnaise per day; chocolate; cream and whipping cream; duck and goose; fish packed in oil; french fries; fried foods; greasy gravies; ice cream; luncheon meats; nuts; peanut butter; potato chips; rich desserts; rich or highly seasoned sauces; sausage; whole milk

5. LOW-RESIDUE DIET

The Low-Residue Diet consists of soft, easily digestible foods. "Residue" refers to indigestible material in food, sometimes called fiber. When the intestines are irritated, as in diarrhea, fiber may add to the irritation. The purpose of the low-fiber, low-residue diet is to minimize stool output.

Foods Allowed white breads, rolls and

LOW-FAT/HIGH-PROTEIN FOODS

	Calories	Protein (grams)
buttermilk, 1 cup (250 mL)	100	8
custards and puddings made with nonfat milk, ½ cup (125 mL)	205	9
egg, 1 (2 per week)	81	6
eggnogs made with nonfat milk	250	10
fish, lean meat, poultry (without skin), baked, broiled, roasted or stewed	165	21
high-protein diet supplements made with nonfat milk, juice or water	400	13
nonfat milk or fortified milk	103	10
nonfat yogurt	122	8
tofu (soybean curd), 4 oz. (125 g)	75	8

SAMPLE MENU FOR FAT-RESTRICTED DIET

	Calories	Protein (grams)
Breakfast (472 calories, 19 g protein)		
fruit juice, 1/2 cup (125 mL)	60	0
egg, boiled or poached, 1	81	6
cooked cereal, 1/2 cup (125 mL)	67	3
toast,1 slice, with 1 tsp. (5 mL) butter and 1 tsp. (5 mL) jelly	15	2
nonfat milk, 1 cup (250 mL)	88	8
coffee/tea, 1 cup (250 mL), with 1 tsp. (5 mL) sugar	19	0
Midmorning Snack (400 calories, 13 g protein)		
high-protein supplement made with water, nonfat milk or juice, 1 1/2 cups (375 mL)		
Lunch (675 calories, 35 g protein)		
broth, 1 cup (250 mL)	23	2
meat, poultry or fish (roasted, baked, boiled or stewed), 3 oz. (75 g)	225	21
potato (boiled, baked, or mashed), 1/2 cup (125 mL)	70	2
cooked vegetables, 1/2 cup (125 mL)	25	0
bread, 1 slice, with 1 tsp. (5 mL) butter	107	2
applesauce, 1 cup (250 mL)	119	0
nonfat milk, 1 cup (250 mL)	88	8
coffee/tea, 1 cup (250 mL), with 1 tsp. (5 mL)sugar	19	0
Midafternoon Snack (350 calories, 10 g protein)		
sherbet shake, 1 1/2 cups (375 mL)		
Dinner (525 calories, 28 g protein)		
meat, poultry or fish (roasted, baked, boiled or stewed), 3 oz. (75 g)	225	21
boiled rice, 1/2 cup (125 mL)	82	2
cooked vegetables, 1/2 cup (125 mL)	25	2
bread, 1 slice, with 1 tsp. (5 mL) butter	107	2
Jell-O or fortified Jell-O, 1/2 cup (125 mL)	65	1
coffee/tea,1 cup (250 mL), with 1 tsp. (5 mL) sugar	19	0

biscuits; refined grain products; plain bagels; plain cake and donuts; cookies without nuts; cold cereals such as corn flakes, Rice Krispies and Cheerios; cream of wheat; instant oatmeal; cooked peeled seedless fruits; ripe bananas, applesauce; canned fruit; fruit juices without pulp; jellies without seeds; meats and other ground or well-cooked protein foods including tender beef, lamb, ham, pork, poultry, organ meats, fish, eggs and cheese; pasta, white rice, tortillas; sherbet; cooked peeled seedless vegetables; vegetable juice without pulp

Foods Prohibited whole-grain products and baked goods; raw fruits and vegetables; seeds, nuts and legumes

Milk is restricted to 2 cups (500 mL) per day, including that used in cooking, and is prohibited entirely if you have diarrhea.

6. NEUTROPENIA DIET

During chemotherapy or radiation therapy, there may be a decrease in blood counts—white blood cells, red blood cells and platelets.

SAMPLE MENU FOR LOW-RESIDUE (HIGH-CALORIE/HIGH-PROTEIN) DIET

	Calories	Protein (grams)
Breakfast (450 calories, 16 g protein)		
orange juice without pulp, ½ cup (125 mL)	60	1
egg, boiled or poached, 1	81	6
cooked cereal, ½ cup (125 mL)	65	3
toast, 1 slice, with 1 tsp. (5 mL) butter		
and 1 tsp. (5 mL) jelly	157	2
milk (if tolerated), ½ cup (125 mL)	80	4
coffee/tea, 1 cup (250 mL)	50	0
Midmorning Snack (595 calories, 21 g protein)		
lactose-free liquid high-protein supplement,		
1½ cups (375 mL)	535	21
canned mandarin orange, ½ cup (125 mL)	60	0
Lunch (565 calories, 31 g protein)		
broth, 1 cup (250 mL)	23	4
potato (boiled, baked or mashed),		
½ cup (125 mL)	70	2
meat, poultry or fish (roasted, baked,		
boiled or stewed), 3 oz. (75 g)	225	21
green beans, ½ cup (125 mL)	16	1
bread, 1 slice, with 1 tsp. (5 mL) butter	107	3
applesauce, ½ cup (125 mL)	119	0
coffee/tea, 1 cup (250 mL)	3	0
Midafternoon Snack (200 calories, 6 g protein)		
custard or pudding, ½ cup (125 mL)		
Dinner (700 calories, 34 g protein)		
meat, poultry or fish (roasted, baked,		
boiled or stewed), 3 oz. (75 g)	225	21
boiled rice, ½ cup (125 mL)	82	2
cooked carrots,½ cup (125 mL)	15	1
bread, 1 slice, with 1 tsp. (5 mL) butter	107	3
plain cake, 1 slice	140	3
milk (if tolerated), ½ cup (125 mL)	80	4
coffee/tea, 1 cup (250 mL)	50	0
Evening Snack (185 calories, 3 g protein)		
Jell-O or fortified Jell-O, ½ cup (125 mL)	65	1
plain cookies, 2	120	2

Neutropenia is a lack of special white blood cells called neutrophils or polymorphonuclear cells (PMNs or polys), which fight infections caused by bacteria, fungi or viruses. Neutropenic patients are more susceptible to serious infections.

See "Reduce Your Risk of Infection" in Chapter 5 for general and diet guidelines.

7. VEGETARIAN DIETS

Special thanks to Sherri Thibeaux, RD
A vegetarian diet generally refers to a diet that omits meat, fish and poultry. However, a number of variations exist.
◆ A vegan or total vegetarian diet includes only plant foods.
◆ An ovo-vegetarian diet includes eggs.
◆ A lacto-vegetarian diet includes dairy products.
◆ A lacto-ovo-vegetarian diet includes dairy products and eggs.
◆ A semivegetarian diet may include fish and poultry as well as dairy products and eggs.

A well-planned vegetarian diet has been associated with lower blood pressure, less obesity and less constipation as well as reducing risk for several diseases, among them colon cancer, coronary artery disease and adult-onset diabetes.

A poorly planned vegetarian diet can result in many nutrient deficiencies. The more restrictive the diet is, the more danger for deficiency diseases. There are many "self-proclaimed" nutritionists, who may be unqualified and may make claims and suggestions that can be dangerous. A registered dietitian is the expert on nutrition and can assist you in planning a safe and well-balanced vegetarian diet. It is especially important to plan vegetarian diets for children and adolescents carefully, to ensure that their growth and development needs are met.

The Vegetarian Food Pyramid

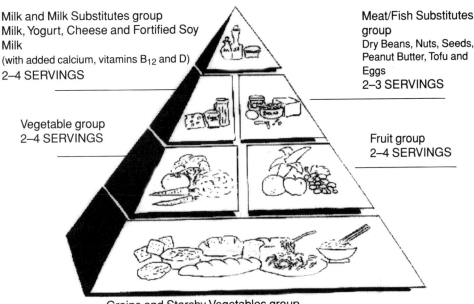

Milk and Milk Substitutes group
Milk, Yogurt, Cheese and Fortified Soy Milk
(with added calcium, vitamins B_{12} and D)
2–4 SERVINGS

Meat/Fish Substitutes group
Dry Beans, Nuts, Seeds, Peanut Butter, Tofu and Eggs
2–3 SERVINGS

Vegetable group
2–4 SERVINGS

Fruit group
2–4 SERVINGS

Grains and Starchy Vegetables group
Bread, Cereal, Rice, Pasta, Potatoes, Corn and Green Peas
6–11 SERVINGS

If you opt for a vegetarian diet of any type, choose a wide variety of nutrient-dense foods, which may include fruits, vegetables, whole grains, nuts, seeds, legumes, low-fat dairy products or fortified soy substitutes, and a limited number of eggs. To improve the value of the vegetable protein sources, your dietitian can show you how to combine complementary proteins (see below). Special attention should be given to ensuring adequate intake of protein, calcium, riboflavin, iron, zinc and vitamins A, D and B_{12}.

Complementary Proteins Proteins are made up of amino acids. There are eight essential amino acids, which must be obtained from the diet. Animal foods such as meat, fish, poultry, dairy products and eggs contain all eight essential amino acids in one food. This makes them a

VEGETARIAN DAILY FOOD GUIDES

(number of servings)

	Lacto-Vegetarian	Lacto-Ovo-Vegetarian	Vegan
Breads and Cereals	4–6	6–7	7–10
Fats/Oils	0	1 tbsp. (15 mL)	1 tbsp. (15 mL)
Legumes (dried beans and peas, lentils)	1+	1+	2+
Milk and Milk Products	2–4	0	0
Nuts	1+	1+	1+
Vitamin–A–Rich Fruits/Vegetables (beet greens, broccoli, brussels sprouts, carrots, escarole, pumpkin, spinach, sweet potato, V-8 juice; apricots, cantaloupe, mango, nectarines, papaya, peaches)	1–2	1–2	1–2
Vitamin–C–Rich Fruits/Vegetables (bell peppers, broccoli, cauliflower, kale, spinach, tomatoes, V–8 juice; cantaloupe, grapefruit, mango, orange, citrus juices)	1–2	1–2	1–2
Other Fruits and Vegetables	2+	2+	2+

Note: One egg can be substituted for 1 serving of milk/milk products for the lacto-ovo-vegetarian.

Breads/Cereals: 1 serving=1 slice bread; 1 cup (250 mL) cooked grain/pasta; ¾ cup (175 mL) cold cereal

Legumes: 1 serving=1 cup (250 mL)

Milk: 1 serving=1 cup (250 mL) milk or yogurt; 1 oz. (25 g) cheese

Nuts: 1 serving=¼ cup (50 mL) nuts or ⅓ to ½ cup (75–125 mL) seeds

Fruits/Vegetables: 1 serving=½ cup (125 mL) cooked or 1 cup (25 mL) raw vegetable or ½ to 1 whole fruit "complete protein." Plant foods do not contain all eight essential amino acids in one food, but with complementary combining, a complete protein can be formed. Complements can be eaten over the course of the day. It is not required that they be eaten at the same meal. The following combinations result in a complete protein.

Grains and Legumes
◆ barley-bean soup
◆ bread and baked beans
◆ brown rice and tempeh
◆ corn and beans
◆ corn tortillas and black beans
◆ cornbread and black-eyed peas
◆ crackers and split-pea soup
◆ flour tortillas and pinto beans
◆ millet and tofu
◆ pasta and kidney beans
◆ rice and beans
◆ rice and bran casserole
◆ rice and lentil curry

Nuts, Seeds and Legumes
◆ chopped nut/tofu vegiburgers
◆ dry-roasted soybean and seed snack mix
◆ hummus (blended seasoned tahini and garbanzo beans)
◆ nuts with any bean dish
◆ seed/nut tempeh
◆ sesame seeds on a bean dish
◆ sunflower seeds in bean chile

Grains and Dairy Foods
Dairy foods are complete proteins by themselves. In addition, they contain extra lysine, an amino acid that is low in grains. When grains and dairy products are eaten together, there is enough lysine from the dairy to complement the grain.
◆ cereal and milk
◆ cheese and crackers
◆ cottage cheese and wheat germ
◆ flour tortillas with cheese pizza
◆ macaroni and cheese
◆ milk and toast
◆ ravioli, manicotti
◆ rice and cheese casserole

◆ rice pudding
◆ yogurt and oats

8. ALTERNATIVE NUTRITION
Tube Feeding and Parenteral Nutrition
To treat serious malnutrition, enteral nutrition (tube feeding) and parenteral (intravenous) nutrition have been used. Nutritional support can help reduce the risk of malnutrition as well as help improve the quality of life.

Sometimes you may not be able to eat, which means you can't maintain your weight or take in an adequate amount of calories, protein and fluids. A short-term feeding by tube will provide your body with enough nutrition to enable you to fight your illness and keep your immune system strong until you can eat normally again. Tube feeding also frees you from pressure or anxiety around eating. The tube is passed through the nose, down the throat and esophagus into the stomach. The procedure, although somewhat unpleasant, fortunately goes quickly.

In some cases, depending on your health or the location of your cancer, tube feeding may be more permanent.

Parenteral nutrition may be needed when your digestive system is not functioning or does not absorb nutrients properly.

9. NUTRITIONAL SUPPLEMENTS
Recipes for cooking with nutritional supplements (see chart on page 214) are in Chapter 20.

To obtain the protein and calorie contents of diet supplements contact:

Ross Laboratories
Columbus, Ohio 43215
1-800-544-7495
or
Mead-Johnson and Company
Evansville, Indiana 947721

HIGH-CALORIE SUPPLEMENTS

	Calories (per cup/250 mL)	Protein (grams)	Lactose
Ensure, Sustacal	250	9	No
Fortified milk	220	14	Yes
Häagen-Dazs Honey Vanilla Ice Cream	426	8	Yes
Homemade milkshake	405	13	Yes
Raspberry and cream sorbet	300	0	No
Resource Plus, Instant Breakfast (made with whole milk)	280	14	Yes
Resource, Ensure Plus, Sustacal HC	350	13	No
Scandishake (lactose free)	420	7	No
Scandishake (with soybean mix)	520	15	No
Whole Milk	160	8	Yes

20
RECITES

◇

BEVERAGES

These beverages are high in protein and calories and make nutritious additions to your diet as between-meal snacks. You will also find them soothing when you have a sore or dry mouth.

◆ To increase the protein and calorie content of recipes calling for milk, add 2 tbsp. (25 mL) nonfat milk powder (50 calories, 5 g protein) or 2 tbsp. (25 mL) protein powder (70 calories, 15 g protein). If you must restrict the fat content of your diet, use skim milk instead of whole or 2% milk. If you are lactose-intolerant, use a milk substitute such as Mocha-Mix or Dairy Rich, or you can make milk lactose-free by adding Lactaid.

Fortified Milk

Use this extra-high-protein milk for drinking and in all recipes calling for milk.

1 cup (250 mL)	nonfat milk powder
1 quart (1 L)	whole milk

Combine ingredients and stir until smooth.

Per 1 cup (250 mL): 220 calories, 14 g protein

Fortified Skim Milk

If you must restrict the fat content of your diet, you can make fortified milk with skim milk.

1 cup (250 mL)	nonfat milk powder
1 quart (1 L)	skim milk

Combine ingredients and stir until smooth.

Per 1 cup (250 mL): 149 calories, 14 g protein

Berry Milk

1 cup (250 mL)	milk
½ cup (125 mL)	fresh or thawed frozen strawberries
¼ cup (50 mL)	blackberry nectar
1 tbsp. (15 mL)	sugar

Put all ingredients in a blender and blend until smooth.

Serves 1.
Per serving: 200 calories, 9 g protein

Milkshake

¾ cup (175 mL)	milk
¾ cup (175 mL)	vanilla ice cream
1–2 tbsp. (15–25 mL)	chocolate or strawberry syrup OR

½ ripe banana, sliced

Put all ingredients in a blender and blend to desired thickness.

Serves 1.
Per serving: 405 calories, 13 g protein

Variation: Omit syrup or fruit and substitute your favorite flavored ice cream for the vanilla ice cream.

Sherbet Shake

This shake is lighter than the milkshake and is a good snack for a fat-restricted diet.

1 cup (250 mL)	lemon sherbet or sorbet
¾ cup (175 mL)	nonfat milk mint leaves for garnish

Put sherbet and milk in a blender and blend to desired thickness. Pour into a glass and garnish with mint leaves.

Serves 1.

Per serving: 325 calories, 8 g protein

Root Beer Float
| ½ cup (125 mL) | vanilla ice cream |
| ¾ cup (175 mL) | root beer |

Put ice cream in a tall glass and add root beer until glass is almost full. Serve with a straw.

Serves 1.
Per serving: 230 calories, 3 g protein

Orange Juice Float
| ¾ cup (175 mL) | orange juice |
| ½ cup (125 mL) | orange sherbet |

Pour orange juice into a tall glass and top with orange sherbet. Serve with a straw.

Serves 1.
Per serving: 215 calories, 2 g protein

Variation: If desired and tolerated, add ½ cup (125 mL) champagne.

Peach Yogurt Shake
1 cup (250 mL)	skim milk
½ cup (125 mL)	plain yogurt
½ cup (125 mL)	drained sliced peaches
2 tbsp. (25 mL)	honey

Put all ingredients in a blender and blend until smooth.

Serves 1.
Per serving: 265 calories, 10 g protein

Variations: Replace peaches with ½ cup (125 mL) sliced bananas, drained fruit cocktail, strawberries, raspberries or blackberries. If you use raspberries or blackberries, strain after blending to remove seeds.

Apricot Yogurt Smoothie
| 1 cup (250 mL) | chilled apricot nectar |
| 1 cup (250 mL) | plain yogurt |

Put ingredients in a blender and blend until smooth.

Serves 1.
Per serving: 265 calories, 12 g protein

Variations: Replace apricot nectar with peach or pear nectar or your favorite fruit juice. Add honey to taste.

High-Protein Smoothies
These smoothies are like milkshakes, thick or thin depending on the temperature.

Blend until smooth:
| ½ cup (125 mL) | cottage cheese |
| ½ cup (125 mL) | plain yogurt |

Add one of the following:
½ banana + some strawberries + 1 tsp. (5 mL) vanilla + honey to taste

½ peach + 1 mango or papaya + 1 tsp. (5 mL) vanilla + honey to taste

½ banana + 1 tbsp. (15 mL) peanut butter + ½ tsp. (2 mL) vanilla + honey to taste

Serves 1.
Per serving: 240 calories, 21 g protein

Variations: Substitute your favorite fruit or fruit puree. Substitute chocolate, malt or other flavoring for vanilla. If you want it thinner, add more milk or more yogurt. If you want it colder, blend with a cracked ice cube. If you want it higher in protein, add wheat germ. If you want it higher in fiber, add bran.

BREAKFASTS
Breakfast can be your best meal of the day. Most breakfast foods are easy to eat because they are soft, moist, bland and light. They make good meals at any time of the day. Remember them when you are not feeling up to heavier food.

You can increase the protein and calorie content of recipes calling for milk by using fortified milk (see recipe on page 214) or cream in place of regular milk. If you must restrict the fat content of your diet, use skim milk or fortified skim milk instead of regular milk. If you are lactose-intolerant, use a milk substitute such as Mocha-Mix or Dairy Rich, or you can make milk lactose-free by adding Lactaid.

Cooked Cereal

When making oatmeal, farina or other cooked cereals, add extra protein and calories by using fortified milk or half and half instead of water. Top cereal with a pat of butter and serve with fortified milk or half and half.

1 cup (250 mL) fortified milk adds 220 calories, 14 g protein.
1 cup (250 mL) half and half adds 324 calories, 8 g protein.
1 tbsp. (15 mL) butter adds 100 calories.

Bran Muffins

These hearty bran muffins add bulk and fiber to your diet.

2 cups (500 mL)	whole-wheat flour
1 ½ cups (375 mL)	bran*
2 tbsp. (25 mL)	sugar
¼ tsp. (1 mL)	salt
¼ tsp. (1 mL)	baking soda
2 cups (500 mL)	buttermilk
1	egg, beaten
½ cup (125 mL)	molasses
¼ cup (50 mL)	margarine, melted
1 cup (250 mL)	raisins (optional)

May be irritating.

In a large bowl, mix together well the flour, bran, sugar, salt and baking soda. In a separate bowl, beat together the buttermilk, egg, molasses and melted margarine. Add to dry ingredients, stirring just until mixed. Stir in raisins. Fill well-greased muffin cups ⅔ full and bake 25 minutes at 350°F (180°C) until a tester comes out clean.

Makes 20 muffins.
Per muffin: 100 calories, 3 g protein

High-Protein, High-Vitamin Crunchy Granola

5 cups (1.25 L)	old-fashioned (not instant) oatmeal
1 cup (250 mL)	soy flour
1 cup (250 mL)	wheat germ
1 cup (250 mL)	nonfat milk powder
1 cup (250 mL)	slivered almonds*
1 cup (250 mL)	unsweetened shredded coconut
1 cup (250 mL)	unrefined sesame seeds*
1 cup (250 mL)	hulled sunflower seeds*
1 cup (250 mL)	safflower or soy oil
1 cup (250 mL)	honey

May be irritating.

Combine dry ingredients in a large bowl. In a separate bowl, stir together oil and honey. Stir into dry ingredients. Spread on cookie sheets and bake at 250°F (120°C), stirring occasionally, until lightly browned. Mixture burns very easily, so watch it closely.

Makes 15 cups (3.75 L).
Per ½ cup (125 mL): 270 calories, 8 g protein

Avocado and Cheese Omelet

2 tsp (10 mL)	butter
2 eggs	
¼ cup (50 mL)	sour cream
½ cup (125 mL)	grated cheese
½	avocado, sliced

In frying pan over medium heat, melt butter. Beat together eggs and sour cream. Pour into frying pan. When eggs are half set, sprinkle with cheese and layer avocado slices on top. Cover and cook a few more minutes until eggs are set and cheese is melted. Fold omelet in half and slide onto warm plate.

Serves 1.
Per serving: 790 calories, 31 g protein

MAIN DISHES

Meat, poultry, fish, dairy and eggs are your chief sources of protein. The following recipes give you interesting ways of preparing these foods so they are soft, moist and high in calories.

Ground Beef Stroganoff
Serve this softer version of beef stroganoff over noodles, rice, mashed potatoes or toast.

1/4 cup (50 mL)	butter
1/2 cup (125 mL)	minced onions
1 lb. (500 g)	ground beef
1 clove	garlic, chopped*
2 tbsp. (25 mL)	flour
2 tsp. (10 mL)	salt
1/4 tsp. (1 mL)	pepper
1/2 lb. (250 g)	mushrooms, sliced
1 can	condensed cream of mushroom soup
1 cup (250 mL)	sour cream

May be irritating.

Melt butter in a frying pan over medium heat. Cook onions until soft, stirring occasionally. Add ground beef and garlic, stirring until meat is slightly browned. Stir in flour, salt, pepper and mushrooms and cook 5 minutes. Stir in soup and simmer, uncovered, 10 minutes. Stir in sour cream and heat through (do not let boil).

Serves 4.
Per serving: 622 calories, 25 g protein

Mongolian Beef
You may especially enjoy this spicy recipe if you are experiencing taste blindness.

1 cup (250 mL)	water

1/2 cup (125 mL)	sliced green onions
1/2 cup (125 mL)	soy sauce
1/4 cup (50 mL)	chopped parsley
1 tbsp. (15 mL)	sugar
2 cloves	garlic, crushed*
1 lb. (500 g)	flank, sirloin, T-bone or top round steak, 1 in. (2.5 cm) thick, scored and pounded

May be irritating.

Combine all ingredients except steak in a shallow bowl or zip-top plastic bag. Add steak, turning to coat well, and marinate 30 minutes. Drain steak, and grill. Cut into 4 portions.

Serves 4.
Per serving: 163 calories, 24 g protein

Oriental Beef Tomato
This spicy dish may be appealing if you are experiencing taste blindness. Serve it over boiled rice or soft noodles for extra calories.

1 lb. (500 g)	beef, top round or flank
1	green pepper
2	stalks celery
1	medium onion
2	green onions
2 tbsp. (25 mL)	vegetable oil
1 small piece	ginger, crushed*
1 clove	garlic, crushed*
2	tomatoes, cut in wedges

Seasonings	
3 tbsp. (45 mL)	reduced-salt soy sauce
1 tbsp. (15 mL)	cornstarch
1/2 tsp. (2 mL)	sugar
1 tbsp. (15 mL)	dry sherry

Gravy	
1 cup (250 mL)	water or beef broth
1 tsp. (5 mL)	cornstarch
1/4–1/2 tsp. (1–2 mL)	salt to taste

To taste. May be irritating.

Combine seasonings ingredients in a shallow bowl or zip-top plastic bag. Slice beef thin and marinate in seasonings 15 minutes. Meanwhile, cut green pepper, celery, onion and green onions in 1-in. (2.5 cm) lengths. Combine gravy ingredients and set aside.

Heat 1 tbsp. (15 mL) oil in frying pan or wok and brown ginger and garlic lightly, stirring constantly. Add drained beef, stirring quickly, and cook to medium rareness. Remove from pan. Heat remaining 1 tbsp. (15 mL) oil in pan and fry onion, green pepper and celery for 10 minutes. Add beef and tomatoes and stir for another minute. Stir in gravy and bring to a boil. Stir in green onions.

Serves 4.
Per serving: 200 calories, 25 g protein

Honey-Glazed Chicken
Honey and butter add extra calories and flavor to this easy recipe.

1	store-bought barbecued chicken, quartered
½ cup (125 mL)	butter
¼ cup (50 mL)	honey

Put chicken in a baking pan just large enough to hold it. Top with pats of butter and drizzle with honey. Bake at 350°F (180°C) until chicken is glazed, about 15 minutes.

Serves 4.
Per serving: 581 calories, 23 g protein

Tuna Casserole

1 can	cream of mushroom soup
¼ cup (50 mL)	milk
7-oz. (198 g) can	tuna, drained
2	hard-cooked eggs, sliced
1 cup (250 mL)	green peas, cooked
½ cup (125 mL)	crumbled potato chips

In a 1-quart (1 L) casserole, mix soup and milk together. Stir in tuna, eggs and peas. Bake, uncovered, 25 minutes at 350°F (180°C). Top with crumbled chips and bake 5 minutes more.

Serves 4.
Per serving: 200 calories, 18 g protein

Variations: Shrimp or diced cooked chicken may be substituted for tuna.

Noodles and Cheese

1 lb. (500 g) package	noodles (spinach noodles are good)
1 cup (250 mL)	cottage cheese
8 oz. (250 g)	cream cheese
½ cup (125 mL)	sour cream
½ cup (125 mL)	chopped green onions
1 clove	garlic, crushed, or garlic powder*
1 tsp. (5 mL)	salt
	pepper
¼ cup (50 mL)	freshly grated Parmesan cheese

*May be irritating.

Cook noodles according to package directions. Meanwhile, in a bowl combine remaining ingredients except Parmesan cheese. Drain noodles and stir into cottage cheese mixture. Turn into buttered 2-quart (2 L) casserole. Bake, uncovered, 20 minutes at 375°F (190°C). Sprinkle with Parmesan cheese and bake 10 minutes more.

Serves 4.
Per serving: 581 calories, 23 g protein

Noodle Casserole

8 oz. (250 g)	broad noodles
½ tsp. (2 mL)	salt
1 tbsp. (15 mL)	margarine or

3	vegetable oil stalks celery, cut into small pieces
1	medium onion, cut into small pieces
2	eggs, well beaten
1 cup (250 mL)	grated or diced Cheddar cheese

Cook noodles in boiling water to which oil and salt have been added. Drain and rinse in cold water. Transfer to a bowl. In a frying pan over medium-high heat, melt margarine. Sauté onion and celery for 8 to 10 minutes, until softened. Add to noodles. Stir in eggs and cheese. Transfer to a well-greased casserole. Bake 15 to 20 minutes at 375°F (190°C).

Serves 8.
Per serving: 110 calories, 8 g protein

Variations: Add mushrooms, diced cooked chicken, turkey or beef, tofu, chopped ham or tomato sauce. Adding meat, poultry or tofu increases the protein content.

Deviled Eggs
Because it is moist, a deviled egg is much easier to eat than a plain hard-boiled egg if you have a dry mouth or some swallowing difficulties. Use as a snack or a light entree.

6	hard-boiled eggs
3 tbsp. (45 mL)	mayonnaise
½ tsp. (2 mL)	dry mustard or curry powder*
½ tsp. (2 mL)	salt
¼ tsp. (1 mL)	pepper

*May be irritating.

Cut eggs in half lengthwise. Slip out yolks and in a small bowl mash with fork. Mix in remaining ingredients. Fill whites with egg yolk mixture.

Per 2 filled halves: 142 calories, 6 g protein

Variations: Make a deviled-egg spread by chopping eggs and combining with other ingredients. Spread on crackers or bread.

Sesame Rolls

½ cup (125 mL)	wheat germ
¼ cup (50 mL)	sesame paste (tahini)
¼ cup (50 mL)	sunflower seeds, ground in blender
3 tbsp. (45 mL)	honey

Thoroughly combine all ingredients and form into a roll 1 in. (2.5 cm) in diameter and 12 in. (30 cm) long. Wrap in foil or waxed paper and refrigerate.

Per 1-in. (2.5 cm) slice: 78 calories, 3 g protein

COOKING WITH NUTRITIONAL SUPPLEMENTS

The following recipes use commercial high-calorie and high-protein supplements for added nutritional value. Ask your dietitian about these supplements. Ensure and its equivalent, Sustacal, add both protein and calories. Because they are lactose-free, they can be used even if you are lactose-intolerant. Use Ensure Plus or its generic equivalent for an additional calorie and protein boost.

Polycose is a tasteless and odorless source of calories. It can be added to foods and drinks without significantly changing their flavor or volume.

You can increase the protein and calorie content in recipes calling for milk by using fortified milk (*see* the recipe on page 214) or cream in place of regular milk. If you must restrict the fat content of your diet, you can use skim milk or fortified skim milk instead of regular milk. If you are lactose-intolerant, use a milk substitute such as Mocha-Mix or Dairy Rich, or you can make milk lactose-free by adding Lactaid. Ensure and Polycose recipes are from *Nutrition: A Helpful Ally in Cancer*

Therapy, courtesy of Eaton Laboratories.

Cocoa Diablo

1 tbsp. (15 mL)	sugar
1 tbsp. (15 mL)	instant coffee
1 tbsp. (15 mL)	cocoa
pinch	salt
pinch	cinnamon (may be irritating)
1/4 cup (50 mL)	water
3/4 cup (175 mL)	vanilla Ensure

In a saucepan, combine dry ingredients with water, stirring until dissolved. Stir in Ensure and heat to serving temperature, stirring frequently.

Serves 1.
Per serving: 280 calories, 8 g protein

Ensure Pancakes

1 cup (250 mL)	flour
1 tbsp. (15 mL)	baking powder
1/2 tsp. (2 mL)	salt
1/2 tsp. (2 mL)	cinnamon (may be irritating)
1	egg, lightly beaten
1 1/4 cups (300 mL)	vanilla Ensure
2 tbsp. (25 mL)	vegetable oil
1/2 cup (125 mL)	finely chopped apple

In a bowl, combine flour, baking powder, salt and cinnamon. In a small bowl mix together egg, Ensure and oil. Stir liquid ingredients and chopped apple into dry ingredients only until moistened. Fry pancakes on dry griddle.

Serves 2.
Per serving: 429 calories, 10 g protein

Ensure Shake

1/2 cup (125 mL)	vanilla Ensure
1/2 cup (125 mL)	instant coffee
1/2 cup (125 mL)	frozen vanilla Ensure creamer
6 tbsp. (90 mL)	Polycose powder

Combine all ingredients in a blender and blend to desired consistency.

Serves 1.
Per serving: 756 calories, 11 g protein

Variation: For additional flavor and color, add 2 tbsp. (25 mL) sundae topping (50 calories).

Polycose Shake

1 1/2 cups (375 mL)	ice cream
1/4 cup (50 mL)	whole milk
6 tbsp. (90 mL)	Polycose powder
2 tbsp. (25 mL)	sundae topping

Combine all ingredients in a blender and blend to desired consistency.

Serves 2.
Per serving: 358 calories, 6 g protein

Fruit Eggnog

1 1/4 cups (300 mL)	whole milk
1/2 cup (125 mL)	drained canned peaches
1 cup (250 mL)	Polycose powder
1/4 cup (50 mL)	sugar
1	egg
1 tsp. (5 mL)	fresh lemon juice
pinch	salt

Combine all ingredients in a blender and blend until smooth and creamy. Chill before serving.

Serves 3.
Per serving: 363 calories, 7 g protein

Fortified Fruit Juice

1/2 cup (125 mL)	fruit juice
1/4 cup (50 mL)	Polycose liquid

Stir ingredients together.

Serves 1.
Per serving: 180 calories

Polycose Gelatin

1 tbsp. + 1 1/4 tsp. (22 mL)	flavored gelatin
1/4 cup (50 mL)	boiling water
1/4 cup (50 mL)	Polycose liquid

Dissolve gelatin in boiling water. Stir in Polycose liquid and refrigerate until set.

Serves 1.
Per serving: 205 calories, 2 g protein

High-Calorie Chocolate Pudding
1 cup (250 mL)	Polycose powder
9 tbsp. (140 mL)	chocolate pudding powder
11 tbsp. (165 mL)	nonfat milk powder
2 cups (500 mL)	half and half
1 cup (250 mL)	chocolate syrup
1 cup (250 mL)	whipping cream

In a saucepan, blend all dry ingredients in half and half. Stir in chocolate syrup. Heat until thick and creamy, stirring frequently. Cool completely. Whip cream and fold into cooled pudding. Chill before serving.

Serves 8.
Per serving: 365 calories, 6 g protein

High-Protein Rice Pudding
2½ cups (625 mL)	whole milk
⅔ cup (150 mL)	Polycose powder
3 tbsp. (45 mL)	sugar
¼ cup (50 mL)	hot water
¼ cup (50 mL)	nonfat milk powder
¼ cup (50 mL)	cooked rice
2 tbsp. (25 mL)	margarine
pinch	salt

Put milk in top of double boiler. Mix Polycose powder and milk powder with hot water. Stir into milk. Add remaining ingredients and cook over simmering water until thick and creamy, stirring frequently. (Pudding may also be baked in a casserole for 2 to 2½ hours at 275°F/140°C.)

Serves 3.
Per serving: 438 calories, 11 g protein

Macaroni and Cheese
½ cup (125 mL)	milk
1 tbsp. (15 mL)	margarine
1 tbsp. (15 mL)	flour
½ cup (125 mL)	shredded Cheddar cheese
	salt and pepper to taste
½ cup (125 mL)	Polycose powder
½ cup (125 mL)	macaroni

Mix Polycose powder with 2 tbsp. (25 mL) milk and set aside. In a saucepan, melt margarine over medium-low heat. Stir in flour and cook, stirring constantly, 3 minutes. Whisk in remaining milk and cook until thickened, stirring constantly. Remove from heat and stir in cheese, salt and pepper. Return to low heat, stirring until cheese is melted. Remove from heat and beat in Polycose mixture. Cook macaroni in boiling salted water until tender. Drain well. Stir macaroni into cheese sauce and place in a casserole. Sprinkle with additional shredded cheese, if desired. Bake 30 minutes at 350°F (180°C).

Serves 1.
Per serving: 742 calories, 16 g protein

SWALLOWING TRAINING PROGRAM RECIPES
These recipes were developed by Caroline Cassens, RD, Clinical Dietitian, Rose Medical Center, Denver, Co., formerly Clinical Dietitian Leon S. Peters Rehabilitation Center, Fresno Community Hospital, Fresno, CA, and by Gaylee Amend, MA, CCC, Senior Speech Pathologist, Leon S. Peters Rehabilitation Center, Fresno Community Hospital, Fresno, CA.

STIFF JELLED CONSISTENCY

Stiff Jelled Fruit
2 jars	baby fruit, any kind
1 package	Knox plain
1 tbsp (15 mL)	unflavored gelatin
2 tbsp. (30 mL)	dry Jell-O powder
½ cup (125 mL)	hot water

Combine Knox gelatin, Jell-O powder and ½ cup hot water by whipping. Heat mixture until boiling. Add baby fruit and whip lightly until thoroughly mixed. Refrigerate.

Serves 4.
Per serving: 85 calories, 2 g protein

Stiff Jelled Yogurt

1 cup (250 mL)	plain unflavored yoghurt
4 tbsp (50 mL)	dry Jell-O powder any flavour
1 package (1 tbsp./15 mL)	Knox plain unflavored gelatin
½ cup (125 mL)	hot water

Combine Knox gelatin, Jell-O powder, and ½ cup hot water by whipping. Heat mixture until boiling. Add yogurt and whip lightly until thoroughly mixed. Refrigerate.

Serves 4.
Per serving: 89 calories, 5 g protein

Stiff Jelled Cottage Cheese

1 cup (250 mL)	cottage cheese
1 cup (250 mL)	orange juice
2 packages (2 tbsp./30 mL)	Knox plain unflavored gelatin

Combine orange juice and gelatin by whipping. Heat mixture until boiling. Pour into a blender and add cottage cheese. Puree until liquid. Strain liquid to remove lumps. Refrigerate.

Serves 3.
Per serving: 137 calories, 14g protein

Stiff Jelled Meat

2 jars	baby meat, any kind
2 packages (2 tbsp./30 mL)	Knox plain unflavored gelatin
1½ cups (375 mL)	evaporated milk seasoning as desired

Heat meat in double boiler. Combine gelatin with cold evaporated milk by whipping and heat until hot. Add meat and mix thoroughly. Add seasoning if desired. Refrigerate.

Serves 5.
Per serving: 151 calories, 13g protein

Stiff Jelled Casserole

1 jar	baby meat
1 jar	baby vegetables
½ cup (125 mL)	mashed potatoes
1 package (1 tbsp./15 mL)	Knox plain unflavored gelatin
¼ cup (50 mL)	hot water seasoning as desired

Heat baby meat, baby vegetables, and potatoes together in double boiler. Combine gelatin and water. Add meat mixture to heated gelatin mixture, whipping constantly. Add seasoning if desired. Refrigerate.

Serves 4.
Per serving: 64 calories, 6g protein

Stiff Jelled Vegetables

2 jars	baby vegetables
4 tsp. (50 mL)	Knox unflavored gelatin
½ cup (125 mL)	hot water

Combine gelatin and water by whipping. Heat mixture until boiling, Add vegetables and whip lightly until thoroughly mixed. Refrigerate.

Serves 4.
Per serving: 33 calories, 3g protein

Stiff Jelled Tomato Aspic

2 cups (500 mL)	tomato juice
½ tsp. (2 mL)	onion salt
3 tbsp. (45 mL)	vinegar
½ tsp. (2 mL)	Worcestershire sauce
2 packages (2 tbsp./30 mL)	Knox plain unflavored gelatin

Combine gelatin and tomato juice by whipping. Add onion salt, vinegar, and Worcestershire sauce and heat until boiling. Refrigerate.

Serves 4.
Per serving: 35 calories, 3½g protein

STANDARD JELLIED CONSISTENCY

Standard Jelled Fruit

2 jars	baby fruit, any kind
½ tsp. (2 mL)	Knox unflavored gelatin
4 tbsp. (50 mL)	dry Jell-O powder, any flavour
½ cup (125 mL)	hot water

Combine Knox gelatin, Jell-O powder and ½ cup hot water by whipping. Heat mixture until boiling. Add baby fruit and whip lightly until thoroughly mixed. Refrigerate.

Serves 4.
Per serving: 106 calories, 2g protein

Standard Jelled Yogurt

1 cup (250 mL)	unflavored yogurt
3 tbsp. (45 mL)	dry Jell-O powder, any flavor
½ cup (125 mL)	hot water

Combine Jell-O powder and ½ cup hot water by whipping. Heat mixture until boiling. Add yogurt and whip lightly until thoroughly mixed. Refrigerate.

Serves 4.
Per serving: 70 calories, 3g protein

Standard Jelled Cottage Cheese

1 cup (250 mL)	cottage cheese
1 cup (250 ml)	orange juice
2 tsp. (25 mL)	Knox plain unflavored gelatin

Combine orange juice and gelatin by whipping. Heat mixture until boiling. Pour into a blender and add cottage cheese. Puree until liquid. Strain liquid to remove lumps. Refrigerate.

Serves 3.
Per serving: 125 calories, 11g protein

Standard Jelled Meat

2 jars	baby meat any kind
3 tsp. (45 mL)	Knox unflavored gelatin
1½ cups (375 mL)	evaporated milk
	seasoning as desired

Heat meat in double boiler. Combine gelatin in cold evaporated milk by whipping and heat until hot. Add meat and mix thoroughly. Add seasoning if desired. Refrigerate.

Serves 5.
Per serving: 146 calories, 11g protein

Standard Jelled Vegetables

2 jars	baby vegetables
3 tsp. (45 mL)	Knox unflavored gelatin
½ cup (125 mL)	water

Combine gelatin and water by whipping. Heat mixture until boiling. Add vegetables and whip lightly until thoroughly mixed. Refrigerate.

Serves 4.
Per serving: 30 calories, 2½g protein

Standard Jelled Tomato Aspic

2 cups (500 mL)	tomato juice
4 tsp. (50 mL)	Knox unflavored gelatin
½ tsp. (2 mL)	onion salt
½ tsp. (2 mL)	Worcestershire sauce
3 tbsp. (45 mL)	vinegar

Combine gelatin and tomato juice by whipping. Add onion salt, vinegar, and Worcestershire sauce and heat until boiling. Refrigerate.

Serves 4.
Per serving: 30 calories, 2½g protein

Other Foods That May Be Served
◆Regular Jell-O
◆Custard
◆Danish Pudding
◆Baked winter squash

APPLESAUCE CONSISTENCY

Thickened Cream Soup
| ½ cup (125 mL) | strained cream soup |
| 8 squares | saltine crackers, finely crumbled |

Stir finely crumbled crackers into soup. Allow thickened soup to stand a few minutes before serving.

Serves 1.
Per serving: 125 calories, 3g protein

Finely Ground meat
Grind cooked meat using fine attachment of a meat grinder. If no fine attachment is available, meat may be ground twice using regular attachment. Serve with hot broth or gravy if desired.

A meat grinder is required to produce proper consistency. A blender will not produce correct consistency.

Thick Mashed Potatoes
Serve well-mashed but very thick mashed potatoes.

Riced Vegetables
Using a spoon, mash cooked vegetables through coarse sieve or ricer.

Carrots, beets, wax beans, green beans or turnips are the only vegetables that will produce the desired consistency using this recipe. No other vegetables should be used.

Riced Fruit
Pears: Using a spoon, mash pears through a coarse sieve or ricer.

Bananas: Using a fork, mash a banana very finely. May be served covered with a small amount of orange juice.

Applesauce: Canned applesauce may be served with no special preparation.

These are the only fruits that will produce the desired consistency. No other fruit should be used.

Blended Cottage Cheese and Fruit
| ½ cup (125 mL) | cottage cheese |
| 1 jar | baby fruit |

Blend cottage cheese and fruit together until mixture has applesauce consistency. Mixture should not be smooth.

Serves 1.
Per serving: 222 calories, 15g protein

Other Foods That May Be Served
◆Very thick refined cereal, e.g., Cream of Wheat, Cream of Rice, Malt-O-Meal, Farina
◆Plain tapioca pudding

THICK SOUP CONSISTENCY

Thickened Cream Soup
Combine equal amount of strained cream soup and well-mashed potatoes. Mix well. Strain through sieve before serving.

Thick Souplike Pureed Meat
¼ cup (50 mL)	baby pureed meat or blended cooked meat
¼ cup (50 mL)	well-mashed potatoes
2 tbsp. (25 mL)	broth

Combine baby pureed meat or blended cooked meat and the well-mashed potatoes. Add the broth. Mix well. Strain through sieve before serving.

Thick Souplike Mashed Potatoes
| ⅓ cup (75 mL) | mashed potatoes |
| ¼ cup (50 mL) | warm milk |

Combine the mashed potatoes with warm milk. Mix well. Strain through sieve before serving.

Thick Souplike Pureed Vegetables

1 jar	baby pureed vegetables or blended cooked vegetables
¼ cup (50 mL)	strained cream soup or broth

Combine baby pureed vegetables or blended vegetables with the strained cream soup or broth. Mix well. Strain through sieve before serving.

Thick Souplike Pureed Fruit

1 jar	baby fruit or blended canned fruit
¼ cup (50 mL)	strained fruit juice or strained fruit (such as nectar or apple juice)

Combine baby fruit or blended canned fruit with strained fruit juice or strained fruit. Mix well. Strain through sieve before serving.

Other Food That May Be Served
◆Smooth yogurt (plain or without pieces of fruit)
◆Smooth pudding

NECTAR CONSISTENCY

Thin Pureed Meat
Use baby meat or blended cooked meat. Add broth to the pureed meat until mixture is consistency of nectar. Mixture should pour freely. Strain through sieve before serving.

Thin Mashed Potatoes
Add warm milk to well-mashed potatoes until mixture is consistency of nectar. Mixture should pour freely. Strain through sieve before serving.

Thin Pureed Vegetables
Use baby vegetables or blended cooked vegetables. Add broth or strained cream soup to pureed vegetables until mixture is consistency of a nectar. Mixture should pour freely. Strain through sieve before serving.

Thin Pureed Fruit
Use baby fruit or blended canned fruits. Add strained fruit juice (such as nectar or apple juice) to pureed fruit until mixture is consistency of a nectar. Strain through sieve before serving.

Other Foods That May be Served

◆Nectar, any kind
◆Tomato juice
◆Strained cream coup
◆Refined cereal with cream, e.g. Cream of Wheat, Cream of Rice, Malt-O-Meal or Farina.

COOKING WITH CONVENIENCE FOODS

You may sometimes feel too ill from your disease or your therapy to do much cooking. However, with the help of the many convenience foods available, you can still prepare appetizing, nutritionally adequate meals with little time and effort.

Many canned, frozen and packaged foods have a high salt content and may not be suitable for people with water-retention problems or people who must otherwise be on a salt-restricted diet. Check the label! Frozen dinners and canned or frozen main dishes and vegetables require minimal preparation. Serve them with milk, bread and fruit or juice for a satisfying and nutritious meal.

For economy, and to build up a resource to fall back on, cook larger quantities and freeze the leftovers in individual serving sizes. A microwave can dramatically shorten heating and cooking times.

Shortcuts

Many canned and frozen convenience foods can be combined with other foods to make quick, easy and appetizing meals. For example:

◆ Melt cheese over broccoli or asparagus; or mix cheese into a white sauce, add broccoli or asparagus and serve on toast or crackers.

◆ Make a patty out of canned corned beef hash, top with a drained canned pineapple slice, and grill.

◆ To canned spaghetti, add cooked ground meat, tuna, diced chicken or ham, dried beef or sliced frankfurters.

◆ Mix canned gravy or canned white sauce with canned tuna or shrimp or diced cooked chicken or turkey.

◆ Add tuna or chicken and chopped onion and green pepper to undiluted condensed chicken soup. Top with an unbaked baking powder biscuit and bake until biscuit is brown and dish is heated through.

Frozen Foods

Keep commercially frozen food on hand. You can also freeze individual servings of uncooked foods, such as hamburger patties, chops, chicken pieces and fish fillets. Homemade stews, casseroles and other mixed dishes can be put into individual serving containers and kept in the freezer. You can have a week's basic meals prepared and frozen for daily use. Then you need only heat the major entree and prepare the side dishes.

Grocery Shopping

Stock up on nonperishable foods and foods with a long shelf life. A supply of canned, frozen and packaged foods will save you shopping trips and offer you a ready variety of foods to meet whatever your taste preference may be at the moment. Many of these products now come in a one-serving size and are especially good for between-meal snacks to increase your calorie and protein intake.

Some foods you might want to stock up on are listed below.

Beverages

canned and dry milk
carbonated drinks
fruit and vegetable juices such as nectars, V-8 and tomato juice
fruit-ades (Kool-Aid, Gatorade, etc.)
instant beef and chicken broth
instant breakfast mix
instant cocoa mix
instant coffee
tea, regular and herbal

Breads, Grains and Cereal Products

bread-machine mixes
crackers (saltines, grahams, etc.)
dry cereal
instant mashed potatoes
instant pancake mix
muffin mix
packaged grain mixes such as rice, couscous, lentils, risotto
Pop-Tarts
regular and instant hot cereal

Fruits and Vegetables

canned fruit
canned vegetable soups
canned vegetables
dried fruit
pureed baby foods

Meat and Other Protein Foods

canned meat, poultry and fish
canned mixtures of meat, poultry and fish with vegetables, noodles, spaghetti, rice, macaroni or beans
canned soups made with meat, poultry or fish, peas, lentils or other dried beans
grated cheeses such as Parmesan and Romano
peanut butter

Desserts

cake and cookie mixes
canned pudding
instant pudding
Jell-O
unflavored gelatin

Snacks and Sweets
granola bars
hard candy
honey
instant breakfast bars
jam and jelly
nuts
plain chocolate
power bars

From the Freezer Case
burritos
frozen vegetables and fruits
lasagna

macaroni and cheese
pancakes
pot pies
soups
TV dinners
waffles
whipped topping

Sauces and Seasonings
canned gravy
canned sauces
gravy mixes
seasoning mixes

21
REHABILITATION EXERCISES

*Francine Manuel, RPT, Ernest H. Rosenbaum, MD, Jack LaLanne,
Isadora Rosenbaum, MA, Eric Durak, MS, Gary M. Abrams, MD
Demonstrations by Jack LaLanne*

———◇———

Physical fitness is a matter of movement. In everyday life, we undertake many activities that use and maintain normal muscle tone. When we are healthy, we need no special training or assistance for such common activities as walking, making the bed, shopping, climbing stairs or running for a bus.

But people with an acute or chronic illness can't take even minimal exercise for granted. Prolonged bedrest—which is often essential or unavoidable—can lead to muscular weakness, tissue breakdown and poor functioning of vital organs. To preserve these vital functions during and after your treatment, you must make regular physical activity—including supplemental exercises aimed at maintaining muscle tone, normal joint motion and physical strength—part of your routine, starting as early as possible.

Many forms of exercise can improve your fitness, stamina, muscle strength and endurance, including

◆ isotonic exercises (moving a limb through a full range of motion);
◆ isometric exercises (resistance against a nonmoving object); and
◆ rhythmic repetitive movements and activities of daily living (ADL): household tasks, moving the body through space and other functional chores (*see* Chapter 22).

Massage therapy (*see* Chapter 23) is also a valuable aid to physical fitness, since it improves circulation and relaxes your mind and body.

If you exercised regularly before you became ill, you will probably be open to the idea of getting involved in an active program all through your recovery. But if you have never been involved in an organized exercise routine, you may need some encouragement and instruction. Welcome this encouragement if you get it. If you don't get it, seek it out, because becoming and staying physically fit should be one of your primary goals.

While you should think of your program as being as much a part of your recovery as visits to the doctor, try to enjoy yourself. Exercise can be a lot of fun. And it can be very stimulating. If you have days when depression and boredom get you down and exercising seems like too much of a burden, just remind yourself of all the benefits of exercising regularly. The more you exercise, the better you will feel. Don't say, "I'm too tired" and wait for tomorrow. Tomorrow may be no better than today. Start now, and keep up a reasonable exercise schedule for better health.

THE BENEFITS OF EXERCISE

Physical fitness is healthy for everyone, of course, but it is essential for cancer patients. Even though it's harder to find the energy to exercise when you are sick, the benefits of keeping active are too great to ignore. Participating in a daily exercise program will help you in several important ways:

◆ You will improve your prognosis. If you are in good physical condition, you may be better able to tolerate cancer therapy. This, in turn, may allow you to have more aggressive treatments, thus standing a better chance of remission or cure.

◆ You will improve your quality of life. Exercise can help you tolerate pain more readily, recover more quickly from surgeries and medical procedures and feel more in control of your situation. Exercise also reduces fatigue and increases appetite. Having the energy to remain functionally independent and to continue to fulfill social roles is important to quality of life.

◆ You will stop your muscles from wasting away. When we are healthy, we usually exercise our muscles by walking up and down stairs, doing housework, shopping, taking part in athletic activities like golf and tennis or simply by walking as we go about our business. Even a low level of activity helps maintain muscle tone and strength. But during an acute or chronic illness, prolonged bedrest is often necessary. When muscles aren't used, they shrink (atrophy) and lose strength. Muscles can atrophy after only 96 hours (four days) of disuse. Moderate exercise aimed at strengthening the large muscles, as described later in this chapter, will prevent this from happening to you, so that you can return to active living more quickly.

◆ You will recover faster. If you do not exercise after surgery or while you're undergoing radiotherapy or chemotherapy, the tissues that may get broken down by therapy will not repair as quickly as they should. Exercising can help your tissues rebound and minimize any deterioration in your joints. It may also help prevent complications such as bone softening, blood clots and bedsores. And you'll get some welcome relief from the boredom and depression that often come with being confined in bed. Exercising can become a vital part of your fight for your life.

Regular exercise also offers many general health benefits. Exercise also decreases stress, controls weight by burning calories and generally promotes a greater sense of well-being. Flexibility exercises alleviate general aches and pains, including those from arthritis. Strengthening your abdominal muscles can also help relieve back pain.

Resistance training and other activities can maintain and increase your bone density, thus reducing your chances of developing osteoporosis (weak bones). Impact exercises such as jogging or strenuous aerobics are also believed to play a part in preventing this disease of gradual bone loss. In cases of fatigue, weakness, severe osteoporosis or progressive illness, high-impact exercise programs such as jogging can be detrimental. Then, gentler activities such as brisk walking can help maintain bone density and health. Remember, although activity is good, moderation is essential. Overdoing exercise—going beyond your limits—can actually reverse your progress.

The most important benefit of all is that you can live longer if you exercise. Many studies have conclusively shown that an inactive (sedentary) lifestyle leads to an appreciably shorter life. Exercise has been shown to maintain youthfulness, promote longevity and help prevent heart disease—as well as certain types of cancer.

Along with the general health benefits, studies on prevention and survival rates in cancer patients have shown that regular moderate physical activity can help protect against some cancers, while also improving the clinical course—at least in the early stages of the disease. Several studies conclude that in the late stages of cancer, exercising improves quality of life right up to death. In one study, cancer patients who included moderate exercise in their routine reported decreased discomfort; after five weeks of moderate exercise, there was a strict connection between improvement and frequency of exercise. They also reported that their satisfaction with life was enhanced.

There is strong evidence that even beginning exercise late in life is beneficial, whereas stopping exercise is harmful. Having exercised as a child has no effect, but more recent activity in life definitely has an impact on the risk for developing cancer.*

Components of the immune system's white blood cells are believed to have a powerful inhibiting effect on tumor growth and to be able to destroy cancer cells. Intense exercising, such as the heavy training of professional athletes, has a negative effect on the immune system. But research suggests that moderate exercise actually enhances the immune system. Low-intensity exercise (e.g., walking) has positive effects on the body's ability to fight infections. So moderate programs, such as walking, using aerobic machines, tai chi, etc., may be the best way to enhance general fitness and may have an impact on the development of cancerous tumors.

Several studies have shown that people with more active lifestyles experience fewer breast, ovarian, prostate and colon cancers.

Researchers believe that exercise may decrease breast and ovarian cancer by affecting ovarian hormonal levels and the percentage of body fat. Women athletes, who have decreased estrogen levels and low percentages of body fat, also have a decreased incidence of breast and ovarian cancers.

Incidence of colon cancers is also lower among more active people. Again, the mechanism may be associated with decreased adipose (fatty) tissue, especially in the abdomen, or the fact that exercise tends to decrease constipation and increase the speed with which waste passes through the intestines.

One study compared "highly active" people (defined as those whose activities burn more than 2,500 calories a week above resting metabolism) with inactive people (those who expend fewer than 1,000 calories a week above resting metabolism). The highly active people had an estimated 40 to 50 percent reduced risk of developing colon cancer. Below are some sample activities that produce this result.

Recent studies have also found an association between exercise and decreased risk of prostate cancer. Lower testosterone levels are believed to be one mechanism behind this result. Diet may also play a role.

HOW MUCH EXERCISE IS NECESSARY?

Fortunately, you don't have to turn yourself into a marathon runner to achieve the active lifestyle that experts recommend. The Centers for Disease Control (CDC) and the American College of Sports Medicine (ACSM) have endorsed a prescription for "moderate activity" developed by Dr. James M. Rippe, an associate professor at Tufts University. This approach calls for 30 minutes of accumulated exercise per day. You do not need to

Event	Duration	Times/week
Aquajogging	40 minutes	3–4
Biking	40–60 minutes	3–4
Jogging	1.5–2 miles	3
Swimming	2,000 meters	3–4
Tennis	2–3 sets	2
Weightlifting	1 hour	3–4

*References for the studies cited in this chapter are available on request from Keren Stronach, Cancer Resource Ceneter, UCSF/Mount Zion Cancer Center, 2356 Sutter Street, San Francisco, CA 94143-1705.

go to a gym: a brisk walk at a speed of between 3 and 4 miles (roughly 5 to 6.5 km) an hour can do it, and so can many common activities of daily living, such as climbing stairs, raking leaves, gardening or dancing.

Although evidence shows that a person needs to exercise only on at least five days out of the week to reap the health benefits of physical fitness, the CDC and ACSM recommend that every American should engage in 30 minutes or more of some type of physical activity daily.

Furthermore, you can benefit from exercise even when you don't do it all in a single session; that is, you can spread out the 30 minutes of walking or gardening over the course of the day. Just making a habit of walking a little farther to the grocery store, or climbing stairs instead of taking an elevator, can produce important physiological changes. (Note, however, that for cardiac fitness, it is still recommended that a person do 20 minutes of continuous aerobic exercise three to four times a week. Both types of exercise are beneficial.)

DESIGNING THE RIGHT EXERCISE PROGRAM FOR YOU

How do you decide which activities to pursue if you want a well-planned fitness program? To answer that, you should first be aware of the three different types of exercise:

◆ Activities that increase your flexibility. The older you get, the more important stretching is, especially if you tend to be inactive. Simple stretches, such as reaching to touch your toes, will keep you limber. Many books have been written on stretching, some of them specifically for bicyclists, soccer players and other athletes. Other activities that can improve your joint mobility include yoga, tai chi and any type of dancing. Skiing, surfing

and soccer are good movement sports.

◆ Activities that build strength and endurance in your muscles. Strength building requires working against progressive resistance, whether with weight machines or other workout equipment at a gym, dumbbells, elastic tubing or even your own body weight. When applied to specific parts of your body, these kinds of activities increase the size of your muscle fibers and give your muscles definition. To increase strength, you must lift a maximum load—as much as you can bear—for only six to eight repetitions at a time. To build muscle endurance, you can decrease the load and increase the number of repetitions to 20 or 30 times. You can also boost your endurance by going through your general exercise routine with 2- to 5-pound (1 or 2 kg) Velcro weights strapped onto your legs or arms.

◆ Activities that improve heart and aerobic endurance. Exercises in this category involve the body's large muscles (those in the hips, thighs, chest, back and shoulders). Walking, swimming, jogging, bicycling, aerobic dancing and ballroom dancing all enhance the ability of your heart and lungs to deliver nutrients and oxygen to your body, as well as to remove waste products via the blood.

Although you can concentrate on any one of these three exercise types, you might want to try a workout program that draws from each category. You can start on a standard workout routine, or be creative.

When to Start Become physically active as soon as possible after your cancer surgery or other treatment. At first you may have some restrictions on your level of activity (*see* "When to Avoid Exercising" below). But it is now the general practice within one day of surgery to get patients out of bed and at least sitting in a chair. Even this minimal activity helps to reduce the loss of muscle mass and to increase strength.

Pain can limit physical exercise after a mastectomy, bowel surgery or some other major operation. Depression, brought on by changes in your body image, may also make you feel like not doing anything. You may need help to get going. Get a family member, friend, coach or trainer to help you. For some people, exercising alone is boring. Using music or a video-taped program may help.

Begin a gentle exercise program while you are still in the hospital. This may involve simple muscle tightening while you lie in bed. As your strength returns, different forms of physical activity—isometric and isotonic exercises, and rhythmic repeated movements for various muscles—will help get you on the path to improved fitness. Massage therapy (*see* Chapter 23) can complement these activities, helping you to relax your mind and body and to improve your circulation and your health.

Making an effort while you're still in the hospital may seem difficult. But you will feel much more confident when you go home if you have already started to regain your strength. You will also be less prone to falls or other accidents that might result from a weakened condition.

Before you leave the hospital, a physical therapist can assess your physical condition and help you develop an appropriate set of exercises. Everyone has different wants and needs, so such programs are usually customized. One sample progressive program is described later in this chapter (*see* "A Sample Progressive Exercise Program" below). The staff of the hospital's Physical Therapy Department can also instruct you, your family and other caregivers on how to proceed with your program at home. Their recommendations on an appropriate program may be essential to your recovery.

Once you leave the hospital, you have many options to choose from. If you aren't comfortable with a formal program, you can choose something as simple as walk-ing every day or every other day. (Ask your physical therapist about the Winningham program, a simple exercise routine based primarily on walking, either alone or in a group. Designed for patients at all stages, it encourages the use of a walking diary to help make exercise one of your prescriptions for medical treatment.) Or you can go up and down stairs at home or at work for 15 to 20 minutes every other day.

On days when the weather is forbidding, you can exercise on a treadmill, stationary bike, rowing machine, Health Rider or stair climber in your home. Home equipment is worthwhile if you have a busy schedule and want to exercise at your own pace and convenience. The January 1996 issue of *Consumer Reports* magazine lists the top exercise machines on the market, and gives information about their durability, safety and costs. You can join a health club if you want a variety of equipment to choose from and to be with people who are also exercising.

If you like classroom-type aerobics, you could join a group, attend a class or purchase one of the widely available exercise videos. These videos offer an ideal way to work up to a full routine: some show a slower group on one side of the screen and a more athletic group on the other, but you can also stop the tape or limit the number of times you repeat an exercise. A variety of TV shows can also take you through an aerobic workout. To avoid boredom, you may even alternate programs.

When to Avoid Exercising Discuss your exercise plans with your physician. If you are ill or are in the first phases of recovery, your physician should instruct you about your limits and about the medical effects of exercise.

Dr. Meryl Winningham, who has pioneered research on low-intensity aerobic conditioning with cancer patients, often discusses precautions that must be taken by cancer patients when planning exercise. The following chart shows two scales that measure a patient's condition and capabilities. The Zubrod scale is scored from 1 to 10, with 10 being the lowest. The Karnofsky scale runs from 0 to 100, with the 90-to–100 range being the highest rating. If your score on the Zubrod scale falls below the 1–to-2 range, or if your score on the Karnofsky scale falls anywhere below 90, your physician will need to decide whether you may exercise.

Many breast cancer patients who have lymph nodes removed find that the nerve endings to this tissue are still active. The electrical impulse that is generated after surgery, known as a shooter, can cause pain in certain movements, especially when lifting the arms over the head. Shooters occur because an arm-stretch-ing program was not instituted after surgery. If you have had surgery for breast cancer, discuss range-of-motion limitations with an exercise professional, especially if you experience shooters. Several options are available to avoid causing further pain, including ice massage on the affected areas after exercising. Using a modified cardiac support hose over the length of the arm may help with blood supply, reducing stimulation to the nerve and reducing the swelling in the hands that often happens after exercise.

Other medical contraindications for exercise include abnormal levels of sodium and potassium (electrolytes) in the blood, abnormal protein metabolism, and platelet counts under 30,000 to 40,000. When your platelet count is low, gentle exercise, muscle tightening, etc., can help

Karnofsky Scale

100 percent	No evidence of disease
90 percent	Normal activity with minor signs of disease
80 percent	Normal activity with effort; signs of disease
70 percent	Cannot do normal activity, but cares for self
60 percent	Requires occasional assistance
50 percent	Requires considerable assistance and frequent medical care
40 percent	Disabled; requires special care
30 percent	Severely disabled; hospitalization may be indicated
20 percent	Very sick; hospitalization necessary for supportive treatment
10 percent	Moribund

Zubrod Scale

0	Asymptomatic; normal activity
1	Symptomatic but fully ambulatory
2	Symptomatic; in bed less than 50 percent of time
3	Symptomatic; in bed more than 50 percent of time; not bedridden
4	100 percent bedridden

Approximate relationship of Karnofsky scale to Zubrod scale:

0 Zubrod	= 100 percent Karnofsky
1 Zubrod	= 85 percent Karnofsky
2 Zubrod	= 65 percent Karnofsky
3 Zubrod	= 40 percent Karnofsky
4 Zubrod	= 15 percent Karnofsky

maintain function and avoid regression. But vigorous exercise may cause bleeding.

Your doctor will also want to assess your pulmonary function: if tests show that your lungs are operating at less than 50 percent of their capacity, you should not do any aerobic exercises.

Patients with metastatic bone cancer who have less than 50 percent bone cortex involved should not be doing any weight-bearing exercise.

KNOWING WHEN TO STOP

If your physician decides that you may begin an exercise program, you will still need to pay close attention to how you feel during an exercise session. Be aware of the following alarm signals:

1. Shortness of breath (difficulty breathing, either when resting or when exercising). If an exercise is hard to perform without your becoming short of breath, exercising for even a minimal amount of time can be hazardous. See your physician before continuing.

2. Dizziness. This is usually a sign of pushing too hard, but it can also occur if you are fatigued, if you have low blood pressure, if you are dehydrated and for other reasons. Check with your physician. Back off exercise until the symptoms have subsided for a few days.

3. Chronic muscle soreness that interferes with daily routines. Stop exercising for a few days. You may need to rest your muscles.

4. Bruises or swelling. These may be caused by chemotherapy; they can also arise when a bacterial or viral infection is not healing well. Check with your physician.

In general, when you exercise, it's important not to get too tired or to hurt yourself. Here are some more rules for safe, comfortable exercising.

◆ When doing exercises for flexibility and muscle strength, try to repeat each exercise three to five times at first. If you feel too tired or too weak, do only one or two repetitions. Gradually increase to between 10 and 20 repetitions.

◆ Try to exercise at least twice a day, and more often if you like it.

◆ Keep a daily record of your progress, using the Exercise Progress Chart on page 262. The repetitions and periods will vary for each person, depending on the person's strength and medical problems.

EXAMPLE OF EXERCISE PROGRESS CHART

Date	Exercise Stage	Repetitions Each Exercise	No. of Exercise Periods per Day	Total Minutes Exercised
10/5	I	3	2	3
10/6	I	3	2	5
10/7	I	5	3	10
10/8	I	5	4	10
10/9	I	10	4	20

Age	Target Heart Rate	Perceived Exertion Ceiling
20–29	140–148 bpm	6–8 (out of 10)
30–39	132–140 bpm	6–7
40–49	125–132 bpm	6–7
50–59	115–122 bpm	5–6
60–69	108–116 bpm	5–6
70+	(consult with your physician)	

With any exercise program, always warm up a little before starting, and cool down when you finish. When engaging in aerobic exercise, stay within the following recommended heart rates during exercise, and monitor your perceived exertion (how hard you feel the exercise is) during the activity. The chart above gives ranges for each, based on your age.

Always take your pulse before, halfway through and at the end of any aerobic routine. Aim to roughly double your heart rate if you can, unless your physician sets a specific rate that you should not exceed. The rule is moderation—take it easy.

If your pulse is slow and you become short of breath, don't keep pushing, even if your pulse is within your age-group limits. Have a medical evaluation to prevent harming yourself from exercise. If your heartbeat becomes irregular or you develop chest pain, stop and consult your doctor soon.

BREATHING

Proper breathing techniques are essential to exercise and can be both therapeutic and relaxing. The techniques have been around for thousands of years and are practiced in the martial arts and used for meditation purposes. Breathing affects the parasympathetic nervous system— the part of the central nervous system that controls our relaxation responses.

Perhaps the best way to breathe when doing heavy exercises is in and out through the nose. This produces a sensa-tion of "fullness" of breath and does not dry the throat. If you can breathe in or out only through your mouth, go ahead—just keep a glass of water handy.

Breathe with as much relaxation as possible. Try to let go of any tension in all the muscles in your neck and shoulders, and fill your lungs all the way.

It is important to keep blowing out and breathing in as you perform any exercise. Many people tend to forget to breathe, especially when doing muscle-strengthening or endurance exercises. Never hold your breath during an exercise: holding your breath increases pressure on the heart and may cause dizziness or fainting.

In our culture, only babies generally breathe correctly. After years of being told to "sit up straight" and "suck in your stomach," many of us develop the bad habit of chest breathing: inhaling by lifting our chests instead of by pushing down our diaphragm. A good relaxation routine centers on slow breaths. The easiest way to make sure you're doing this slow breathing correctly is to press your hand over your abdominal region when you inhale, concentrating on pushing the air into your belly. This will cause distension and a feeling of fullness in the abdominal region. This "diaphragm" breathing also results in inhaling and exhaling more air than does chest breathing.

Bed-bound patients risk collecting mucus in their lungs, which can cause pneumonia. Deep breathing followed by coughing can help prevent this complication.

Deep-breathing exercises can help you improve your breathing habits so that you use your entire lung, not just the upper part. Begin each exercise session with a deep-breathing exercise. Deep breathing is also a good way to rest between exercises.

Here are two exercises that help promote breathing and relaxation:

◆ Slow deep breaths. Using the technique described above, breathe in for a count of four seconds and breathe out for a count of eight seconds. When your capacity improves, you may be able to breathe in for a count of 10 seconds and out for a count of 20 seconds.

◆ Short, fast deep breaths. This exercise helps you learn the rhythm of using your diaphragm instead of your rib muscles to breathe with. Concentrate on pushing the air out through your nose from the diaphragm, and then relax and allow your lungs to fill back up with air, making sure that your belly expands at the same time. Aim for a rate of one push every second.

Deep-Breathing Exercise The following deep-breathing exercise may be done standing up or lying down.
1. Leave your arms at your sides, keeping your hands loose.
2. Slowly take in a deep breath through your nose while raising your arms over your head.
3. Slowly breathe out through your mouth while bringing your arms back down to your sides.

Breathing Blow Bottle (Incentive Spirometer) The following exercise uses a breathing blow bottle (also called a breathing incentive spirometer) to increase your lung capacity and help avoid pulmonary complications. If you do not breathe deeply, especially after lying on your back for prolonged intervals, you become increasingly susceptible to bronchitis and pneumonia, because fluid tends to collect in the lungs.

Coughing is also good for you; take a deep breath and cough three to five times to clear your lungs.

Increasing Lung Expansion
1. Blow out your breath (exhale).
2. Inhale through the breathing tube, causing the ball to rise as high as possible.
3. Repeat steps 1 and 2 from 5 to 10 times.

A SAMPLE PROGRESSIVE EXERCISE PROGRAM

The exercise program described in this chapter (*see* "Sample Exercises" below) has been devised to increase your strength and endurance. The program, which takes you from your bed to being up and around in three stages, can be started as soon as your physician says you are able to exercise.

◆ Stage I exercises are simple exercises to help you maintain and increase your range of motion. They require little exertion and can be done in bed.

◆ Stage II exercises use a small added weight to increase resistance and can be done when you are spending part of the day out of bed. Once you have gotten back to your normal activities, you will need to establish an exercise routine that includes exercises like these to build up your body's reserves so that temporary bouts with bedrest will not deplete your energy stores.

◆ Stage III exercises provide you with a strengthening and maintenance program for when you are able to spend the whole day out of bed.

This series of exercises is a progressive and comprehensive physical rehabilitation program for people with acute or chronic illness. With your doctor's permission, you can begin these exercises even while you are recovering from surgery and while you are undergoing radiation or chemotherapy.

Start with light warmup exercises several times a day, gradually increasing both the difficulty of the exercises and the number of times you repeat them. Your maximum physical capacity will improve with time and with use of the program. When you reach the level of more advanced exercises using muscle resistance, you will also need to add a deceleration or "cooldown" period to your program. Suddenly stopping exercise after a 10- to 20-minute period could be dangerous. (Nevertheless, if you experience irregular heartbeats, chest pain, lightheadedness or nausea, stop exercising immediately. Do not continue until you have clearance from your doctor.)

These exercises will need to be modified for each individual. Often you will have limits dictated by your physical condition. Your physician and your physical and occupational therapists can help you set up a program that matches your abilities. In addition, you may need to adjust your exercise program daily depending on how you feel, what tests are ordered, or medical necessities such as special diets, x-rays or specific medical therapies.

The exercise program we present here is completely flexible. It can be done at times convenient to you. You can do only part of the program if your energy level is low, or change the pace several times a day so that by the end of the day you have accumulated several 1- to 10-minute periods of exercise for various parts of your body.

The Medi-Gym Some of the exercises in Stage I and Stage II require simple items of exercise equipment to help you increase your muscle strength by making you work against a slight resistance. These items may be purchased together in the Medi-Gym kit described below, or you can make your own kit using the substitutions suggested.

◆ Elastic sheet: a paper-thin elastic sheet made of the same material as a dentist's rubber (30 in. x 6 in., or roughly 76 cm x

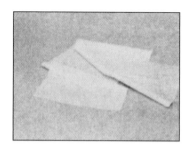

15 cm) or a surgical rubber Penrose drain (1 in. x 30 in., or roughly 2.5 cm x 76 cm). Used for added resistance in Stage I's general strengthening exercises.

◆ Breathing incentive spirometer: a breathing appliance with a mouthpiece. Used to increase lung capacity and to

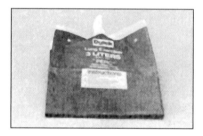

avoid pulmonary complications in Stage I. You can substitute a soft balloon or a surgical glove with a mouthpiece.

◆ Exercise putty (Theraplast): elastic putty. Used in Stage I to strengthen and

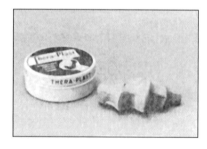

coordinate hands and fingers. You can substitute clay or Silly Putty.

◆ Sponge ball: a lightweight sponge ball, about 4 inches (10 cm) in diameter. Used in Stage I's general limbering, strength-

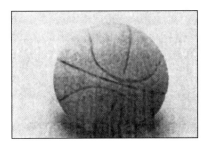

ening and coordination exercises. You can substitute a small Nerf ball, available in toy stores.

◆ Clothespin: an ordinary wooden clothespin. Used in Stage I to coordinate hands and fingers. For added resistance,

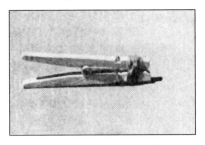

wrap a rubber band around the clothespin's tip.

◆ Ankle weight: a 3-pound (1 kg) ankle weight with a Velcro closure, used for added resistance in Stage II's general strengthening exercises. There are sever-

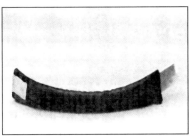

al possible substitutes for this item: (1) Purchase sinkers from a fishing-tackle store, and pin or sew them to heavy material; purchase Velcro from a store that carries sewing supplies. (2) Put canned goods in an old purse that has a handle. (3) Sew sandbags.

◆ Exercise stretcher: an elastic rope with looped handles. Used in Stage II exercises for stretching and strengthening the large muscles. You can construct a stretcher from elastic shock cord (also called

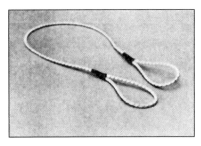

bungee cord), available in outdoor supply stores; make loops at the ends by tying knots. Or you can substitute a piece of surgical rubber Penrose drain.

◆ Jump rope: any type of rope will suffice. If you are bed-bound, you can tie the rope to the foot of the bed and use it to pull yourself up to a sitting position. Also used in jump-rope exercises. You can substitute a piece of rope or clothesline.

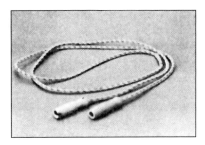

SAMPLE EXERCISES

This section offers some sample progressive exercise programs. Some of the exercises use equipment described earlier (*see* "The Medi-Gym"); some use equipment (such as an over-the-bed trapeze) that may be provided by the hospital while you are recovering from surgery. In Stage II, some exercises call for a cane or broom handle, and several require a chair.

STAGE I: BEGINNING TO MOVE

Stage I exercises are simple range-of-motion exercises that require little exertion and can be done when you are bedridden. Even if you are very ill, you will probably be able to do some or all of these exercises. Remember, it is important to exercise in order to maintain your muscle tone and your joint mobility.

Begin by taking 10 deep, relaxing breaths. Remember, do not hold your breath while you do any exercise. Breathe rhythmically in and out.

Shoulders and Chest The following exercises increase the mobility of your shoulder joints and strengthen your chest muscles.

Straight Arm Lifts

1. Lie on your back, and place your arms down by your sides.
2. Keeping your elbows straight, lift your arms up and as far back over your head as you can.
3. Keeping your elbows straight, lower your arms to your sides.

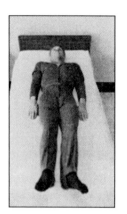
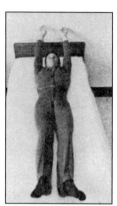

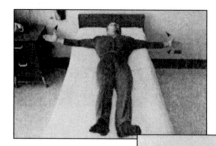

Side Arm Lifts

1. Lie on your back, and place your arms down by your sides.
2. Keeping your elbows straight, bring your arms out to the sides and up over your head until your hands touch.
3. Keeping your elbows straight, lower your arms back to your sides again.

Elbow Touches

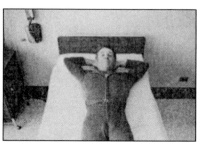

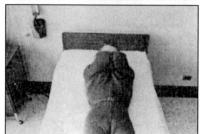

Elbow Touches
1. Lie on your back, and place your hands behind your head with your elbows flat on the bed.
2. Bring your elbows together in front of your body.
3. Lower your elbows back down to the bed. (This exercise can also be done sitting up.)

Straight Arm Crosses
1. Lie on your back, and put your right arm straight out to the side at a right angle to your body.
2. Keeping your elbow straight, bring your arm across your chest to your left side.
3. Keeping your elbow straight, return your arm to its original position.
4. Repeat steps 1 to 3 with your left arm.
5. Try using both arms at once, criss-crossing them in front of you.

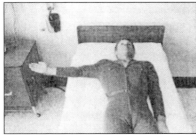
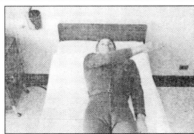
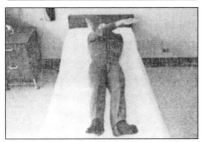

Elbows and Wrists
The following exercises help preserve the mobility of your elbow and wrist joints.

Elbow Bends
1. Lie on your back, place your arms down by your sides and make a fist with each hand.
2. Bring your fists up to your shoulders, bending your elbows.
3. Lower your fists to their original position.

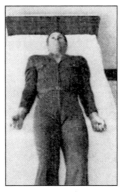
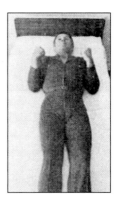

Wrist Rotation
1. Lie on your back, and make a fist with each hand.
2. Make small inward circles with your fists.
3. Reverse direction, and make small outward circles with your fists.

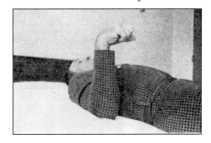

Now is a good time to stop and rest. If you are tired, pause and take 10 to 20 deep, relaxing breaths. Try to relax your neck and shoulders. If you let tension build up, you'll get tired more easily. Place your hand on your stomach and try to make it rise when you breathe in. Blow out as long as you can.

Hips, Knees and Ankles
The following exercises mobilize and strengthen your walking muscles.

Knee-to-Chest Lifts
1. Lie on your back, placing your legs together and flat on the bed.
2. Bend your left leg, and bring your knee up toward your chest.
3. Straighten your knee while lowering your leg slowly to the bed.
4. Repeat steps 1 to 3 with your right leg.

Don't forget to breathe. Do not hold your breath. Breathe in when you lift your leg, and blow out as you lower it back down.

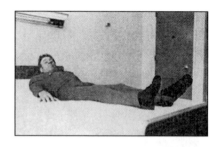

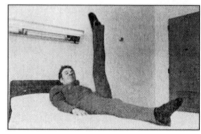

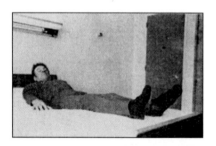

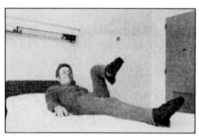

Knee Touches
1. Lie on your back with both knees bent, keeping your feet flat on the bed.
2. Relax and let your knees fall slowly outward as far as they will comfortably go.
3. Bring your knees back up together.

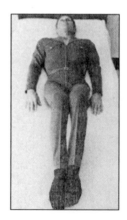

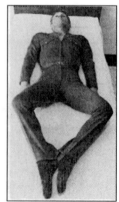

Straight Leg Lifts
1. Lie on your back, placing your legs together and flat on the bed.
2. Keeping your knee straight, lift your left leg as high as you can.
3. Keeping your knee straight, lower your leg slowly to the bed.
4. Repeat steps 1 to 3 with your right leg.

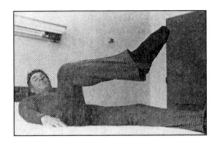

Ankle Rotation
1. Lie on your back, lift your right heel a little off the bed and make small inward circles with your foot.
2. Reverse direction, and make small outward circles with your foot.
3. Repeat steps 1 and 2 with your left foot.

Now is a good time to stop and rest. Take 10 to 20 relaxing breaths before starting the next series of exercises.

Trunk
The following exercises strengthen your trunk.

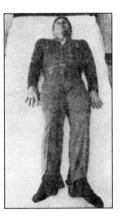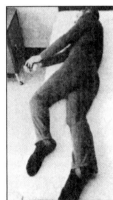

Side-to-Side Rolls
This exercise helps prevent bedsores.

Caution: If you are in a hospital bed, do this exercise with the bedrails raised. If there are no bedrails, have someone stand beside the bed to make sure you do not roll out of bed.

1. Lie on your back, with your knees and elbows slightly bent.
2. Lift your left shoulder and roll to the right, reaching with your left arm for the bedrail or the side of the mattress.
3. Roll back.
4. Repeat steps 1 to 3 on your other side.

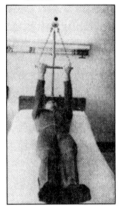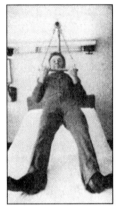

Trapeze-Bar Pullups
1. Lie on your back, and place both hands up on the trapeze.
2. Lift your buttocks up off the bed.
3. Try to get your nose or chin up to the bar.
4. Lie back again, and repeat steps 1 to 3.

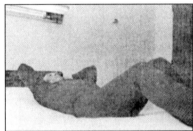

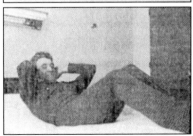

Partial Situps

1. Lie on your back, with your hands clasped behind your head.
2. Try to lift your head off the pillow.
3. Now try to lift your head and shoulders up.
4. Lie back down, and repeat steps 1 to 3.

The next set of exercises uses the Medi-Gym equipment for added resistance. If you are tired, take a rest before proceeding. Breathe deeply 10 to 20 times.

STAGE I MEDI-GYM

In the following exercises, you will use the clothespin, rubber band, exercise putty, sponge ball, elastic sheet and breathing incentive spirometer from your Medi-Gym.

Clothespin and Rubber Band

These exercises use a clothespin and a rubber band to strengthen your hands and fingers. They can be done lying down, even if you have an intravenous feeding tube in your arm.

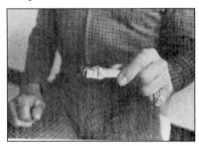

Finger Squeeze

1. Squeeze the clothespin between your thumb and your first two fingers. If this is too difficult, squeeze the clothespin between your thumb and all four of your fingers.
2. For added resistance, wrap a rubber band around the tip of the clothespin and repeat step 1.

Advanced Finger Squeeze

1. Hold the clothespin between your thumb and first finger, trying to keep your thumb and finger in a circle.
2. Open the clothespin as wide as it will go, and hold it open for a few seconds.
3. Repeat steps 1 and 2 with your thumb and each of your other fingers.
4. For added resistance, wrap a rubber band around the tip of the clothespin and repeat steps 1 to 3.

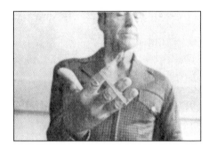

Finger Spread

1. Place a rubber band over the fingers of one hand, stretching the rubber band.
2. Spread your fingers apart.
3. Repeat steps 1 and 2 with your other hand.

Exercise Putty

The following exercises use exercise putty to strengthen your hands and your coordination control. The putty can be pulled, worked in a ball, or bounced. Use your imagination to invent your own exercises in addition to those described here.

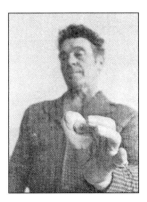

First-and-Second-Finger Pinch
1. Place a ball of putty between your thumb and your first finger.
2. Squeeze through the ball until your thumb and finger meet.
3. Repeat steps 1 and 2 with your thumb and each of your other fingers.

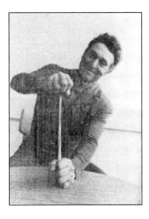

Wrist Pullups
1. Place your left forearm on a table, and hold a piece of putty in your left hand.
2. Hold the other end of the putty in your right hand.
3. Pull the putty up with your right hand.
4. Repeat steps 1 to 3, starting with your right forearm on the table.

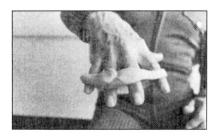

Finger Spread
1. Make a loop out of putty.
2. Place the loop around the fingers of your left hand, between the top two joints.
3. Spread your fingers apart against the loop.
4. Repeat steps 1 to 3 with your right hand.

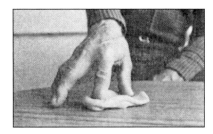

Finger Opening
1. Smash the putty flat with the palm of your hand.
2. Stick your thumb and first finger into the putty, close together.
3. Push your thumb and first finger apart.
4. Repeat steps 1 to 3 with your thumb and each of your other fingers.
5. Change hands, and repeat steps 1 to 4.

Hand Squeeze
Squeeze the putty in your hand like a ball,
moving it around at the same time.

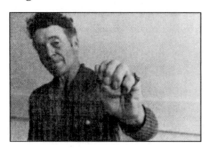

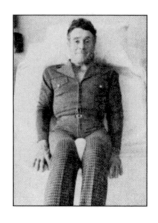

Sponge Ball
The sponge ball is light, easy to handle
and safe—it won't bruise your skin if it
hits you. Some of the following exercises
are done lying down; for others, you will
sit up.

Knee Squeeze
While either lying down or sitting up, put
the ball between your knees and try to
hold it there.

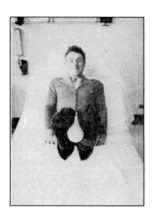

Leg Lift
Lie down, put the ball between your feet
and try to lift it off the bed. (Breathe in
when you lift. Blow out as you lower the
ball back to the bed.)

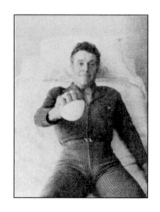

Hand Squeeze
Squeeze the ball in your hand, moving it
around at the same time.

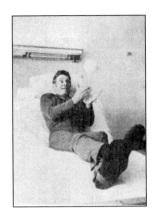

Up-and-Down Toss
Sit up (make sure your bedrails are raised); throw the ball up and catch it.

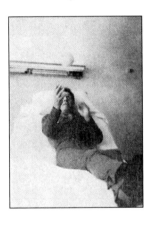

Side-to-Side Toss
Toss the ball from one hand to the other, leaning from side to side to catch it.

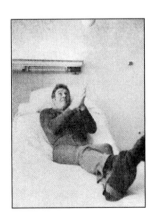

Clap and Catch
Toss the ball back and forth with a friend. For more coordination, try clapping your hands just before catching the ball.

Elastic Sheet

The following exercises use an elastic sheet
for resistance. The sheet is very thin and
easy to stretch. All of these exercises may
be done either lying in bed or sitting up.

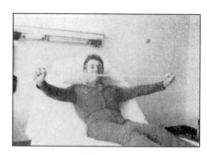

*Caution: Never use the elastic sheet close
to your face. If you lose your grip on it, it
could injure your face or eyes. Do not do
these exercises if you have any weakness
or tremor or if your grip has been injured.*

Arm and Chest Stretch

Grab both ends of the elastic sheet and
stretch it sideways.

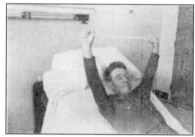

Chest and Shoulder Stretch

Stretch the elastic sheet apart behind your
head or back.

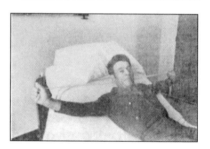

Wrist Stretch

1. Hold both ends of the elastic sheet in
    your left hand.
2. Loop the sheet around your right
    wrist.
3. Try to push your right wrist up
    against the elastic sheet.
4. Repeat steps 1 to 3 with the elastic
    sheet looped around your left wrist.

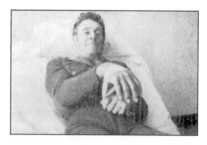

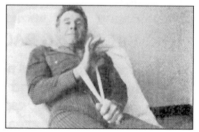

Calf Stretch

1. Hold one end of the elastic sheet in each hand.
2. Bend your knees and loop the sheet over the bottom of your feet.
3. Push the sheet down with your feet while pulling the sheet up with your hands.

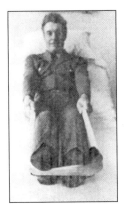
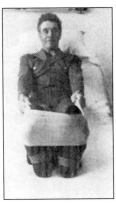

Leg and Thigh Stretch

1. Hold one end of the elastic sheet in each hand.
2. Loop the sheet over the bottom of your left foot.
3. Bend your left knee toward your chest.
4. Push your left leg straight out against the elastic sheet while pulling the sheet up with your hands.
5. Repeat steps 1 to 4 with your right foot.

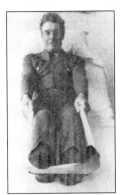
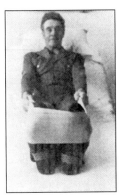

Thigh Stretch

1. Hold one end of the elastic sheet in each hand.
2. Loop the sheet over the bottom of your feet.
3. Try to spread your legs apart against it.

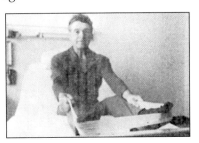

STAGE II: BED/CHAIR WITH RESISTANCE

Neck

The following exercises strengthen your neck muscles. If you have head and neck disease, either omit these exercises or check with your physician before trying them.

Chin Tuck I

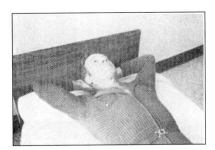
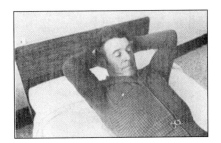

Chin Tuck I

1. Lie on your back and place your hands behind your head, with your elbows bent and pointed out to the sides.
2. Holding your hands behind your head, bring your chin up to your chest.
3. Push your head back against your hands.
4. Lower your head back against your hands.

Chin Tuck II

1. Lie on your back and place your hands on your forehead, with your elbows bent and pointed out to the sides.
2. Pushing against your head with your hands, bring your chin to your chest.
3. Relax and lower your head back down to the bed.

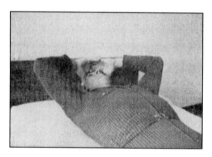

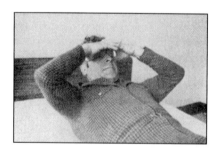

Side Neck Bends

1. Lie on your back, bending your right elbow and putting your right hand on the side of your head.
2. Bend your head to the left.
3. Bend your head to the right while pushing against your head with your right hand.
4. Repeat steps 1 to 3 with your left hand.

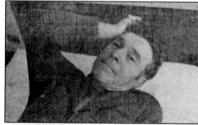

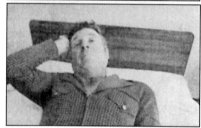

Shoulders and Chest

The following exercises strengthen the muscles of your shoulders and chest.

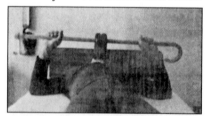

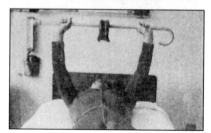

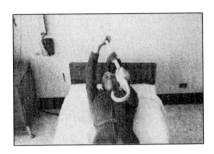

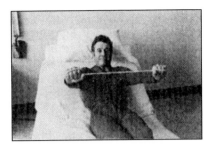

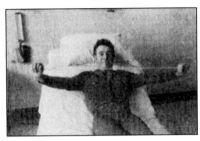

Straight-Arm Cane Lift

This exercise uses the 3-pound (1 kg) weight to strengthen the shoulders, expand the rib cage and exercise the chest muscles. Lifting your arms over your head greatly expands your rib cage, giving you an excellent opportunity to breathe deeply as you raise your arms.

1. Loop the 3-pound (1 kg) weight around the middle of a cane or broom handle.
2. Lie on your back, and take the cane in both hands.
3. Keeping your elbows straight, lift the cane up and as far back over your head as possible.
4. Keeping your elbows straight, lower the cane slowly to the original position.

2. Lie on your back, and take the cane in both hands.
3. Keeping your elbows straight, hold the cane up over your head.
4. Twist the cane slowly to the left, and then slowly to the right.

Side Arm Stretch

This exercise uses the exercise stretcher to strengthen your chest muscles.

1. While either sitting up or lying down, take the ends of the exercise stretcher in your hands.
2. Stretch your arms out to the sides, pulling against the exercise stretcher.

Overhead Arm Stretch

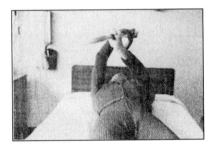

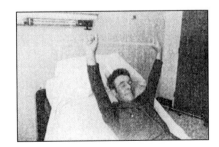

Straight-Arm Cane Twist

This exercise uses the 3-pound (1 kg) weight to strengthen your shoulder muscles.

1. Loop the 3-pound (1 kg) weight around the middle of a cane or broom handle.

This exercise uses the exercise stretcher to strengthen your shoulder muscles.

1. While either sitting up or lying down, take the ends of the exercise stretcher in your hands.
2. Holding your arms over your head, stretch sideways.
    Stop and rest before proceeding. Take 10 to 20 deep breaths. If you are not too tired, start the next group of exercises.

Walking Muscles
The following exercises strengthen your walking muscles.

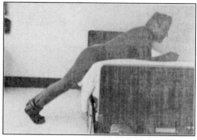

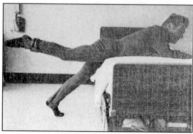

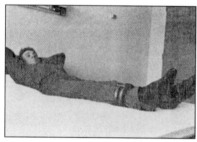

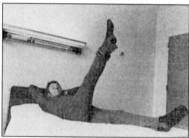

Straight Leg Lifts
This exercise strengthens your knees and thighs.

1. Strap the 3-pound (1 kg) weight around your right ankle.
2. Lie on your back. Keeping your knee straight, lift your right leg straight up as far as you can.
3. Keeping your knee straight, slowly lower your leg to the bed.
4. Repeat steps 1 to 3 with your left leg.

Backward Leg Lifts
This exercise strengthens your buttocks.
1. Strap the 3-pound (1 kg) weight around your right ankle.
2. Lie on your stomach, with your abdomen on the bed and your feet touching the floor.
3. Keeping your right knee straight, lift your right leg up and back.
4. Repeat steps 1 to 3 with your left leg.

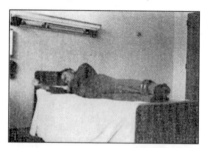

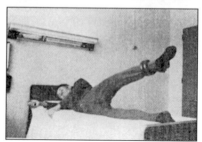

Sideways Leg Lifts

This exercise strengthens your thighs.

1. Strap the 3-pound (1 kg) weight around your left ankle.
2. Lie on your right side, with your right arm under your head. Brace yourself against the bed with your left arm in front of your chest.
3. Keeping your knee straight, lift your left leg up.
4. Keeping your knee straight, lower your left leg slowly to the bed.
5. Repeat steps 1 to 4 on your other side.

Arms and Legs

The following exercises strengthen your arms and legs.

Elbow Bends I

This exercise uses the exercise stretcher to strengthen your arms and back.

1. Sit on the bed, placing the loops of the exercise stretcher around the bottoms of your feet and holding the middle of the exercise stretcher in your hands.
2. Sit up with your legs straight out and your arms straight out in front of you.
3. Bending your elbows, bring your arms to your chest.
4. Relax, allowing your arms to return to their original position.

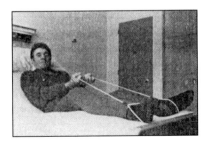

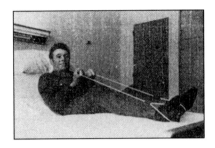

Upward Arm Stretch

This exercise uses the exercise stretcher to strengthen your upper arms.

1. Lie on your back with the exercise stretcher underneath your back.
2. Holding the ends of the stretcher in your hands, extend your arms straight up, pulling the ends of the stretcher toward the ceiling.

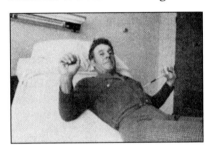

Trapeze Arm Stretch

This exercise uses your bed trapeze to strengthen your upper arms.

1. Loop the exercise stretcher over the trapeze.
2. While sitting up, take the ends of the exercise stretcher in your hands and pull down as far as you can.
3. Raise your arms, and repeat step 2.

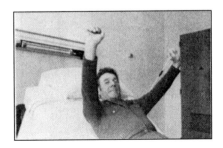

Downward Arm Stretch

1. While sitting up, place the exercise stretcher around the back of your neck like a scarf.
2. Taking the ends of the exercise stretcher in your hands, pull down until your arms are straight.

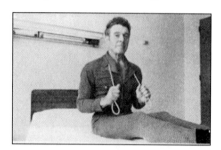

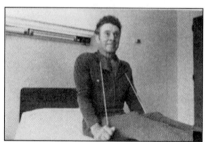

The following exercises are done sitting on the side of the bed or in a chair. If you are not used to standing up and walking around, be sure to have someone with you to help if you get dizzy.

Elbow Bends II

This exercise uses the 3-pound (1 kg) weight to strengthen your arms.

1. Loop the 3-pound (1 kg) weight around the middle of a cane or a broom handle.
2. While sitting in a chair or on the edge of a bed, hold the cane in both hands, palms up.
3. Bending your elbows, lift the cane to your chest.
4. Lower the cane to your knees, straightening your elbows.
5. Repeat steps 3 and 4 while holding the cane in both hands, palms down.

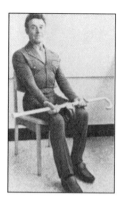 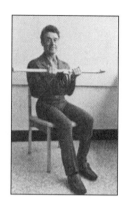

Knee Lifts

This exercise uses the 3-pound (1 kg) weight to strengthen your knees.

1. Strap the 3-pound (1 kg) weight around your left ankle.
2. While sitting in a chair or on the edge of a bed, extend your left leg, straightening your knee and lifting your foot off the floor.
3. Repeat step 2 with the weight strapped around your right ankle.

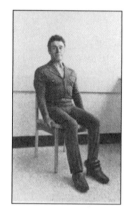 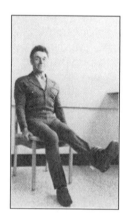

Stand Up–Sit Downs
This exercise strengthens your whole set of walking muscles and your hips, knees and buttocks.

1. Sit on the edge of either a bed or a chair that has arms.
2. Stand up slowly.
3. Sit down slowly.
4. Use the arms of the chair at first; then try to not use the arms.

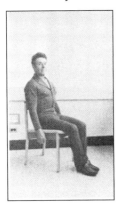 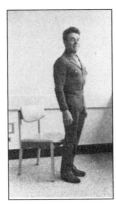

STAGE III: UP AND AROUND

Once you start spending the whole day out of bed, walking around the house and resuming your normal daily activities, you are ready for Stage III activities. These are vigorous exercises, and safety precautions should be observed when using a chair. Take your pulse when you begin and after you finish. Your pulse should return to its resting rate within five minutes.

Try to exercise four to five times a week. As with Stages I and II, begin with 3 to 5 repetitions of each exercise; try to work your way up to between 10 and 20 repetitions.

Once again, especially with vigorous exercise routines like the following ones, proper breathing is very important. Be careful not to hold your breath. Breathe in and blow out regularly during all the exercises.

Outlined below are two types of exercise routines: one for aerobic conditioning and the other for improving strength. You may perform activities from either or both, depending on your medical condition and exercise goals.

Not all patients should perform all types of machine exercises. If you have had surgery for breast cancer in the upper chest/armpit area, you may use rubber tubing at first for the chest pulls and rowing exercises. Your goal is to progress to light dumbbell or hand-weight exercises for chest work and flies (pendulum exercises moving the arms to the front and sides). Rubber tubing allows you to experience the feel of progressive resistance and to control how much force you exert. Over time, you will increase your strength enough to move on to other strength stations.

Circulation Enhancers
Vertical Arm Swings
1. Stand with your feet apart.
2. Clasp your hands together, keeping your elbows straight.
3 Swing your arms up over your head, and then bring them back down toward the floor again.

Finish up your exercise session with 10 to 20 deep breaths.

SPORTS AND RECREATION

When you are able to do Stage III exercises comfortably, think about adding some sports and recreational activities to your exercise program. You can work up to these gradually:

◆ Climb stairs four or five times daily.
◆ Take walks. Pace yourself: go one block the first time, and then try to increase your distance daily.
◆ Gardening is an excellent exercise if you enjoy it. At first someone may have to assist you with the heavier work. Even a small plot will provide you with exer-

cise, as well as fresh air, sunshine and a sense of accomplishment.

◆ Bicycle. Plan your routes to be more or less strenuous to fit your needs.

◆ Jump rope. This vigorous exercise gives overall muscle toning and coordination.

◆ Swim. If you feel energetic, join a health club and use the saunas and steam rooms as well as the pool. Water is much easier

SAMPLE PROGRAM I: AEROBIC CONDITIONING

These exercises will produce modest improvement of cardiovascular capacity and improved functional abilities (enhanced energy, reduced fatigue, better breathing capacity), with possible improvement in the immune system over time.

AEROBIC CONDITIONING ACTIVITIES

Exercise	How Performed	Times/week	Length/ Intensity
Aqua aerobics	self/class	2–3	20–40 min., 50–70%
Aqua deep-water walking	self	2–4	10–25 min., 50–70 %
Breathing/Slow	self	daily	5 min.
ITP (interval training program) walking		1–2	fast for 10–15 min. slow for 5–10 yd. (4.5–9 m) sets during the same 2-mi. (3 km) walk
Qi gong, with tai chi centering	1-on-1	daily or alternate days	depends on style
Stationary bike (treadmill, rower, upper-body arm crank, etc.)	self	3–6	10–40 min., 50–70 %
Tai chi	self	daily	depends on style
Walking	self/partner	3–6	20–60 min., 50–60%

SAMPLE PROGRAM II: STRENGTH AND CONDITIONING
Goals: Improve posture, strength, range of motion, flexibility

STRENGTH AND CONDITIONING ACTIVITIES

Exercise	How Performed	Times/week	Length/ Intensity
Body part ◆ Work on movements in postsurgery areas that have pain and decreased motion	self/partner	3–6	10–15 min.
Elastic bands ◆ Increase isotonic strength and range of motion in major muscle groups; learn principles of progressive resistance.	self/1-on-1	2–4	10–20 min.
Light dumbbells ◆ Increase range of motion in upper body.	self/1-on-1	2–4	10–20 min.
Manual ◆ Perform resistance movements with instructor, to improve function postsurgery.	partner/1-on-1	2–4	10–15 min.
Weights ◆ Improve general strength through specific ranges of motion.	self/class	2–4	20–60 min.

A typical strength-training program for cancer patients should consist of a specific exercise routine. One such routine is detailed below:

	Sets	Repetitions
Warmup, 5 minutes		
Resistive exercises:		
Bench press, lateral pulls	2–4	10–8–6*
Shoulder press, T-rows	1–2	10 each
Biceps, triceps, abdominals	1–2	10 each
Leg press, extensions	2–3	10–8–6*
Leg curls, calf raises	1–2	10 each

Stretching component, 5–10 minutes

*Increase weight as you become comfortable at each weight level and are ready to increase the weight by a fixed amount (e.g., 2, 5 or 10 pounds [1, 2 or 3 kg]) to provide progressive resistance with major muscle groups.

to exercise in because it supports your limbs, making it easier to move about.

POSTMASTECTOMY REHABILITATION

You can enhance your physical and psychological recovery following a mastectomy by returning as quickly as possible to the normal activities of your daily life.

Your first step is to better understand postmastectomy problems by talking about your concerns with members of your medical team, family and friends, and if possible with a volunteer from the American Cancer Society's Reach to Recovery program.

Your next step is active participation in a structured exercise program, such as the American Cancer Society's Reach to Recovery postmastectomy exercise program, the YWCA's ENCORE (Encouragement, Normalcy, Counseling, Opportunity, Reaching Out and Energies Revived) program, or a similar exercise program, such as the one given here. (For information about Reach to Recovery and ENCORE, see the Resources at the end of the book.)

In this section, we will first describe the Reach to Recovery and ENCORE programs. We will then present a series of postmastectomy exercises to help you increase your muscle strength and range of motion. (In Chapter 22, we will give suggestions on coping with the activities of daily living and using them as helpful exercises.)

Beginning a regular exercise program (e.g., as presented in Stage III, above, or the Winningham walking program) has been proven effective in overall disease control.

Reach to Recovery

Reach to Recovery's approach offers strong support and aid at the most crucial time during the immediate post-surgery period. The program's volunteers have a depth of understanding, since they have also experienced a mastectomy and have returned to the mainstream of life. They offer their personal experience and emotional support to help you maintain your self-esteem and self-confidence and to reduce your fears.

Volunteers supply the Reach to Recovery booklet, a temporary breast form (prosthesis) and helpful hints about self-image, sexuality and clothing. A free demonstration of exercises with necessary tools is provided, so that you can begin exercising as soon as you have permission from your physician, usually a few days after surgery.

A member of your health care team can help you contact your local Reach to Recovery chapter. There is no charge for this volunteer visitor program.

ENCORE

The ENCORE program complements Reach to Recovery and is available in approximately 24 YWCAs across the United States. You may enroll in ENCORE about three weeks after surgery, with your doctor's permission. The program includes group exercises and discussion groups where you can air problems.

POSTMASTECTOMY EXERCISES

Thanks to Lisa Glassberg

Here is a program of standard exercises, many similar to those used in the Reach to Recovery program, that can be used along with videotapes, cassette recordings and the Medi-Gym (*see* the Resources at the end of the book). The most important thing is to involve yourself in a program on a regular basis. Appoint yourself your personal health instructor and go to work. You can gain satisfaction in your achievement. You know best how hard to try, how hard to push and how much pain you can tolerate.

The following exercise program will help initiate your recovery. It can be used in conjunction with the Reach to Recovery or ENCORE programs. If you had breast reconstruction at the same time as your mastectomy, do not begin this program without your surgeon's approval.

Postmastectomy Stage I: Beginning to Move

The following exercises are done with your affected arm and do not require much motion.

Upper-Arm Isometrics

1. Start with shoulder shrugging, ten repetitions, holding for a count of six.
2. Tighten the muscles of your upper arm by slightly bending the elbow and pulling the arm in toward your body.
3. Hold for a count of six; relax for one to two seconds before repeating.

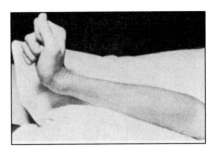

Hand Squeeze

In your Medi-Gym kit, you will find some exercise putty and a sponge ball. Squeeze them in your hand.

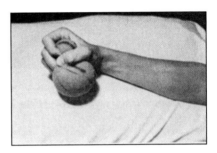

Fingers

Use the exercise putty, the sponge ball and the clothespin from your Medi-Gym kit for gentle finger work.

Postmastectomy Stage II: Increasing Physical Activity

Crawling the Wall

1. Stand facing a wall, about 6 to 8 in. (15 to 20 cm) away from it.
2. Reach toward the wall, and "walk" your fingers up as far as you can. Mark the place where you stop each day to encourage you to go higher the next time.
3. Repeat steps 1 and 2, but begin by turning so that the side of your body faces the wall.

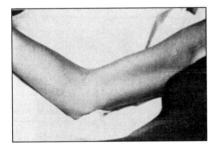

Lower-Arm Isometrics

1. Turn your hands palms up.
2. Make a fist and curl up your wrist.
3. Hold for a count of six; relax for one to two seconds before repeating.

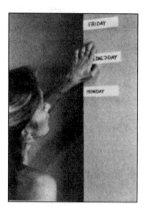

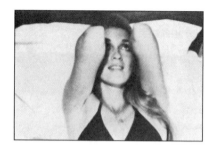

Cane Exercises
1. Put a cane (a broom handle or a yardstick is also good) behind your back and put both hands on it. Pull from side to side.
2. Put the cane behind your neck, and repeat as above.

Pendulum Exercise
1. Begin by sitting in a chair. Bending forward, let the arm hang straight down. Move it in small circles, the way a clock's pendulum moves.
2. Progress to a standing position. (Hold on to a chair or place your hand on a counter or table for stability.) Swing your arm forward and out to the side as well as making circles.

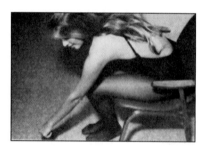

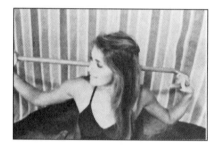

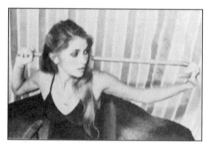

Elbow Touches
1. Lie on your back, placing your hands behind your head with your elbows flat on the bed.
2 Bring your elbows together in front of your body.
3. Lower your elbows back down to the bed. (This exercise can also be done sitting up.)

Pulley Exercise

1. Place the exercise stretcher from your Medi-Gym or a jump rope over a door. (You can hammer a nail at the top of the door to keep the rope from falling off.)
2. Stand with your back to the edge of the door. (You can also face the edge of the door. This exercise can also be done sitting down.)
3. Use your good arm to pull your affected arm as high over your head as possible. Go only slightly into the painful range.

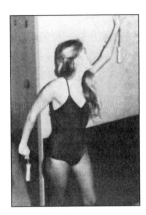

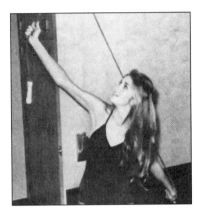

EXERCISE PROGRESS CHART				
Date	Exercise Stage	Repetitions Each Exercise	No. of Exercise Periods per Day	Total Minutes Exercised

22
SELF-CARE AND ACTIVITIES OF DAILY LIVING

Judy Bray, OC

⬦

Attention to self-care and daily living skills, such as brushing your teeth, shaving, combing your hair, getting dressed, etc., serves three purposes: it increases your ability to perform these activities, provides overall muscle toning and increases your range of motion.

Performing as many self-care tasks as possible will also help you develop independence and self-esteem. Feeling dependent on others can be defeating, and a certain satisfaction can be gained from setting objectives in life and accomplishing them. Recovering from an illness or injury is certainly one of these accomplishments.

Consider the degree of physical effort required for self-care tasks in terms of graduated levels based on how much mobility and energy each activity requires. Feeding yourself requires the least amount of effort. When you are stronger, you will be able to graduate to the activities of hygiene and grooming; still later, you'll be able to bathe and dress yourself. Your overall goal is to return to your former activities as fully as possible. Keep a Self-Care Progress Chart on page 269. Make a list of all the activities you perform daily in caring for yourself, and then add each new accomplishment to the list along with the date on which you achieve it.

Many assistive devices or gadgets are available to help you retrain yourself, making certain tasks easier to accomplish. You must conserve energy, using it appropriately to achieve both short-term and long-term goals. In addition, you should consider safety in the home. When you are tired and weak, it is all too easy to have an accident that could slow your recovery or even reverse your physical status dramatically.

ASSISTIVE DEVICES

An assistive device compensates for loss of function and enhances your ability to take care of yourself more comfortably and safely. Such devices can be as simple as a long-handled bath brush or as complex as a wheelchair. Assistive devices can be obtained from medical and surgical supply stores, listed in your yellow pages telephone directory, or by mail order from self-help companies such as the ones listed in Resources at the end of the book. Your local hospital will also have the names of supply companies in your area. Some commonly used devices are described below; many can be improvised at home.

Occupational Aids
◆ One-handed bread and vegetable board
◆ One-handed vegetable basket for straining cooked vegetables
◆ One-handed electric can opener
◆ One-handed "Spill Not" bottle and jar holder
◆ Spill Not and rubber twister for unscrewing lids of bottles and jars
◆ Multipurpose clamp that provides good leverage for small items, or for turning knobs (e.g., on a TV or radio)
◆ Electric plugs with handle

◆ One-handed suction nail brush
◆ One-handed suction nail file

Eating and Drinking Aids
Special cups with lids will help you avoid spilling liquids.

◆ If you have poor coordination or trouble swallowing, the Tommee Tippee cup is useful.

◆ The Wonder-Flow vacuum cup (Figure 1) allows you to drink while lying flat on your back or on your side. These cups can be used with straws. Use extra-long (18 in./46 cm) straws if you tire while trying to hold a cup. You can also improvise with foam cups that have plastic lids, such as those used in take-out food places.

◆ Serve soup in a cup for ease and safety.

◆ If you have trouble swallowing, a plastic glass with a cutout for the nose (Figure 2) will allow you to drink without tipping your head back, as a precaution against choking. The Tommee Tippee cup is also helpful.

◆ If your grasp is weak, a stretch-knit coaster clipped around a glass (Figure 3) will give you a firmer grip. You can also use adhesive-backed bathtub safety treads or similar rubber decals wrapped in a spiral around the glass.

◆ The Mac Mug (Figure 4) has an easy-to-grasp T-shaped handle that is insulated to protect heat-sensitive skin. Two-handled cups, such as children's cups or the Tommee Tippee cup, are also helpful.

◆ Built-up handles on knives, forks and spoons (Figure 5) will help if you have difficulty in grasping. You can improvise these by using foam-rubber hair curlers, sponge rubber or washcloths.

◆ If you have difficulty with coordination, a plate guard will prevent food from being pushed off the plate. The guard clips onto the edge of the plate and acts as a stable surface to push against. You can also use a dish with a high edge, such as a pie plate, or a special plate that is raised on one side (Figure 6).

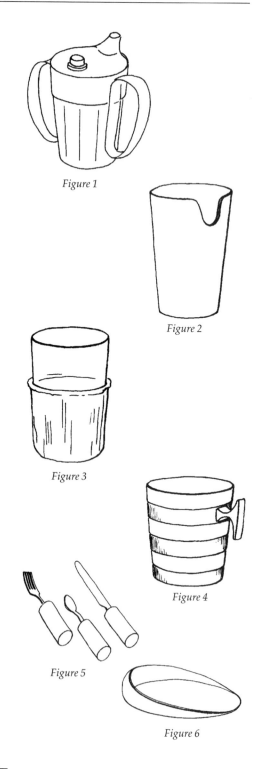

Figure 1

Figure 2

Figure 3

Figure 4

Figure 5

Figure 6

◆ If you must have your meals in bed, a firm wedge-shaped cushion (Figure 7) behind your back will place your body in a more comfortable position, especially for swallowing.

◆ Use a breakfast tray with legs (Figure 8) or a serving tray, or improvise with a cardboard box with spaces cut out on the long sides for your legs (Figure 9). Cover the tray's surface with a damp towel or some other material to keep dishes from sliding.

Bathing Aids
◆ Grab bars (Figure 10) can be fastened to the bathtub or attached to the wall for safety and ease in getting in and out of the tub or shower.

◆ A bath seat will help you get in and out of the bathtub and allow you to sit in the shower.

◆ A combination grab bar and bath seat (Figure 11) is available in many styles to fit all needs and types of bathroom fixtures.

◆ A portable showerhead can be used with a bath seat to shower in the bathtub.

Toilet Aids
A raised toilet seat (Figures 12) makes coming to a standing position more comfortable (especially if you are bothered by hip pain). Easy-to-clean padded-vinyl toilet seats (Figure 13) are also available.

ENERGY CONSERVATION
Conserving energy in small tasks will help you to have the stamina necessary to do daily self-help and other, more pleasurable activities. By eliminating unnecessary steps or movements, you will build up an energy reserve that lets you enjoy a more productive and fulfilling day.

Analyze your day, and pace yourself so that work is in accordance with your energy level. Do heavier tasks when your energy is high, and save lighter tasks for rest times.

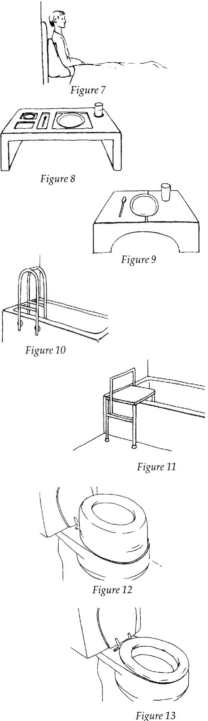

Figure 7

Figure 8

Figure 9

Figure 10

Figure 11

Figure 12

Figure 13

Dressing

◆ Try to do the major part of this task while seated in a chair, preferably one with arms.

◆ Long-handled reachers (Figure 14) will eliminate your having to bend over and will help you get garments started over your feet.

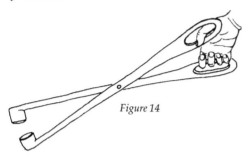

Figure 14

◆ It is easier to put your weak arm or leg in first when dressing and to take your strong arm or leg out first when undressing.

◆ Loose-fitting tops with front-closing zippers, ties or buttons are most convenient.

◆ A buttonhook (Figure 15) may help you with manipulating small shirt and trouser fastenings.

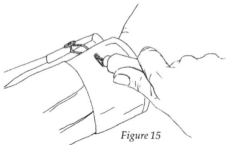

Figure 15

◆ If you are not ready to dress in street clothes, an attractive lounging outfit or muumuu will give you and those around you a boost in morale.

Housework

◆ Where possible, sit rather than stand. Bar stool height is a compromise between standing and sitting.

◆ Have work in front of you rather than at the side.

◆ Reduce effort when moving by mov-

ing more slowly and by not lifting as much as before.

◆ Slide rather than lift objects.

◆ Try to maintain good posture when standing, bending or sitting.

◆ To reduce fatigue, use fitted bedsheets to eliminate energy spent on bed-making.

◆ To decrease the need for bending, use long-handled dustpans and self-wringing mops.

◆ Store frequently used items close to you.

◆ Containerize: put everything needed for a task in a basket or box—an example would be grouping together items for morning care (Figure 16).

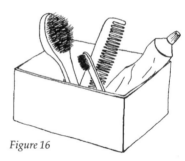

Figure 16

◆ Wear a cobbler's apron (Figure 17) or similar garment for carrying small lightweight items to reduce unnecessary trips about the house.

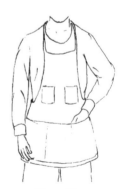

Figure 17

◆ Use a wheeled cart for moving items from one room to another.
◆ Alternate work and rest periods.
◆ Plan a basic itinerary each day in order to reduce unnecessary motions and steps.
◆ Pace your work schedule. Don't try to complete all tasks in one day. Have a weekly plan for scheduling major tasks such as washing, ironing, shopping and cleaning, so that one task can be done each day.

Cooking

◆ Plan ahead with meal preparation. Write menus for a week's meals at a time. Shop for staples once a week and for fresh produce twice weekly.
◆ Assemble all ingredients and utensils before beginning to prepare a dish.
◆ Make larger quantities, and freeze portions for later use.
◆ Plan how to use leftovers when cooking.
◆ Don't be reluctant to use frozen or convenience foods. You can add your own seasonings.
◆ A Crock-Pot slow cooker will allow you to cook a one-pot meal with minimum preparation time and effort. Your dinner will cook safely in it throughout the day, allowing you to rest.
◆ Use small tabletop appliances to eliminate unnecessary standing or bending.
◆ Use lightweight cookware to conserve energy.
◆ Use nonstick cookware for ease in cleaning up.
◆ Use paper plates or plastic cups for snacks or lunches to eliminate dishwashing.

SAFETY

◆ Remove scatter rugs.
◆ Clear floors of all small objects, such as bathroom scales or doorstops, to reduce the risk of slipping or tripping.
◆ Install additional phones to avoid tripping over extension cords.
◆ Avoid loose or floppy slippers or shoes.

◆ Check all stair treads and thresholds for loose hardware.
◆ Since most falls occur on the bottom step of stairs, make that step highly visible by painting it a different color or having it well lit.
◆ Whenever railings are present, hold on to them. Railings can also be easily installed when there are none.
◆ Have a lamp beside your bed so you don't stumble in the dark.
◆ To prevent dizziness when you first get out of bed, sit and dangle your feet for a moment before standing up.
◆ Use an electric heating pad with caution: you may misjudge the heat.
◆ Check the bathroom. Put adhesive-backed rubber strips in the tub or shower to prevent slipping. Buy soap on a cord and hang it around the faucet or your neck.
◆ When in the kitchen, do not reach across a hot burner.
◆ Survey your own living situation and take precautions that would benefit you.
◆ Have a large, easy-to-read list of emergency numbers, including fire, police, relatives and friends, near your telephone.

ACTIVITIES OF DAILY LIVING FOR POSTMASTECTOMY PATIENTS

Specific daily living and self-care skills should be incorporated into your exercise program. Your goal is to resume your normal way of life by gaining progressive independence in daily personal care, household responsibilities, work, active hobbies and sports. You can help yourself reach that goal by steadily increasing your range of motion, strengthening your muscles and decreasing pain and swelling.

Initially, you may need to adapt some tasks to your level of active motion and comfort. Pace yourself to accomplish a task, and then work on gradually increasing your strength and range of motion. The most difficult daily living activities will be those requiring you to reach up, out and around (especially a two-handed task).

The following suggestions will help you cope with activities of daily living; you can also use them to gradually increase your range of motion and muscle strength.

◆ Continue to use both hands as you did before the mastectomy. It is often tempting to avoid using a sore limb. To encourage yourself to use your sore arm, wear a cotton glove on your opposite hand to decrease its ability to feel accurately. If you have had surgery on the left side, wear the glove on your right hand. If you have had surgery on the right side, wear the glove on your left hand.

◆ Towel drying with both hands after bathing will help you increase your range of motion.

◆ When blow-drying and styling your hair, it may be more comfortable initially to support the affected arm on a telephone book or other prop until range of motion and strength have been restored.

◆ To fasten a bra, begin by fastening it in front and then turning it around. Progress to reaching behind your back to fasten it, first with straps off, then with straps on your shoulders.

◆ When putting on a blouse, shirt or sweater, put the affected arm in first. When undressing, take the affected arm out last. To remove slip-on clothing, draw it over your head first, and then slide it off your arms.

◆ When closing a zipper at the back of a garment, use a zipper pulley. As you achieve more active arm motion, you can

discontinue using the pulley. Hanging up clothes in a closet provides you with movement similar to that obtained when using a pulley. Begin by hanging up a lightweight garment using your affected arm. As you gain strength and range of motion, try hanging up heavier garments, such as slacks or a coat.

◆ When cooking, do the stirring with your affected arm. At first you may prefer to slide rather than lift cookware off the stove or counter; try lifting and reaching, using both hands, as soon as you are able.

◆ Plan your marketing to eliminate heavy lifting or carrying.

◆ General household activities you may use as exercises to increase your range of motion include sweeping; making the bed; mopping; polishing mirrors, silver, etc.; turning doorknobs and keys; folding laundry; washing walls and windows; vacuuming, and reaching up to high shelves.

◆ When watering plants, use both hands to hold the watering can. As your strength increases, try using your affected arm, especially for watering plants in high spots.

◆ Gardening offers many opportunities to help you increase your range of motion, such as raking, hoeing, cutting and planting. Caution: Wear gloves to avoid cuts or injuries to your hands or fingers, because your affected arm is more susceptible to infection after surgery.

◆ Sports that offer more vigorous exercise, such as swimming, tennis, bowling and ping-pong, may be attempted when you have already achieved a good range of motion. Remember to reach up, out and around.

YOUR SELF-CARE PROGRESS CHART	
Activity	**Date/ Notes**
Eating	
Drinking from straw	
Drinking from glass	
Using napkin on face and hands	
Eating finger food	
Eating with spoon or fork	
Cutting with knife	
Opening and pouring liquids	
Hygiene	
Using handkerchief	
Brushing or combing hair	
or putting on wig	
Shaving	
Brushing teeth or dentures	
Using bedpan or urinal	
Sponge bath—face and upper body	
Sponge bath—lower body	
Make-up, nail care, etc.	
Dressing	
Assisting with putting on sleepwear	
Putting on robe	
Putting on slippers	
Putting on street clothing (sitting)	
Putting on street clothing (alternating sitting and standing)	

23
MASSAGE

Francine Manuel, RPT, Ernest H. Rosenbaum, MD, Isadora R. Rosenbaum, MA

◇

One of the most soothing treatments for a bedridden person is massage. In Europe and elsewhere, it is used frequently to promote relaxation, decrease pain and speed healing. It may also help reduce or eliminate the need for certain medications.

Unfortunately, in this country the practice has fallen by the wayside. The advent of HMOs and strict cost-cutting measures have labeled this treatment as frivolous and nonreimbursable as a medical treatment. That does not mean it is not helpful or therapeutic. It simply is a wonderful experience that insurers do not want to pay for.

If you can afford it, find a professional to come into your home, or take advantage of the massage therapist at your health club. If you have a willing family member or friend, massage can be a pleasant way for others to participate in your recovery and gain satisfaction from being able to help.

Massage therapy can help prevent bedsores. By turning over, you release pressure on the areas you have been lying on. Massaging the pressured areas encourages more blood to flow into the tissue. If massage is done frequently, it will prevent skin breakdown. The buttocks, tail bone (coccyx), wings of the shoulder blades (scapulae), hips, heels, elbows and bumps (malleoli) around the ankles are susceptible spots for pressure sores.

GIVING A MASSAGE
The following instructions can be used by a friend or family member to give you a massage. It is very important that you find a comfortable position at the start; no matter how soothing the stroke, an uncomfortable patient will not be able to tolerate the massage for very long.

There are four basic massage strokes:
1. Effleurage (light or deep stroking)
2. Petrisage (kneading)
3. Tapotement (hacking or slapping)
4. Friction

Effleurage Effleurage is the very slow stroking with which you begin and end every massage. The two types of effleurage are light stroking, which is used to relax the patient, and deep stroking, which empties the blood and lymphatic vessels.

Begin by placing your hands very light-

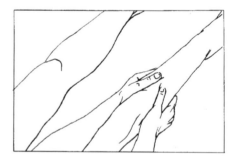

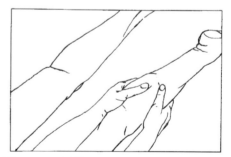

Figure 1. Effleurage

ly on the area to be massaged. With the lightest pressure that you can apply, run your hands slowly over the area. Make full contact with the skin with both hands. All strokes should be done in a continuous motion: once you begin, never take your hands off the patient's body until you are finished a stroke. After five minutes of light stroking, begin to deepen the strokes in the direction toward the heart, gradually increasing the pressure. Lighten the strokes going away from the heart.

Be careful: if the patient complains, you are doing it too hard. Massage should never hurt—that defeats the purpose of relaxation. Some people can tolerate only the lightest effleurage. Deep effleurage can be used to decrease edema (swelling from fluid collecting in tissues), but only with a physician's approval.

Petrisage Petrisage (kneading the muscles) can be done in two ways: with the palms or heels of your hands, or with your fingertips. In this stroke you actually pick up the muscle tissue away from the bones and work on the affected areas to decrease muscle spasm. Again, it should not hurt, although the patient may tell you that it "hurts good"—a common response to an effectively given petrisage.

Tapotement Tapotement is done by hacking with the sides of your hands or by cupping your hands and using them to percuss (tap sharply) an area of the body. This stroke, while pleasing to most muscle-bound athletic stars, is not usually very pleasing to a seriously ill patient. It should never be used without a physician's approval. People have been known to fracture ribs by pounding on the chest. Tapotement can also be dangerous for anyone with kidney disease.

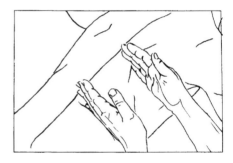

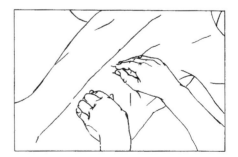

Figure 3. Tapotement

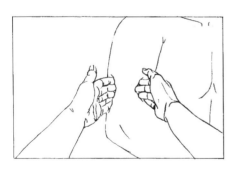

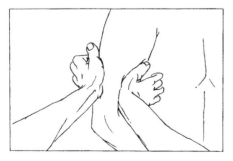

Figure 2. Petrisage

Friction The last massage stroke is friction, which is done with one or two fingertips. Apply pressure in a circular manner over bony prominences, such as the pelvic bones, shoulders, vertebrae (backbones), and kneecaps. Do not move around with this stroke. Instead, stay in one spot for a prolonged time and then move on to another spot.

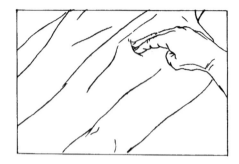

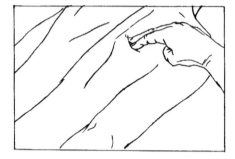

Figure 4. Friction

24
SEXUALITY AND CANCER

Jean M. Bullard, RN, MS, David G. Bullard, PhD, Ernest H. Rosenbaum, MD, Isadora R. Rosenbaum, MA

Sexuality can sometimes be affected by a serious illness, such as cancer, and its treatment. By "sexuality," we mean the feelings we have about ourselves as sexual beings, the ways in which we choose to express these feelings with ourselves and others and the physical capability each of us has to give and experience sexual pleasure. Sexuality can be expressed in many ways, including how we dress, move and speak, as well as by kissing, touching, masturbation and intercourse. Anxieties about survival, family or finances, along with changes in body image and the ability to tolerate different levels of activity, can place a strain on the expression of sexuality and create concerns about sexual desirability.

If you were comfortable with and enjoyed your sexuality before your illness, chances are excellent that you will be able to keep or regain a healthy sexual self-image despite the changes brought about by cancer. Many people who have cancer or who are the partners of persons with cancer may experience no change in sexual feelings or behavior. Others may find that increased closeness and communication resulting from the experience of illness enhances their sexuality. Still others may never have considered sexuality to be of great importance in their lives, or may consider it less important now than previously.

If, however, you are experiencing some changes or stresses in your sexuality because of cancer or its treatment, the material presented here is designed to help you explore ways to deal with these changes. We do not intend to present a course in sex counseling or a list of "how to's" about sexual functioning. Nor do we intend to suggest that everyone with cancer will have sexual problems. Sexual problems frequently arise not so much from changes imposed by a medical condition or its treatment but from how we feel about and deal with those changes.

We will present concepts and principles that have been found useful by many people who have handled changes in sexuality. We hope that this information will help you become more aware of your attitudes about your sexuality; that it will form a basis for you to begin to communicate your sexual feelings and needs more directly to people important to you, including those responsible for your health care; and that it will help you decide how sexuality fits best into your own life at this particular time.

Remember, you are the expert on your own sexuality. We hope that the material presented here will validate your sexual concerns and stimulate your thinking about how best to handle them. For more information on specific concerns or questions, see the Resources at the end of the book.

SEXUALITY ISSUES FOR PATIENTS AND THEIR PARTNERS

Sexuality has long been a matter of great interest and concern in our culture. We have moved from one extreme, in which our puritanical views made public discussion about sexuality totally unacceptable, to the current extreme, in which explicit sexuality is commonplace, exploited in popular advertising and as the main theme of many books and films. Feelings about sexuality tend to be intense ones, closely tied to moral and religious beliefs, as well as to deep feelings about self-esteem and desirability. Sexuality has different meanings and importance for each of us, and we each have our own ways of expressing ourselves as sexual beings.

Until recently, little accurate information about sexuality has been available. Most of us have been exposed to a wide assortment of myths and misinformation about sexuality handed down through generations or gained from discussions with our friends. The popular media have "told" us what sexuality is and have set many standards for being "sexually attractive."

Unfortunately, these ideas tend only to reinforce much of the misinformation we grew up with and make it difficult for us to feel secure about our own unique sexuality. There are as many different ways of expressing sexuality as there are people, and most people experience concerns about their sexuality at some time during their lives. Consequently, health care providers are beginning to recognize that addressing sexuality is an important part of health care.

"We are all sexual beings." This simple statement makes the important point that sexuality is part of who we are, not just what we do. Sexuality is expressed in many ways—how we dress, how we talk, how we work and how we play. Furthermore, each of us is uniquely sexual in the sense that we choose whether or not to be actively sexual, and in what ways, how often and with whom. If sexuality were something people could easily discuss, we would no doubt discover that the importance of sexuality varies tremendously from person to person.

One problem that can get in the way of a comfortable discussion of sexuality has to do with the words we use. Some "labels" that supposedly describe sexual problems are demeaning and embarrassing. It would be difficult to feel good about being described as "impotent" or as a "premature ejaculator." One of the more degrading ways to describe a woman with sexual concerns is to label her "frigid." These labels say nothing about what someone is actually experiencing and may in fact lead to false assumptions about that person's specific problems.

Anxiety about sexuality often comes from trying to make ourselves fit a stereotype of what is supposed to be "normal," "super sexual," "masculine" or "feminine." One problem that may arise from comparing our sexuality against some external standard is that expectations about how we should be, feel or act sexually may prevent us from discovering and enjoying what is right for us. Trying to live up to the pressure of these expectations can lead to fear of failure or of not being as "sexual" as someone else.

Our ideas about the "right way" to be sexual, which often stem from the myths or expectations we grew up with, may hinder expression of our sexuality.

COMMON MYTHS ABOUT SEXUALITY

◆ *"Sex is only for the young and able-bodied."* We seldom see older people or physically disabled people in "sexy" commercials or movies. We are thus led to believe that the only way to be attractive to others is to have a young and "perfect" body. Although most of us know that this is not true, we can still be influenced by the myth. We are sexual beings from birth to death, capable of sexual pleasure regardless of our age or our body's condition.

◆ *"Sex means intercourse."* This myth makes it difficult to enjoy the special pleasures of touching, kissing and stroking for their own sakes. If we view them only as steps toward the goal of intercourse, we may not consider them as options for sexual expression and satisfaction when intercourse is not desired or is difficult because of fatigue, illness or anxiety. If we avoid touching for fear that it must lead to intercourse, we may cut ourselves off from forms of sexual affection that can be warm, comforting and satisfying.

◆ *"The goal of sexual activity is orgasm."* While many people enjoy orgasm, every sexual experience does not have to include it. In fact, trying too hard to have an orgasm can create pressures that prevent orgasm from happening. Satisfaction can come from a variety of pleasurable experiences, and it is usually enhanced when the expectation and goal of orgasm are removed.

◆ *"Sexual performance equals love."* You don't have to prove your love with sexual prowess. (Moreover, being able to perform sexually with someone does not necessarily prove anything about your feelings for that person.) Sharing your sexuality in a variety of ways can be an important part of loving, but there are many other ways of expressing love as well. Showing how much you care in these other ways can help take the pressure off sexual activity.

◆ *"Sexual activity is natural and spontaneous."* "You shouldn't have to talk about it" is a phrase we often hear. When sexual activity feels good, there is often no need to talk about it. But when questions or concerns arise, as they do at some time for most people, it is important to be able to communicate feelings and needs, likes and dislikes. None of us is a mind reader. No matter how well we know another person, talking about what makes us feel good is usually necessary to prevent incorrect assumptions from being made. Remember that assumptions are built on the past; it is important to be able to find out if your partner wants to try something

new or different. Talking about sex can also help to reduce anxiety and can be one more way of sharing.

◆ *"Masturbation is harmful."* Many people have grown up hearing warnings about the "evils" of masturbation or self-stimulation—an activity that has been humorously described as "the world's worst-kept secret." Although most of us don't talk about our masturbation patterns, many of us, including people in happy relationships, continue masturbating throughout our lives. It is not surprising that people continue activities that they have found pleasurable in the past. Whether or not masturbation is an acceptable practice for you is, of course, a personal choice based on your own values and preferences.

The important thing to remember is that medical evidence has shown that masturbation not only is harmless but also can be a very healthy part of sexuality. It provides an opportunity to learn about how our bodies respond—information that can be important for sexual pleasure with a partner. For example, research has found that women were more likely to have orgasms with intercourse if they had previously had orgasms through other means, such as masturbation.

Read through some of the above myths again to see if any are important for you, and spend a few moments thinking or talking about other expectations that you are aware of that were not mentioned. Do your expectations help you enjoy and feel more comfortable about your sexuality, or do they hinder your enjoyment and comfort? Answering that question for yourself can be useful in beginning to make changes for the better.

THE SEXUAL RESPONSE CYCLE

How do our bodies respond sexually? Sexual response is a natural total-body response involving more than just our genitals. With stimulation from thoughts, touch or other sources, general muscle tension begins to build up, and blood begins to flow toward and accumulate in the genitals and other sensitive areas. If stimulation continues and we are relaxed, comfortable and able to focus on our pleasurable body sensations (rather than on anxiety or worry), the level of body tension and blood flow continue to increase, and orgasm may then occur.

Orgasm is a reflex. It happens by itself under the right circumstances—much like a sneeze. We can't directly will an orgasm to happen any more than we can will a sneeze to happen. If orgasm does occur, blood then flows back from the genitals to the rest of the body, muscle tension diminishes and our bodies return to their pre-excitement state. If orgasm does not occur, these same changes happen, but more slowly.

The natural sexual response cycle can be interrupted in a number of ways. If, for example, a man becomes anxious about his "performance," he may lose his erection or climax sooner than he wishes. If a woman is worried about being able to have an orgasm, her anxiety may make it impossible to have one.

Each of us has particular conditions that are necessary if we are to enjoy sexual activity. The more aware we are of what is right for us, the greater are our chances of enjoying sexual pleasure. Most of us have learned one way of obtaining sexual satisfaction or orgasm—through various kinds of genital stimulation such as masturbation, intercourse and oral or manual stimulation.

Many people, however, are able to experience sexual excitement, even orgasm, through stimulation of other sensitive body areas. Since it is the brain, rather than the genitals, that interprets and experiences this stimulation as pleasurable, it has been said that the brain is the real "sex organ." This means that we do not have to depend on our genitals for

our sexuality. Our options for sexual pleasure are as varied as our imaginations.

Many people with serious illnesses find that the circumstances they need in order to enjoy their sexuality have been altered in some way because of the illness and its treatment. Under the stress and worry of a life-threatening illness, expression of sexuality frequently takes a back seat. It is difficult to feel sexual when you are fighting to survive, are in pain or constantly tired. Treatment for cancer may involve lengthy hospitalizations and separations from those you love. Hospitals or convalescent facilities usually do not provide much privacy, and hence there may be little opportunity for sexual expression.

Being in a hospital may mean separation from sources of feedback about your worth and desirability. Wearing hospital gowns and being deprived of familiar means of enhancing your appearance, like makeup, aftershave lotion and your own clothes, can temporarily lower your self-esteem and make you feel uncomfortable in the presence of others. Physical examination and diagnosis often involve exposing portions of your body that are normally considered private. Feelings of shame and embarrassment can result if hospital staff neglect to ensure adequate privacy during these procedures. The attitudes of staff, the numerous examinations and procedures, and lack of privacy may make you feel asexual: that is, they may temporarily deprive you of any sense of yourself as a sexual person.

Many hospitals are beginning to encourage ways of minimizing this depersonalization and to provide space and opportunity for people to have privacy. If your hospital has not yet addressed these issues, there are some things you can do to make your stay there more comfortable. If you want time alone or with someone special, ask for a "Do Not Disturb Until __ O'clock" sign or make one yourself to place on your door. Ask the staff to knock before they enter your room. A "Please Knock" sign may help remind them. If you request it, many hospitals will provide an extra cot in your room for an overnight visitor. If you are on a ward and share a room with other patients, your doctor may know of a way that you can get some private time in another room, a private lounge or sunporch. You may bring special items from home, such as pictures for the wall, plants, personal items, family photos or pillows, to create a more comfortable atmosphere. Wearing your own pajamas, nightgown or robe can help, too.

During illness, the control you usually experience over your body may be lost, and you may feel inadequate and helpless. Serious illness may change the way you experience your body, or actually change the way you look, through surgery, amputation, scarring, weight loss or other events. These changes may create painful anxiety about whether you will be able to function in your accustomed social, sexual and career roles, or about what people will think of you. This anxiety, the depression and fatigue that may accompany it, and the numerous other worries that can occur with serious illness understandably make sexuality assume less importance.

But once the immediate crisis of serious illness has passed, sexual feelings and how to express them may become important to you again. Feeling anxious about resuming sexual activity is normal and natural. It is easy to "get out of practice" when you are away from any activity. You may have questions about whether sexual activity will hurt you in any way or whether you will be able to experience sexual pleasure. Your partner may share the same worries and may be especially concerned about tiring you out or causing you pain.

Starting a new relationship is a task we all face at one time or another, but it can be made more difficult by worries about our worth and attractiveness. If your body has undergone changes as a result of your illness and treatment, you may have questions about whether you are still desirable, how to please your partner or what dating will now be like. Whether you are looking for a new relationship or already have a regular partner, you may find yourself in the position of having to share your feelings about these changes with someone, perhaps for the first time.

This sharing may feel awkward at first. Learning how and when to start talking about sexual issues may not come easily. You may feel shy or nervous about exploring new and different ways of experiencing sexual pleasure. You may be waiting for your partner to make the first move toward sexual activity, while your partner is waiting for you to make the advances. This waiting game is often misunderstood as rejection by both people. To think of breaking the silence yourself may be frightening. Yet the payoff for making the first move—greater understanding of each other's needs and concerns—is usually worth it.

Although health care personnel are now more aware of sexual concerns, many people continue to receive little or no information about sexuality during their treatment for and recovery from illness. You may have no opportunity to ask important questions about these matters. If sexuality has not been discussed with you or if your questions have been avoided, you may feel that your worries and questions are foolish, unimportant or inappropriate. Don't let these feelings prevent you from seeking answers. Ask your doctor, nurse, social worker or another staff person with whom you feel comfortable. He or she should be willing to listen to your questions and either answer them or refer you to someone who can. Help is available. Some university medical centers offer sexual counseling specifically for people with medical illness or physical disability. Your doctor or social worker will know whether such resources are available near you.

The kinds of changes in and concerns about sexuality that we have just discussed are general ones. The next section outlines some of the specific ways that cancer and its treatment can affect sexuality. For information on self-help organizations for specific kinds of cancer, see the Resources at the end of the book.

BODY IMAGE

Cancer and its treatment frequently bring about body changes. For example, surgery may entail removal of a breast (mastectomy); creation of an artificial hole in the abdomen for the evacuation of wastes (ostomy); removal of part or all of the reproductive organs, or removal of a body extremity (amputation). Chemotherapy or radiation therapy may cause such side effects as hair loss or weight loss.

Some people adjust to these changes relatively soon, some take a longer time, and some may never accept them. But acceptance need not mean total comfort with the situation. For some, a sense of outrage and loss may always remain to a certain extent. It is natural to have feelings about these changes, including anger, grief, mourning and anxiety.

Body image—the mental and emotional picture we have of our bodies— may also be altered. Anxiety can arise when there is a conflict between what we think our body should look like or what it has previously looked like and how it actually looks now. This anxiety can influence our interactions with others and affect how we view ourselves sexually. If we see ourselves as less attractive or less lovable, we may avoid social or sexual situations so as not to experience the rejection we may expect from others. Unfortunately, such avoidance may also deny us positive experiences that could contribute to our feeling better.

Dealing with feelings about body changes may be difficult. The support systems we have available to us, our social and career roles and the meanings we attach to a particular loss or change will all influence our ability to cope.

Mastectomy and Sexuality Sexual issues after treatment for breast cancer may include lowered desire, difficulties with physical arousal and concerns about body image. Chemotherapy, by causing premature menopause due to lowered estrogen and androgen levels, may lead to lowered desire or problems with arousal or lubrication problems. Some women report improvement in these difficulties after topical application of testosterone or estrogen cream to the labia and vulvar areas, although the long-term safety of such hormonal creams has not yet been studied. Problems with lubrication and physiological arousal may be helped with artificial lubricants and vaginal moisturizers.

Body image concerns are normal and are especially understandable in view of the overemphasis that our culture places on the sexual significance of breasts. Undressing in front of your partner or sleeping in the nude may feel awkward and uncomfortable. With time and patience, many women are able to overcome their self-consciousness and again feel secure and comfortable with their bodies. Some women have found it helpful to explore and touch their bodies, including the area of the scar, while nude in front of a mirror. You may want to try this alone first and then together with another person—a spouse, lover or close friend—while sharing your feelings about these changes.

After surgery, your partner may just not know what to say or how or when to bring up the topic of sexuality, and may wait for you to bring it up while being afraid of hurting or embarrassing you. Sometimes this "protection" may feel instead like rejection. Although it will probably feel risky to break the ice and approach the topic of sex, most people feel relieved once they've done this. Exercises such as the one just mentioned may be a good way to start.

When you first resume sexual activity, you and your partner may worry about pain. If your incision or muscles are tender, minimizing pressure on your chest area is important. Lying on your unaffected side may give you more control over your movement and reduce irritation of the incision. Don't hesitate to stop if you feel pain. Let your partner know why you are stopping.

If your partner trusts that you will speak up if something is painful or uncomfortable, you will both feel more relaxed and less inhibited in exploring and experimenting. Taking a rest or changing position may help you relax, and relaxing will usually decrease any pain. With communication and cooperation, you and your partner can work together to find the positions and activities that will give you the most pleasure.

Experimentation and time seem to be keys to finding satisfactory ways of adapting sexually after breast cancer. Talking with other women who have had mastectomies—with support groups and with volunteers in the American Cancer Society's Reach to Recovery program, for example—can provide support and encouragement as well as suggestions about clothes and prostheses.

Ostomy and Sexuality An ostomy may represent a new start in your life, removing pain and worry along with the diseased body part. But some new concerns may arise, such as wondering how a partner will react to the stoma or how the risk of odor or spilling during sexual and other activities can be minimized. In the past, our society has treated bowel and bladder concerns as taboo subjects (like the topic of sexuality). With very little open discussion, and even less opportunity to talk with other people with ostomies, it is easy to see how people felt that there was something shameful about having an ostomy. Although we may still hear and feel those negative messages, people today do have access to more supportive attitudes if they seek them out. As a society, we are beginning to increase our realization of how negative social stereotypes and silence about important body functions can be destructive. Concerns about hygiene and cleanliness are natural, but as experience with your ostomy increases, so will your comfort and confidence in social and sexual situations.

Sharing information about your ostomy with certain people may be a way for you to become more comfortable. If the fact of an ostomy is a "secret" that you have felt would be painful to reveal to anyone, you may find that talking about the ostomy for the first time with someone you trust is a real relief. The support and caring you get in return will help you feel less alone. It is also true that when you share something intimate about yourself, other people quite often feel more comfortable in talking about things that are meaningful to them. Being vulnerable and showing your feelings about important things can lead to greater closeness and intimacy.

Talking with other people who have ostomies—such as members of the United Ostomy Association—may be especially helpful in understanding that you are not alone and that you can learn to be more comfortable with the fact of your ostomy. Having someone who can listen to you and understand your questions can be of real benefit. Similarly, talking openly with your partner about your feelings and encouraging him or her to do the same is often the best way to decrease any anxiety that might surround the topic.

Experimenting with the timing of your ostomy management and with different types of appliances may help you to discover when your ostomy is most and least active. Learning about your individual patterns and how best to regulate your elimination may take a month, six months, or longer. There will probably be some spilling or accidents during this learning stage, until your pattern and schedule of evacuation are more regular. Laughing, crying or just accepting these occurrences as inevitable in the beginning is important for both you and your partner.

Laryngectomy and Sexuality After laryngectomy (surgical removal of the voice box), you may worry about odor from the stoma or about the noises made while breathing through the stoma. These worries can be distracting and may make it difficult to enjoy sexual activity. Keeping the area around the stoma clean and using perfume or aftershave lotion can help. Wearing a stoma shield or T-shirt will muffle the sound of your breathing and minimize the amount of air your partner feels being pushed through the stoma. Sharing your feelings with your partner will help you both adjust to the changes that have taken place and will create the best groundwork for a pleasurable sex life. Communication with other people who have had laryngectomies can also be helpful.

Cancer of Genital or Reproductive Organs and Sexuality Surgery or radiation therapy for cancer of the genital or reproductive organs can bring about intense concerns with body image. For some people, such treatments may also directly affect their physical ability to get an erection, ejaculate, have intercourse or reach orgasm. Other people may experience little or no change in sexual functioning after the same treatment. As a result, it is generally impossible to predict the effects of treatment for any one individual. Sexual problems that may appear to stem from physical results of treatment may in fact be due to anxiety and concern about body image and sexual functioning.

Discussing potential problems and possible solutions with your doctor or other members of the health care team before treatment will reduce worry and reassure you that if problems do occur, there are ways of handling them. Since in most situations there are no totally reliable means of sorting out physical from emotional causes of sexual problems, your exploration of and experimentation with what you can do is most important. Your diagnosis does not dictate what is possible for you sexually.

ENERGY LEVEL

Life after cancer treatment may be exhausting. Fatigue, depression and generally feeling sick are common. Treatments for cancer, such as chemotherapy and radiation therapy, may in themselves also create unpleasant and tiring side effects. The amount of energy available to you for the activities of living, including sexual activities, may vary from day to day or week to week. Some people learn to cope with these variations in energy level by planning their activities to coincide with times of the day they feel best. If you are experiencing some of these difficulties, being sexually active may not always be important to you. But for times when it is, planning to have sex when you feel least tired may be helpful.

Remember, too, that sex does not necessarily mean intercourse or orgasm. If you can expand your view of sexuality to include other ways of being close—such as holding, caressing, touching and quiet talking—your options for sexual expression, even while tired, are greatly increased. Talking openly with your partner will help you both to be flexible in dealing with the variable course of your illness. Many people find that, as they become more skillful in communicating about their feelings and needs, their options for sexual satisfaction increase as well.

The important thing is to be patient, both with yourself and with your partner.

Adjustment will not occur overnight. Give yourself time—time to explore and share your feelings about your body changes and time to begin seeing yourself again as a desirable sexual being. When you can grant yourself some acceptance of your body and recognition of your potential for sexual pleasure, it will be easier to imagine someone else doing the same. Sharing feelings about and exploration of a changed body have brought many couples closer together and enriched their relationships in surprising ways.

If there has been an interruption in your accustomed sexual interaction, it is important to realize that there are no set guidelines or timetables for resuming sexual activities. You are unique in your sexuality; only you can decide when and what is right for you. If you need help, ask your doctor to refer you to a competent sex counselor, or contact a nearby university medical center or community mental health center for a list of local resources.

PAINFUL INTERCOURSE

After treatment for genital cancer, some women find intercourse painful. If intercourse has become painful for you, it is important to visit your physician or gynecologist for an examination to determine the cause of the pain. It may be related to surgery, radiation therapy or chemotherapy, or it may be the result of a simple problem, such as an infection. If the cause is insufficient lubrication, try using an artificial lubricant, such as Astroglide, Gyne-Moistrin or K-Y Jelly; a vaginal moisturizer, such as Replens; and vaginal and vulvar

application of estrogen creams.

Shortening of the vagina, or stenosis, a condition in which the vagina loses its elasticity, can result from surgery or radiation therapy and may make intercourse difficult. If this is a problem for you, a physician may recommend the early use of dilators to exercise and stretch the vagina. Early resumption of intercourse can also help to prevent these problems. Different positions during intercourse, especially sitting or lying on top of your partner, may enable you to move in ways that are pleasurable rather than painful.

The most important thing to remember is to stop when you first feel any pain. If you let your partner know ahead of time that you will immediately communicate any experience of pain, he or she will probably feel less worried and more able to enjoy experimenting with you. Stopping to rest, slowing your movements, breathing deeply and sharing your feelings will help you to relax. By exploring together what feels most pleasurable, you and your partner will eventually discover the kinds of sexual activity that suit you best.

GETTING AND MAINTAINING ERECTIONS

Some men who have trouble getting and maintaining erections may suspect that this problem may have been caused by cancer or its treatment. Since some drugs can temporarily interfere with the ability to have erections, you may want to ask your physician about any possible side effects from drugs you are taking. If you get an erection with masturbation or you wake up in the middle of the night or in the morning with one, it is most likely that anxiety or "trying too hard," rather than a physical problem, is keeping you from having erections.

In trying to deal with erection problems, it is important to explore the sensations in and around your penis. Exploring these sensations when you are not distracted by trying to please or perform for your partner will help. Spend some time alone in a comfortable place, such as the bedroom or bathroom, at a time when you will not be interrupted. Undress and begin to explore your entire body, focusing especially on and around your genitals. Touch your penis, scrotum, abdomen, thighs, perineum (the area between the scrotum and anus) and anus. Try different kinds of touch—soft and light, firm and strong. Pay attention to the different kinds of sensations you feel, and notice which touches are most pleasurable. You may find that moistening your hand with oil, lotion or soap makes your touch more pleasurable. Learning about what feels good to you is valuable in showing your partner what pleases you most. Trying some of the exercises described in *The New Male Sexuality* (*see* the Resources at the end of the book), either by yourself or with a partner, can help you explore your potential for erections.

The more options you have for sexual expression, the less emphasis there is on having erections; this lack of pressure in turn makes it more likely that they will occur. There are many kinds of sexual expression and stimulation of your partner that do not require an erect penis. Knowing that many women need or prefer direct stimulation by hand or mouth on or around the clitoris in order to have an orgasm may be reassuring. This is stimulation that even an erect penis in a vagina usually cannot provide. If you explore other kinds of sexual touching and expression for a while, you may discover that erections will return with time or that the increased variety of sexual options satisfies both you and your partner. Patience, communication and time are critical factors in developing pleasurable sexual experiences.

If erections have not returned and you feel that this is important to you and your partner, you may consider asking your doctor to determine whether to refer you to a sex therapist for brief counseling (especially if you get good erections upon awakening or by yourself—just not with a partner) or to a urologist for a medical evaluation of this condition. Sometimes an erectile problem is a symptom of underlying vascular disease, diabetes or other treatable medical conditions. The urologist can make an assessment of whether these other problems are present, and whether one of the following medical treatments would suit your particular needs:

◆ Viagra (sildenafil) is the first oral medication developed and approved to help erections in both men with organic and with psychological-based erectile problems. Taken one hour prior to sexual activity, it has been found to be highly effective and safe, although it is not appropriate for men with certain cardiac problems or who maybe taking organic nitrate medications such as nitroglycerin for heart disease. Additional medications which will enhance erection are currently being tested and may be available in 1999.

◆ The MUSE system administers the medication alprostadil directly into the end of the penis as a urethral suppository, and has been shown to be effective for some men with erectile problems.

◆ External penile vacuum devices. A tension ring is placed around the base of the penis after it has become erect with the aid of a vacuum cylinder. These devices may work better for men who clearly have a major organic component to their erectile problem, such as severe diabetes, multiple sclerosis or spinal cord injury. While this approach does create erections that are functional for intercourse, men whose erection difficulties may be more emotional or psychological may be disappointed when the results are not as firm as they had been expecting. Side effects may include bruising of the penis.

◆ Intracorporeal penile injections were

originally used diagnostically in urologists' offices, but patients can now be taught to inject themselves prior to sexual encounters, resulting in firmer erections that often do not disappear until an hour or more after orgasm or ejaculation. Side effects are pain, a persistent and painful erection (priapism) and scarring.

◆ Penile implant surgery. A variety of implants with semirigid silicone rods or inflatable cylinders are available. Costs are high (from $6,000 to $15,000). Complications are device failure (requiring additional surgery) and infection.

ORGASM

After a serious illness, an interruption in your usual ability to experience sexual pleasure can be perfectly natural. For some women, this interruption may make having orgasms more difficult. If this is a problem for you, learning to re-explore pleasurable body sensations may be helpful. Do this at a time when you can be alone and are not distracted by having to please or perform for your partner.

Find a comfortable place where you can be alone, such as in your bedroom or bathroom, and a time when you will not be interrupted. Undress slowly and stroke your entire body gently. Then focus on the most sensitive areas. These may include your neck, breasts, thighs, genitals or any area that feels good to you. Use different kinds of touch—soft and light, firm and strong. Try touching your body after moistening your hands with oil, lotion or soap. Pay attention to the different kinds of sensations you feel, and notice which ones are most pleasurable. Learning which kinds of touch feel best will help you heighten your sensations and will give you information to share with your partner about what pleases you most. The discussion and exercises in *For Yourself* (*see* the Resources at the end of the book) may help you continue to explore your potential for sexual pleasure and orgasm.

Orgasm is a reflex that results when the right amount of physical and psychological stimulation occurs. It can be felt as a somewhat mild and pleasurable sense of relaxation or as a stronger, more intense sensation, depending on many factors, such as your level of energy, the source of stimulation and the setting. From research and from the reports of many people, we know that men and women can experience orgasm even when the genitals have been removed or when there is no genital sensation (as with some spinal cord injuries), because orgasm and other sexual pleasures are actually experienced in the brain. With exploration, you may discover that other body areas, such as arms, breasts, neck, ears and underarms, can be highly sensitive. With practice, stimulation of these areas may lead to orgasm. Some people have reported that orgasm from these sources feels different, but is pleasurable and satisfying.

Some of the medications mentioned above, especially Viagra and others being tested for male erectile problems, are also being evaluated as to their safety and effectiveness in helping women with arousal or organism difficulties, such as those sometimes experienced after chemotherapy and chemically induced menopause.

CHANGES AND YOUR SEXUALITY

Survival overshadows sexuality. Remember that stress, depression, worry and fatigue may temporarily lower your interest in sex. It is normal and natural for someone who loses good health to experience such feelings. When you are ill, just coping with basic everyday decisions may seem like a burden. Taking one day at a time and being patient with yourself are important. Sexual interest and feelings generally return when the immediate crisis of illness has passed.

Expect the unexpected. The first time you have sexual relations after being treated for cancer may be a new and different experience. Physical limitations or fears about performance, appearance or rejection may initially prevent you from focusing on the pleasure of your sexual contact. On the other hand, you may instead be surprised by enjoying unfamiliar pleasurable sensations. Such new experiences are often reported by people who have recently divorced, lost a job or weathered a family crisis, as well as by people recovering from an illness. If you expect some changes as a natural part of recovery, they will be less apt to distract you from sexual pleasure if they do occur.

Give yourself time. It can be natural at first for you or your partner to be frightened of, perhaps even repulsed by, physical changes such as scars or unfamiliar appliances. Such feelings can be temporary, and talking about them, frightening as they may be, is usually the first step to mutual support and acceptance. Becoming comfortable with changes in yourself and your sexuality will probably not happen overnight. Take the pressure off yourself about having to "work on sex." Reaching a satisfactory and enjoyable sex life will happen gradually, one step at a time. At first you may want to spend some time by yourself exploring your body, becoming familiar with any body changes that have occurred and rediscovering your unique body texture and sensations. Once you feel relaxed doing this, move on to mutual body exploration with a partner, if you wish. (More specific ideas for such exercises are described in the Resources at the end of the book, particularly in *For Yourself* and *The New Male Sexuality*.)

Communication is all-important. The more talking and sharing you can do, the more your awareness of what feels good to you sexually will probably increase. It is rarely easy for anyone to begin talking about sex. You might initially try sharing with your partner some of the myths or expectations you grew up with about sexuality. Discussing this topic is often humorous and may break the ice in starting a frank conversation about your sexual needs and concerns. Make "I statements" about what is important for you and how you feel. Rather than general statements, try something like this: "I would really like to experiment with different positions that would be more comfortable for me. How would you feel about that?" Then ask your partner to try these statements also.

Take the emphasis off intercourse. When you first resume sexual activity, try spending some time in pleasurable activities such as touching, fondling, kissing and being close without having intercourse. Re-experience the pleasure of playing, holding and being held without having to worry about erections and orgasms. Once you feel comfortable with this, you can proceed at your own pace to other ways of being sexual, including intercourse if you wish. Intercourse is only one of many routes to sexual satisfaction. Your own experimentation and exploration can help you discover what feels best and what is acceptable to you.

Don't let your diagnosis dictate what you can do sexually. Your sexuality cannot be "diagnosed." You will never know what you are capable of experiencing in terms of sexual pleasure if you don't explore being sexual—new positions, new touches and above all, new attitudes. You are the sexual expert about yourself; your brain is your best sex organ, and its ability to experience sensation is virtually limitless.

You are loved for your total worth, not just for the appearance of your body. Try not to make the mistake of placing so much importance on the way you used to look or feel that you can no longer appreciate your unique worth. Your partner and friends will continue to love and value you as long as you let them. The crisis of illness often brings people who love each other even closer together and enriches their relationships in ways they never expected.

You don't have to do it all yourself. Don't hesitate to seek counseling or information if problems arise. Help is available from a wide range of sources. If you have questions about sexuality or are experiencing some difficulties you wish to discuss further, we strongly urge you to bring them up with your health care providers or to ask them to recommend competent sex counselors or therapists in your area. Other resources that may be available near your home include persons or groups of people who themselves have had cancer and who have had experience in talking about sexual concerns with others. The Resources at the end of the book may be helpful.

PART IV: SUPPORTIVE AND SOCIAL SERVICES
— FOR LIFE AND DEATH ISSUES

25

IN-HOSPITAL ROUTINES AND HEALTH CARE SUPPORT TEAMS

Ernest H. Rosenbaum, MD, Isadora R. Rosenbaum, MA, Diane Craig, RN Onc, BSHS, Carol S. Viele, RN, MS

———◇———

Today we are witnessing many changes in medicine, including new diagnostic techniques not even conceived of 10 years ago, as well as new methods in surgery, radiation therapy, chemotherapy, immunotherapy and other areas of patient care. Physicians and other members of the health care team—registered nurses (RNs), licensed vocational nurses (LVNs), nurse's aides, residents, interns, medical students, nursing students, social workers, clergy, therapists, mental health consultants and translators—are changing their attitudes toward the ethical and medical responsibilities of the practice of medicine. Training has become more specialized; in many areas, responsibilities are delegated to various members of the health care team. Changes have continued to occur in patient financial payment for third-party medical and office services as well.

THE PATIENT'S RIGHTS

Nearly everyone who has been in a hospital for even the briefest time knows how demoralizing and upsetting hospital routine can be. Until recently, the patient's position has been one of extreme frustration. Feeling trapped, the patient could do little about this, since hospital routine tended to be inflexible except in emergencies.

These days, the patient has much more control over the situation. We are seeing an increasingly humanistic approach to patient care. Members of the medical team

recognize that they are there to serve you and to help you get well and that, no matter how advantageous a smoothly running routine may be, it should be modified to meet your needs.

A hospital has many functions: the prevention of disease, the pursuit of clinical research, the education of health professionals and, increasingly, the education of patients and their families. But all these activities must be conducted with an overriding concern for the patient. Recognizing the patient's dignity as a human being will help ensure that his or her rights as a patient are respected. The complete text of the Patient's Bill of Rights, recognized by many hospitals, is printed in the Appendix.

ADMISSION TO THE HOSPITAL

Admission procedures may vary depending on the type of insurance coverage or managed-care plan you have. Health Maintenance Organizations (HMOs), Preferred Provider Organizations (PPOs) and similar providers may require you to obtain authorization in order to be admitted unless it is an emergency. These third-party payers also control the length of your stay, since many procedures can be done on a same-day basis.

In an emergency, you may have little to do with the details of your admission. A friend or family member may be asked to go through the admitting procedure for you. This person should be familiar with the necessary information about you (described below). In addition, he or she should remember to bring any personal items you'll need.

In a scheduled admission, your first stop is the hospital's Admissions office. You will need identification and health insurance cards. An admissions clerk will ask you questions about your insurance, the reason you are being admitted, your next of kin and so on, to fill out the admission forms required by the hospital.

Your doctor, or his or her staff, will usually have reserved a bed for you. The Admissions office may offer you a choice between a private room and a semiprivate room. The clerk will discuss these options and their cost with you. (Unfortunately, in some hospitals, particularly county or city hospitals, limited availability and cost considerations often restrict choice.)

You should bring necessary personal items—such as a brush and comb, a toothbrush and toothpaste, your bathrobe and slippers—as well as any special items that will make your stay more comfortable or cheer you. You should not bring anything of substantial value or more than five or ten dollars in cash. If you are admitted through the Emergency Department, you may check your valuables with the cashier.

You may not be allowed to keep any medication you bring with you. To help your doctor evaluate your medication program, bring a list of the names and dosages of the medications you normally take.

Coping with Hospital Routine Being admitted to the hospital and becoming a patient are extremely stressful events. You are suddenly placed in a strange environment, with few or none of your familiar supports. Though your role has changed, you do not need to give up everything that is important to you—your

independence, control over your own life or the handling of responsibilities.

It is the message of this book that you can best help your recovery by becoming an active participant in your own medical care. But how can you adjust to being a patient? How can you participate in your medical care?

1. Accept that a hospital stay is a difficult time. You can reduce your stress and fear of the unknown by learning what to expect in the way of hospital routine, understanding the roles of the nurses and other members of the health care team, and knowing what to do about problems.
2. Be aware of your rights, and communicate your needs.
3. Offer your own suggestions, and do not hesitate to ask questions.

Here are some practical suggestions for dealing with common hospital situations. Your fear and frustration can be reduced by learning the roles and procedures of the various staff who will be caring for you.

PATIENT-STAFF RELATIONSHIPS

The Nurse After you have been admitted and taken to your hospital room, one of the first people you will meet is the nurse. Your nurse will greet you, introduce him- or herself and check your weight, blood pressure, temperature and pulse. (In some hospitals, an LVN or nurse's aide will check these vital signs.) He or she should see that you are comfortable, show you how to operate the "call" buttons, ask questions about allergies to medications and ask whether you have any questions or requests.

Nurses are the direct line to the doctor in his or her absence and are a vital link between doctor and patient. They are the primary people to whom patients regularly communicate their needs, frustrations, fears and delights. The principal nurses assigned to each patient within a 24-hour period try to communicate to one another all the things each has learned about the patients in their care. They meet as each shift changes, to ensure that patients' needs, desires, medical history and status are communicated from one nurse to the next.

Nurses are responsible for approximately 80 to 90 percent of patient care in the hospital. In most other areas of patient care, the doctor relies on the nurses' knowledge and judgment, along with input from the patient, to make patient care decisions.

Doctor's Rounds While you are in the hospital, your doctor will visit you during the day. This is the time for you to make requests or discuss problems. Nurses also communicate with the doctor about your condition during the doctor's rounds.

For practical reasons, the doctor's visits cannot be regularly scheduled and often occur at different times. Surgeons often see their patients in the early morning (that is, at 6 to 7 A.M.). If the doctor arrives unexpectedly or awakens you, you may forget several important questions or requests. It may therefore be helpful to make a list of questions to have ready when the doctor sees you. Keep a pad of paper at your bedside, and jot down things you would like to discuss as they come to mind.

Loss of Independence With illness comes varying degrees of dependence on family, doctors, nurses, friends, strangers, machines and medications. For many, the idea of dependence may be accompanied by fear. Feelings about dependence are learned patterns that cannot easily be changed; becoming aware of them may help you decide what areas of life you are willing to delegate control of to others, so that you can expend your energies on what is important to you.

Waiting Having to wait is a frequent problem in the hospital. Waiting can produce anxiety, frustration, exhaustion and anger. Some waiting cannot be prevented, because certain activities or procedures take a long time to complete. At other times, waiting is just one of those inexplicable mysteries of large institutions. Sometimes the waiting can be eliminated by reminding those in charge that you are waiting: you can often help by keeping yourself and others informed.

But you must also put reasonable limits on what you demand of your health care team. Sometimes, answers or help cannot be given immediately. Emergencies must take precedence over routine ward care and may cause delays. Your understanding, patience and cooperation during medical emergencies, or when more time needs to be spent on a critically ill patient, makes good sense; another time, you may be the person needing special emergency care, and you can then expect to be given whatever additional time and efforts are necessary.

Fear of Staff Patients are often afraid to complain, fearing that they may alienate the very people on whom they ultimately depend to give them comfort or to help save their lives. But within reasonable limits, you should communicate your feelings and problems. To help you, your nurses must know both your positive and negative reactions to the care and services you receive. You are in the hospital to help yourself get well, not to please the doctor or the nurses.

Unfortunately, some people you meet during your hospital stay may be rude, unsympathetic or otherwise not the kind of people you usually like or respond to positively. You can help both yourself and other patients by registering a complaint about these people and any problems you encounter with them. Hospital staff need your help in monitoring themselves and in improving the quality of the care they provide. Please speak up.

The Clergy One of the many functions of the clergy is to comfort the sick, at home or in the hospital. Clergy visits in a hospital are not necessarily limited to members of one congregation or even one religion. Some patients may have no religious affiliation. Yet the clergy can still be welcome figures, sympathetic listeners and sources of emotional and spiritual sustenance. If you would like to be visited by one of the hospital chaplains, ask your nurse. Similarly, tell your nurse if you do not want to be visited by the clergy.

DOCTOR'S ADMITTING ORDERS

When you are first admitted to the hospital, your doctor writes admitting orders. These go in the front of your chart, which is kept at the nursing station. The orders are a formal list of directions and precautions that will be the basic guide for your care in the hospital. The format for admitting orders is as follows:

◆ Admit: "to Ward _____" or "to Room _____"

◆ Diagnosis: the name of your disease (e.g., "lung cancer")

◆ Condition: "good," "fair," "stable," "poor," "gravely ill," etc.

◆ Vital signs: the schedule for checking your temperature, pulse, blood pressure and respirations (usually "every four hours"; but if your condition is unstable—for instance, after surgery—the order may be for "every hour" or even "every 15 minutes")

◆ Allergies: any that might be known from your experience (e.g., allergies to codeine, penicillin, sulfa drugs, adhesive, etc.)

◆ Activity: "ad lib" (i.e., as you seem able to accommodate it), "restricted to bed with bathroom privileges," "commode use only," etc.

◆ Diet: "regular," "low fat," "low salt," "high protein," "high roughage," etc., and the number of calories you should be having

◆ Nursing orders: "daily weights," "intake and outputs" (measure all fluids in and out), "guaiac all stools" (check for blood in stools), schedule for changing dressings, etc.

◆ IV orders: information about any intravenous fluids you should be receiving

◆ Medications: information about any medications you should be receiving

◆ Labs: orders for blood tests, x-rays, etc.

◆ Notifications: when the doctor should be notified because of a change in your condition that would indicate a problem (e.g., "call house officer for temperature over 100°F," "… for pulse over 120 or less than 60," "… for respiratory rate greater than 30 or less than 10")

The doctor signs the orders, and they become the legal flow sheet for your care; you cannot receive any care or medications not specified or allowed in the orders, but your doctor will change or adjust them as the need arises, usually in consultation with the nursing staff. Nurses are allowed to add or change orders only with the doctor's permission.

YOUR OWN ADMITTING ORDERS

Your List The best way for you to be comfortable and to maintain control over your life in the hospital is to think about what you like and about what you want to continue to do for as long as you are able, and then do those things. Much is possible if you know what you want and remember to ask for it. If possible, before you go to the hospital, make a list of your likes and dislikes and ask that these be considered in making up your orders.

Diet As a patient, you might consider these important matters: When do you like to eat? Do you like a bedtime snack? Are there foods you do not like?

In most hospitals, the Dietary Department is willing to be flexible in accommodating your desires. Ask to see the dietitian, and let your wishes be known. (Your diet must, of course, conform to your medical needs as determined by your doctor.)

You may be more comfortable with the idea of eating foods prepared at home and brought in for you. Occasionally, a meal ordered from your favorite restaurant can be a pleasant change.

Bathing Do you prefer to take baths or showers? If you are able, continue your bathing habits; the exercise you get is a bonus. Ask for help if necessary. In some hospitals, a doctor's order is necessary for a bath or shower, so be sure to include that need on your list of things to discuss with the doctor.

Hospital Room Hospital rooms can be bleak and dreary, their odors and sounds foreign and sometimes offensive. For a prolonged stay, you may want to bring in a poster for the wall, photographs of your family, a religious picture, or a portable tape recorder or radio with earphones. Sometimes bringing your own bed pillow from home is comforting. If you have a roommate, be as considerate of his or her needs as you would expect him or her to be of yours.

Visiting A special stay with a family member or friend beyond the usual visiting hours is an item you may want to include on your list of needs. A long wait in the X-ray Department, for example, or a particularly difficult period during your illness can be made easier by the presence of someone who provides company and comfort. Ask the nurse what the visiting hours are, but do not hesitate to ask for exceptions if your needs do not fit into the prescribed hours. You have certain rights; again, though, you must also be reason-able and try to work within the structure of your hospital's rules.

Many hospitals will provide a cot for a relative or friend to spend the night, particularly when the patient is critically ill. Children are not the only ones who sleep better with someone close by. Cots are provided only for patients in private rooms.

FEARS

Anxiety Sometimes you may not know exactly why you are afraid; you simply have an overwhelming sense of anxiety. It can be fear of the unknown or fear about your future. Talking with someone is a step toward dealing with your fears, known or unknown.

No matter how silly or uncomfortable you feel, consider asking your doctor or nurse for a few minutes of time. Not every nurse or doctor will be the right person for you to talk with; so as soon as possible, start thinking about the people on your health care team with whom you feel most comfortable. Have a conversation with one of these people and discuss your specific fears if you have identified them, or simply admit that you feel scared. Nurses are familiar with patient fears and can often help relieve them.

Sleep Problems Everyone who faces an illness and its treatment has certain fears—fears of surgery, therapy, pain, even death. These are very real fears to the patient and must be dealt with; some can even be eliminated.

Nighttime, in particular, can be frightening. In unfamiliar surroundings, many people have trouble relaxing and falling asleep. You may be kept awake by the noise of nurses at work, machines operating, or voices or TV sounds coming from another patient's room or from a roommate's portion of your room. After the distractions of the hospital's busy daytime activities have diminished and visitors are gone, patients are left with their own thoughts. Pain sometimes becomes more intense, because there is nothing else to think about.

A hospital functions 24 hours a day. At night, the health care team's members are awake, caring for their patients, and are as available to patients for physical and emotional needs as in the daytime. Nurses are always about; they will try to disturb you as little as possible, but they will check on you, since they need to protect and care for patients and carry out the doctors' orders. If you feel you are being disturbed unnecessarily, or if you have nighttime problems you need help with, talk things over with your nurse or doctor.

We often do little things at home before retiring that help us get to sleep more easily—for example, you may drink a cup of warm milk or read a few pages of a book. Try to continue these patterns while in the hospital. If you are accustomed to taking a sleeping pill, tell your doctor or nurse to ensure that the appropriate order will be written. Your doctor may prescribe a sleeping pill for you to take as needed; do not hesitate to use it if you feel the need. A good night's sleep can help you feel physically refreshed and better able to cope with the stresses of the day ahead.

Before the lights are off, be sure you know how to get the nurse's help if you need it during the night. Know where the nurse's call button is. All hospitals have some system for calling the nurse—use it if you need it. You will be helping your nurse to help you. You might want to ask that a night-light be left on in your room, so that you won't be disoriented by darkness. If you are able to get up, be careful: bedrails are raised at night for your protection, unless otherwise specified by the doctor.

Hospital Tests We can all identify with fear of the unknown. Patients have often said, "If I had only known what to expect,

I could have relaxed or at least tried to cope." Unfamiliar tests and examinations by consulting physicians, residents, interns or even your own doctor can cause fear and anxiety.

The doctor will usually tell you what tests are being scheduled. Ask your nurse what time they are scheduled for. If your doctor has not already made the following things clear, or if you remain unsure about any of them, ask the nurse:
◆ The purpose of the test
◆ What will be done to you
◆ What you will be asked to do
◆ How you will feel both during and after the test
◆ How long the test will last
◆ Any other questions you may have.

You may simply want to know what is likely to hurt and what probably won't, or whether the test has potential risks or side effects. Again, your doctor will probably have told you, but the nurse also knows and can reassure you further. Some hospitals provide literature about tests, such as x-rays, scans and so on.

When you understand and appreciate a diagnostic test's nature and purpose, as well as how the test is performed, much of the fear is dispelled. Not knowing what will happen is what causes the most fear. Once a test is performed, an explanation of the results of the test and how they relate to your therapy will also help alleviate your fears.

Patients are often afraid of receiving test results. Ask to learn about your test results early in order to reduce your anxieties and worries. These are subjects about which you should ask your doctor, but after that you may need to talk about the results numerous times with a nurse or another member of your health care team. They want to help you understand what is happening to your body.

They also understand that there may be times when you are too afraid to discuss the specifics of a painful subject. What you should know is that someone will be available when you are ready to talk.

COMMON PROBLEMS

It would be impossible for this book to cover all the problems you might encounter while in the hospital. Whether a specific problem arises depends on the individual, the illness and how these relate to one another. But we can discuss some of the more common problems that a hospital stay can cause or make worse. For more information on diet and nutrition, see Chapters 16 and 17.

Constipation Lack of activity, an entirely different or significantly changed diet, intravenous feeding or certain drugs (such as narcotics) can produce constipation in hospital patients.

Sometimes constipation occurs simply because your environment has changed, because you have to use an unfamiliar bathroom (perhaps with a roommate not far away) or because someone else is doing the cooking. And having to use a bedpan has caused the system of many a patient to rebel.

Do not suffer. Ask about receiving bran or a glass of prune juice for breakfast. A glass of hot lemon water works for some people. You may add these items to your menu if they are not listed; you will be told if your condition would not tolerate particular foods. Drink lots of fluids of all kinds, and try to keep your level of activity up: take walks in the hall, or ask whether you can have some physical therapy sessions. Tell your nurse that you are constipated, so that your doctor may prescribe laxatives or enemas if needed. Chapter 17 provides more detailed solutions to constipation.

Nausea The medications you receive can cause nausea or an upset stomach. To reduce or relieve this common problem, the medications can sometimes be given late at night (so that you can sleep through the nausea period) or early in the morning on awakening (to help eliminate morning nausea). Tell your nurse or doctor that you are nauseated. Your doctor can order an antinausea medication. Taking antinausea medicine about 30 minutes before meals will help reduce mealtime nausea. Other antinausea techniques are discussed in Chapter 17.

Skin Problems Having a chronic illness and being confined to bed can cause skin problems such as pressure sores (bedsores) or rashes due to the roughness of bed linen. The nursing staff will be working to prevent and care for pressure sores, but you can help too. Good hygiene is extremely important at this time. If you can, take a shower or a tub bath. Try to change your position in bed as often as possible to get the blood circulating to the affected area. Accept the back rub that is offered you at night; not only does it feel good, it also helps prevent and care for skin problems. For further discussion of skin problems and solutions, see Chapters 4 and 5.

Pain Pain is sometimes the main reason for admission to the hospital. It can be both physical and mental. Severe, chronic pain can be a most destructive problem that affects many functions of your life. It often prevents a person from expending energy in personal relationships with loved ones at a time when those relationships are most important.

Pain is often accompanied by anxiety. You may worry about whether the pain will go away; if you have received medication and the pain is ebbing, you may feel anxious about the return of chronic pain. Reducing anxiety often makes it possible to achieve better or complete pain control.

Some patients do well taking pain medications only when pain occurs. But for others, pain control cannot be achieved by treating the pain only when it comes. They do better with a regular schedule of pain medication throughout the day, with additional doses as needed. In all cases, treatment must be individualized.

Anxiety about pain can be reduced by finding an effective pain relief measure. Knowing that your pain medication will be available on request will also reduce fear of suffering. Medications are also available to help decrease anxiety. Thinking positively and trying to relax will help your pain medication give maximum relief. Medications are also available to help decrease anxiety.

We often teach patients how to give their own pain shots, so that they can get faster relief and can be in control of their pain when they go home.

Many patients feel that they are "acting like a baby" if they complain of pain; as a result, they suffer needlessly. It is all right to say that you hurt. The best pain control can be achieved when pain is treated before it becomes severe.

Pain medications that contain narcotics commonly cause side effects; usually these affect the gastrointestinal tract and can be managed. Side effects should therefore not prevent the use of narcotics if the narcotic is working to control pain. Constipation is a common side effect. Daily stool softeners, laxatives and enemas may be needed as long as you are receiving the narcotic. Close attention must be given to treating constipation in order to prevent more serious complications, such as stool impactions (severe constipation with stool accumulation and blockage in the rectum).

Many pain medications are available today. They come in pill and liquid forms, and some are given by injection. It is extremely important to tell your doctor and nurse the location of the pain, what it is like, whether it gets worse and whether the medication you are taking gives relief. Only you can do this.

Since pain medications are often effective only when they are given before the pain gets out of control, it is your responsibility to tell your health care team about the pain early, before it hurts too much. It is also important for you to know that there are stronger and variable forms of medication. Pain control without heavy sedation is possible. Local pain blocks, or neurosurgery to cut the nerves that carry pain fibers, may sometimes help.

Remember, the team wants to see that your pain is relieved before it reaches a high level, because severe pain is devastating and can precipitate other problems. It is your responsibility to communicate your needs to the medical staff. Only by knowing your problems can they help you. Pain control is covered in detail in Chapter 5.

The Role of the Family Traditionally, the patient's family has been overlooked as a resource in care and recovery planning. The idea that health status is a private matter has long been accepted without question. Originally, the family was asked to "wait outside"; the patient was expected to keep the family informed, letting them know "what the doctor said"—an approach that eliminated communication between the family and the health care team.

That concept of the family's role is becoming as archaic as that of the passive patient. Just as patients must take more responsibility for helping themselves get well, so too can the patient's family contribute. Having the family "wait outside" wastes a great deal of valuable "people power" that could be available to facilitate a patient's recovery. Also, many family members want or need to do something to contribute actively to the patient's healing.

Becoming Familiar with the Environment Here are a few examples of the many things a family can do to help:

◆ Know the nurses and doctors in charge of the patient's care, and help the patient remember them.

◆ Learn how to work the bed and how to call the nurse.

◆ Find out what supplies are in the room and where to get others.

◆ Locate the visitors' room, sunrooms, televisions and kitchens nearest the patient's room.

◆ Locate the bathrooms, phones and cafeteria.

◆ Learn how to reach the nursing station by phone, so that family members can call in for updates.

Family Communication with the Nurse and Doctor Tell the nursing staff that as a family member, you wish to participate in the patient's care; otherwise, they will assume that you do not choose to help. Sometimes family members want to help, but fear that they will be in the way. Others may believe that they would not be allowed to help. Be assured that the nursing staff can use all the help they can get: let them know that you want to participate actively in caring for your loved one. Family members can often serve as spokespersons for patients who are either reluctant or unable to speak for themselves.

Here are some questions the health care team might like answered by the family:

◆ Is the patient likely to be outspoken or passive about expressing needs?

◆ Does the patient have any habits or characteristics that might easily be upset by the hospital stay—e.g., difficulty in sleeping, or attitudes about illness?

◆ Does the patient have any fears or anxieties about illness, pain or body image that might not be revealed to a stranger?

◆ Are there outside influences, such as specific worries or joys, that might affect the patient's drive to get well?

The answers to such questions help the health care team understand the patient more fully and take a realistic and more personal approach to the patient's care. The family usually knows how the patient reacts under stress; the nurse does not. Nurses do know that illness and hospitalization are stressful situations for most people, but they need the family's help in minimizing this problem for specific individuals.

Conversely, the nurse can tell the family the following useful information:

◆ When the doctors make rounds, and the best time and place to reach them.

◆ How to help the patient meet special physical needs for therapy, such as nutrition, exercise or mental diversion.

◆ The reasons for tests and treatments.

◆ Where to find aid in financial, disability or insurance matters.

We strongly encourage families to share their feelings with the doctor and the rest of the health care team as much as possible. It is sometimes difficult to be hopeful about a patient's recovery in the face of a life-threatening illness.

When recovery is expected to be limited, or to take a long time, it is normal to become disappointed and discouraged. The nurse's job includes listening to the family's as well as the patient's fears and anxieties. Nurses may help to dispel doubts. More often, they can reassure families that their feelings are appropriate. No one is ever completely positive or without doubts. Talking with the nurse can be helpful, if only to get the feelings out into the open.

It is difficult for family members as well as patients to ask a question about something they know little about. Because of its terminology, medicine can seem like a foreign language. If for any reason you have failed to ask the doctor to explain unfamiliar words, ask the nurses for help. Let them know what you do or do not understand.

Some people prefer to know only the barest details, while others want to know everything. Remember, no question is unimportant or ridiculous. If you take unanswered questions home with you, your anxieties and fears will increase.

When a patient is questioning the doctor, it is often easier if two or more family members are present. Making a list beforehand can help the family remember what they were concerned about and get many questions answered at one time. Patients can benefit greatly from having a family member present at these question-and-answer sessions.

For example, many couples prefer to be seen as a team when one is hospitalized or receiving outpatient therapy. When both are present, the healthy partner can take responsibility for much of the information received by both, recalling it for the patient and communicating it to other family members at a later time.

Some patients do not want their families involved and do not want their physicians to discuss their case with family and friends. The patient has the right to request this and to have the request respected.

A word of caution to the family is important here. Some patients may become completely passive, letting their families give and receive all information. This can lead to two problems:

◆ It is important for the medical staff to hear the patient's account of symptoms and of how he or she views the illness. If the family takes over the entire process, understanding and insight into the patient's attitudes and feelings may be lost.

◆ Active participation in all areas of treatment is necessary for early and optimal recovery. Involvement in their own care helps patients generate the energy needed for their recovery. Family members can help, but letting them do everything will inhibit the patient's progress on the road to recovery.

Family Responsibilities Sometimes another family member falls ill during a patient's long or difficult hospitalization.

Whether through caring for the rest of the family in the patient's absence or through expending much of his or her energy on the patient's behalf, the relative may have neglected his or her own health.

Sharing patient responsibilities with other members of the family is essential. If you as a family member wish to undertake all the responsibilities, that may be fine. If not, or if you need to rest or take care of your own important needs and must therefore be absent from the patient, ask the nurse or the hospital social worker for help. They can contact you should the need arise and can, if necessary, explain why you are away taking care of yourself.

When dealing with patients who show anger or resentment because their family support person is away, the doctor, nurse or social worker can be helpful. These health care team members should always remember that understanding the other person's needs and point of view is essential if they are to deal rationally with both their own feelings and the feelings of others.

Patients must be realistic about their expectations of others. A lot of positive energy is often mobilized within a family by focusing on getting the patient well. But that is not always the case, and patients should neither expect it nor be disappointed if it does not take place. Remember, too, that the family's life goes on outside the hospital, and many family members are at times either totally unavailable or available only at limited times. Resentments should not be allowed to build up.

In short, it is still the patient's responsibility to understand the family's position and to know when to lean and when to stand alone. If necessary, the patient can have a family conference with the health care team.

Discharge Planning It is natural to feel some anxiety when you anticipate release (discharge) from the hospital to go home; there are significant differences in the two environments. You will be leaving the security of the hospital support team—the nurses and physicians, who provided physical care and support; the physical therapist, who began an exercise program and whose firm assurance enabled progressive ambulating; the occupational therapist; the nutritionist, who provided diet instruction; and the medical social worker, who helped you and your family deal with the practical problems relating to your illness, as well as fear and anxieties. But proper discharge planning can assure you of a continuing support system at home, and your rehabilitation will be enhanced by all the additional advantages, both physical and psychological, of being at home.

Discharge from the hospital represents a crucial move and a progressive step in your rehabilitation. Many patients become more alert and better oriented after returning home. You can expect your appetite to improve and your interest in becoming active to increase. As you become physically able, you will find enjoyment in taking up favorite activities once again. Gradually resuming some of your particular roles in the home, as your health allows, will have noticeable effects on your physical rehabilitation, as well as on your attitude about yourself. Even small accomplishments are important in bolstering your sense of being able to cope and your motivation toward as full a recovery as possible. As you mobilize your strength, your accomplishments may surprise you, your family and your health care team.

The transition from hospital to home can be smooth if it's facilitated by early discharge planning, involving the health care team, you and your family and the discharge coordinator. The discharge coordinator, usually a medical social worker or a discharge planning nurse, is the key professional who arranges for any needed home care and acts as a liaison with the patient, the family, the health care team and home health care agencies.

Discharge planning should begin shortly after admission to the hospital, as soon as a diagnosis is made and therapy initiated, even though there are still many unknowns. While you are in the hospital, your health care team will work together to anticipate what your medical and physical needs will be in the home and will discuss these needs with you and your family. You will need to participate in planning your home care by providing information regarding the physical setup at your home (stairs, bathroom facilities, etc.), the availability of people to help you and whether special equipment can be accommodated.

Your doctor, assisted by other members of your health care team, will outline your required at-home plan of care, what side effects to expect following treatment, what limitations to expect because of physical weakness and what problems may result from chronic illness. They will establish guidelines to enable you to handle both temporary and long-term problems. The health care team will help you and your family set realistic goals and suggest ways to obtain assistance when needed.

A call by the discharge coordinator to your insurance company or to your county's social services department will reveal many at-home services that can be provided free to you. These services may include visiting nurses, attendant care, meal preparation and equipment rentals. Certain organizations, such as the American Cancer Society, also provide some services and equipment. You and your family should become aware of the services available in your community as early as possible in your illness, by meeting with the medical social worker or discharge planning nurse.

Discharge planning is simply a continuation of your in-hospital program.

Generally, by closely observing the nursing care you receive in the hospital, you and your family will gain valuable clues about areas of concern. When you participate in organizing and carrying out your hospital care, you also learn how to care for yourself at home. Those who are most involved in their hospital care will make the easiest transition to home care.

Your medications will already be familiar to you from the hospital. But making a written schedule of the amounts and times prescribed by your doctor will prove helpful while you settle into a routine at home. You should also already be aware of the vital importance of good nutrition and regular exercise in your recovery. Planned programs in both these areas should be continued at home. While you are in the hospital, ask the dietitian and the physical therapist to talk to you and your family to help set up your home programs.

Unfortunately, sometimes discharge planning may be sketchy, and many needs may be overlooked. Make it your responsibility to initiate plans for your home needs. List questions to discuss with your doctor, your family, your nurse, the dietitian and the physical therapist. A poorly planned discharge can cause much anxiety for you and your family, and can result in an unnecessary readmission to the hospital.

Even with a well-planned discharge, certain limitations in your home setup or in your own or your family's abilities to cope may not become apparent until you have been home for a while and tested things out. If you have been discharged recently, you can call on the medical social worker or discharge planning nurse for further help in planning your home care. Your doctor and his or her office staff will also be able to help you re-evaluate your home situation and arrange for needed care.

It is reassuring to know that when you are home, help and support are just a phone call away. If you have questions or a need for reassurance, or if a troublesome situation arises, call your doctor. In private medical practice, a physician or a member of the office team is available 24 hours a day to give medical care and advice and to meet your emergency needs. Restrict routine questions and problems to regular office hours, though: evenings and weekends are only for emergencies.

If you cannot reach your doctor, your questions or problems may be solved by someone who knows you and your medical situation. Do not be reluctant to call your hospital ward and speak to one of your nurses. Take their names and the ward phone number with you when you leave the hospital. A nurse is always on duty there. He or she can answer many of your questions, direct you to the appropriate person to call or reassure you by just talking to you. A problem that could wait until morning can also keep you and your family awake all night with worry. Nurses do remember patients and their families, and too often this resource remains untapped after the patient goes home. In an emergency, you can always request an ambulance and go to your hospital's emergency room.

26
IN-HOME SERVICES

Eugenie Marek, RN

A major change in health care over the last decade has been the significant increase in home care services. We seem to be coming full circle, since the concept of home care is as old as medicine itself. In the United States we have developed impressive centers for both inpatient and outpatient treatment of disease, but we are remembering that a great deal of care for an illness is best done at home, where we often heal the most easily. The changes in government guidelines and insurance company policies have highlighted the cost-effectiveness of such care.

Advances in medical technology are making it possible for you to be at home relying on devices or systems that you or a caregiver can easily learn to use. These are real advances in treatment or symptom relief over traditional techniques that would have required you to stay hospitalized. Some of the areas where there has been progress that can benefit you at home are:

◆ More effective and longer-acting medications

◆ IV lines and catheters that are usable for weeks

◆ Small pumps and other devices that allow continuous treatment or continuous delivery of medications

◆ Alert systems and sensing devices for safety when home alone

◆ Advances in wound care for rapid healing

◆ Furniture and equipment to aid rehabilitation and comfort

◆ Transport companies to help access care from home

This list is far from complete. Your home care plan will include many of these and other recent advances to make your in-home care as thorough and effective as possible.

PREPARING TO GO HOME

Hospitalization is not a prerequisite for in-home health care, but it is most often where such care is first ordered. However, services may be ordered at any point during your illness. In the case of chronic problems, your physician will work with the established home care agency to adjust or restart services as needed.

When you are ready to leave a medical center after an illness or treatment, you will be interviewed by a discharge planner, who will be working with your doctor to determine what your continued needs will be. The plan developed will include medications, equipment, personnel and treatments. Many hospitals have developed their own home care programs so the transition to home is a smooth one. The hospital has well-established standards and oversees the workers involved. The range of licensed personnel includes registered nurses, home health aides, medical social workers, physical, occupational and speech therapists, as well as specialists who manage IV infusions, taking blood samples, wound care and x-ray.

When a separate, accredited home care agency is involved, the hospital discharge planner ensures that the required services are in place for when you go home.

Additionally, this planner can assist you if you want to hire additional help for further reassurance or to supplement what is covered by your insurance plan.

While as much as is possible will be worked out beforehand, the final plan for your in-home care will be devised when you are first visited at home. The first-hand observation of the trained nurse is needed to be sure that equipment, personnel and scheduling are appropriate. Small details can make big differences. Try not to feel anxious about leaving the hospital without all the details in place. This is to ensure the best plan for you.

REIMBURSEMENT/ PAYMENT

Insurance companies are glad to explain what in-home services are covered by your plan. Your discharge planner may also be of assistance. Generally, a great deal, if not all, of home care is covered by insurance, although policies differ regarding number of home care visits, degree of illness or disability required and the type of equipment. If you anticipate that you might need such services, finding out about them in advance when you feel well will help you be prepared to make decisions that might come with a price tag later on.

THE FIRST HOME VISIT

The first time that you are visited at home, some important matters will be discussed. This initial assessment will serve as a baseline for your record at the home care agency. Any changes in your condition that may occur later on will be included in this record, resulting in possible changes in your care. The home care nurse that you are now meeting will probably continue to visit you, establishing an important relationship.

During this visit, you and your caregivers will be interviewed about your health history, recent illness, current symptoms and any other problems for which you will need care. Your ability to manage the required care, family and neighborhood resources and the ways in which the home care agency can assist will be explored. You will receive a physical examination to check that you are stable and to collect any new health information that may be important.

This first visit will result in fine-tuning your plan for in-home care, working out details of the type of personnel, frequency of their visits, treatments needed as well as medications, supplies, devices and equipment you require.

Although the home care nurse will be performing specific procedures as needed, his or her efforts will also focus on instructing you and your family or other caregivers in managing your care, providing assistance and support as you learn, and on professionally assessing your response to the care. Home care nurses have daily experience in managing problems of safety, nutrition, elimination, mobility, skin care, medications and pain, as well as troubleshooting in a wide variety of unusual situations. They are known for their flexibility and responsiveness. They want you to speak up, express your worries and ask for their advice and help.

One way that you can begin your own caregiving is to be organized. Designate a place to keep information and items related to your care at home. Be sure to have a list of important telephone numbers, a calendar for noting appointments and home care visits, and a list of your medications and when you will need a refill. This might also be the best place to keep your medications and other supplies. Having everything organized and in one place will give you a better sense of control. It's also important to have what you need available when you need it.

Since your home care nurse will ask about the effectiveness of your treatments, as well as specifics about any changes in your health, keep a log or diary just for this purpose. When you don't feel well, it will be easier to remember details that you have written down.

If you will sometimes be alone, you may want to test yourself while the nurse is still in your home to see if you are able to perform a task. This will contribute to your success later on.

PAIN CONTROL AT HOME

Often the biggest concern for patients as they prepare to go home is pain management. Faced with going home to well-meaning but untrained caregivers or possibly being alone at times, you might understandably worry about what to do if your pain gets out of control. Discuss your concerns with your home care nurse beforehand. He or she can add some practical safeguards to your home care plan to lessen your worry.

Possibly you are worried because you are not fully aware of important recent advances in pain management: more effective medications, dosing devices and alternative and nonmedication treatments. While you may depend on your oncologist's wide range of experience with pain relief, there are now pain specialists that can be consulted if needed. If pain is a problem, you will be leaving the hospital only when a firm medication plan has been set up for your use at home. While you are still hospitalized, there will be a trial to see how well you do with these medications.

You might be surprised by the range of medication possibilities in addition to the traditional "pain pill." You may be prescribed a time-released pill or liquid, skin patch or rectal suppository. It is also possible to administer IV medications at home with a small pump. Even more sophisticated systems are available if needed.

What is most important is that you know that you will not have to suffer needlessly. Your comfort is one of the highest priorities of your physician and other caregivers. There is now so much available that can be offered to bring about effective pain relief. But there are also two important responsibilities that you have to ensure good pain control:
◆ Adhere to the pain management schedule, even when you are not in pain.
◆ Carefully observe how well your medication works, especially when it doesn't.

It is now understood that the best way to control pain is to treat it early. Stopping a little pain is easier than starting to medicate when your pain is no longer tolerable. If you want to be a good caregiver to yourself, don't wait to take a dose of pain medication; take your medication regularly, as prescribed, even if you feel fine.

Types of Pain Generally speaking, there are two types of pain: chronic and acute.
◆ *Chronic* pain is pain that is with you most of the time. You may recognize it as a slight back ache or belly pain, for example. There may be chronic pain with certain types of cancer. This continuous pain responds to continuous treatment. This is why you will be given a medication schedule. If your pain changes so that it is "breaking through" despite the treatment, let your caregivers know so that an adjustment can be made quickly. To simplify the adjustment, keep to your established schedule until you are told to change it.
◆ *Acute* pain may be described as a pain that is new to you, possibly sudden, and sharp or more severe than usual. For example, the term acute is used to describe appendicitis, which is characterized by sudden, strong abdominal pain.

Notify your physician if you experience acute pain. Acute pain should be investigated. But don't panic. Acute pain does not necessarily mean that your cancer has spread or that there is something seriously wrong with you. It may be your body's signal that there is a minor problem that is easily remedied. For example, constipation may be accompanied by pain, but it is easily relieved with appropriate treatment.

Concentrate on being familiar with your pain and what helps to relieve it; make notes in a log so you can share this information with your family, home care nurse and physician. Think of your home care nurse as wanting you to talk about your discomfort. Consider whether your pain is interfering with your sleep or your desire to eat. Have you been ignoring a pain problem hoping it would go away? Have you been consistently following your medication schedule? If not, why not? Your nurse may ask you these and other questions.

Try to understand your pain. Become an expert in a positive way. Pain is a very complex phenomenon, with both a physical and psychological component. It may be worse with anxiety or fatigue, and it may be lessened when approached with consistency and a calm mind.

MANAGING MEDICATIONS AT HOME

You may now have to take medications for the first time or more than before, possibly around the clock or on a complicated schedule. Speak to your discharge planner or home care nurse if you feel anxious or overwhelmed. These professionals have many helpful suggestions that they know work well from their extensive experience. Don't feel that this is "too small" a problem to ask about. Small problems can become very large when you don't feel well. Here are a few general comments on managing medications.

Whether you have a pain medication schedule, or generally must take several pills, use pill organizers to keep you on track. These are small plastic boxes, usu-

ally with seven compartments, one for each day of the week, that you can fill in advance. If you must take medication three times a day, get three separate organizers. Save your memory for more interesting problems! Show your system to your caregivers so they can support you in keeping to your schedule.

Medications come in many forms: pills, skin patches, rectal suppositories. Be sure to ask about specific directions and even a hands-on demonstration if you are trying a new technique.

Most medications are easy to give to yourself. Even IV infusions, such as antibiotics, can now be infused through catheters that are long lasting and low maintenance. If your medications involve any device or equipment, you will be given instruction by a trained caregiver at home, in your physician's office or in hospital. There will always be time for you to practice with a device while supervised.

Several medications that are sometimes used in cancer care require a subcutaneous injection. If you require such medication, you or a caregiver may be asked to learn to give such an injection. Subcutaneous means below the skin. Such an injection uses a very short, thin needle to place a small amount of medication into the soft tissue just below the skin. For example, a diabetic injects insulin subcutaneously several times a day. Your home care nurse will instruct you or a caregiver in this injection technique. You may be surprised how quickly you learn this, although your nurse will give you plenty of time to practice until you feel comfortable.

Using pain-relieving medications that contain narcotics, coupled with less activity, can slow the gastrointestinal tract, causing constipation. Because this happens so frequently, a good home care regime will address this from the start by including stool softeners, laxatives and possibly enemas while narcotics are being used. There is no reason to avoid the use of narcotics for pain relief. Many patients will also adjust their diets to prevent bowel sluggishness. (See "Constipation" in Chapter 17.)

Nausea can be a sign of constipation, or it can be a side effect of your illness or medications. Discuss your nausea with your nurse, noting any details that may explain its cause: when it occurs, how often and how it is relieved. Report nausea to your doctor, but continue to take your medications until told to stop. (See Chapter 17 for dealing with nausea and other medication side effects.)

You and Your Medication Following are a few important considerations with regard to medications. Most errors occur from small oversights that later seem easily avoidable.

◆ Keep an accurate and up-to-date list of your medications. If possible, be able to identify your pills by appearance. Don't transfer medication from one container to another.

◆ Be sure that at least one reliable person knows your medication schedule and can give you your medications if you don't feel well.

◆ Follow instructions on the prescription labels carefully, especially "p.r.n." ("as required") orders. If unsure, consult your pharmacist or home care nurse.

◆ Reorder your prescription medications before they run out. Allow several days, especially for narcotics, which require a "triplicate" form from your physician. Keep handy the name and telephone of your pharmacy.

◆ Keep you medication out of reach of children.

◆ Since medications have such an important effect upon your treatment and symptom relief, always consult your doctor before you stop taking your medications or change your medication schedule.

ACTIVITIES OF DAILY LIVING

One of the real comforts of being home with an illness is having what is most important to you near you. But it can be frustrating to find that your comfortable, familiar home now seems set up to sabotage your convalescence. In planning your care in your home, take some time to think about the location of your bed in relation to the bathroom, kitchen, telephone and a favorite easy chair. Also think about your bed and the furniture nearby in terms of height and convenience for your movement. Talk with family members about temporary changes that will spare your energy.

When home care is first begun, the nurse or physical therapist will assess your living space with a professional eye, making suggestions to increase safety. This is the time to think about your subjective comfort too. Will you be near the bathroom but feel isolated from the others in your home?

You may also require equipment to keep you safe or improve your mobility, such as a walker, an elevated commode or a shower seat. These are usually covered by insurance if deemed appropriate by your physician. The home care agency will process these orders.

EMERGENCIES

Despite the best planning, sometimes emergencies do occur. Your doctor and home care agency will have given you telephone numbers to call to be assessed immediately. If you feel the situation is more serious, call 911 for assistance. Keep a list of important phone numbers handy, near telephones and in your pocket, wallet or purse. (See the sample Emergency Phone Numbers listed in Chapter 27.)

REGAINING OPTIMAL FUNCTIONING

Once the assessments and routines are established for the in-home care that you require, you will begin to see some improvements. As you and your family develop more skill and confidence in attending to your recovery, professional support may be less necessary. You will begin to feel more "at home" with responding to your needs. Your relationship with the home care agency and the services they provide will change, depending upon the demands your ill-ness places upon you. Needs, plans and goals will be revised periodically.

A note of encouragement: even if your health cannot be fully restored, your ability to function as comfortably and fully as possible is a major goal of your medical treatment. The in-home services provided to you will serve to heal you physically as well as restore your optimal well-being. Home support lets you remain with your family and friends, living in the caring situation of your own familiar surroundings.

27
THE DOCTOR'S OFFICE

Ernest H. Rosenbaum, MD, Isadora R. Rosenbaum, MA, Catherine Coleman, RN,
Paula Chung, Betty Lopez, CMA, Anna Hicho, Regina Linetskaya, MA

———————◇———————

The managed-care trend of insurance plans and HMOs is causing the practice of medicine and health care delivery to change rapidly. But much of the primary and continuing care of patients still takes place in the doctor's office. Initially, you may be seen and thoroughly evaluated as a hospital inpatient, but your follow-up care will involve regular appointments as an outpatient.

The doctor's office differs from the hospital in that there is an ongoing one-to-one relationship between the patient and the same health care team. The resulting familiarity and rapport can be an important factor in therapy and recovery. It is also the basis for building trust, confidence and security.

As supportive relationships develop, it will seem easier to discuss physical, emotional, vocational or financial matters that contribute to your total sense of well-being. The medical office team strives to maximize your independence and to minimize the fragmentation of your care.

THE ROLE OF OFFICE PERSONNEL

The Receptionist In most offices, when you phone or come in for an appointment, the first contact you make is with the receptionist. Receptionists can assist you in many ways, for they are the link between you and the rest of the office team. They will give you certain forms for insurance and medical information, which will be important to your physician, the accounting department and the appropriate department in your HMO or managed-care organization.

You or your family and friends may often find it necessary to phone the doctor's office for information or to report a problem. It is extremely important to be open about your reason for calling and to communicate this to the receptionist. One of the receptionist's chief duties is to direct incoming calls to the person best equipped to resolve your concern or problem. It is impossible for the doctor to talk to every patient who calls in, so the receptionist is trained to answer questions whenever possible and to refer your medical problems to the nurse or doctor, according to the need.

When a new patient calls for an appointment and cannot be accommodated immediately, disappointment and sometimes even panic may result ("I'm desperately ill, my life is at stake, and you can't take me until when?"). The receptionist will try to pass your call to an appropriate source of help; rescheduling can be accommodated in an urgent situation.

Another function of the receptionist may be to help you schedule any laboratory tests or x-ray procedures the doctor orders. These tests must often be done at inconvenient times (such as early morning) or may involve specific instructions (such as fasting or taking time for a "prep" for an x-ray or a CT scan). If you discuss your personal needs with the receptionist, he or she will make every effort to arrange tests around your schedule. Remind the receptionist of your insurance provider, so that tests can be scheduled at the location through which your insurance company delivers services.

The receptionist may also need to call you sometimes. Don't panic. Some patients report being terrified when they receive a call from the doctor's office, anticipating that they're about to receive bad news from a lab report. But most such calls are made just to change an appointment date or time.

The Laboratory Technician The laboratory technician is another important member of the medical team (though some offices do not do their own lab work, but instead have you visit an outside lab for your tests). Usually the patient sees the lab technician before seeing the doctor. Often you will have blood tests at each visit, as the results may be needed to establish the progress (improvement or regression) of the disease as well as to provide clearance for chemotherapy or radiation therapy. Other times you will have blood tests every few visits, depending on your treatment plan.

Since the simplest blood count takes time to complete, ask the lab technician or the doctor's receptionist how much time you should allow so that your lab values will be ready before your visit with the doctor. Most labs require at least half an hour to produce results, even for urgent tests.

The Doctor During your initial consultation concerning your diagnosis, your doctor will try to give you a basic understanding of your disease, the reasons for diagnostic and staging tests, and the potentials of the various kinds of treatment. The doctor will also want to listen to your questions and apprehensions so that he or she may allay unnecessary fears and offer help with any practical problems you may face because of your disease.

This first interview may be highly charged emotionally. Faced with a seri-ous, possibly life-threatening illness, you may be shocked, frightened and unable to exercise your normal capacity to express your feelings, ask questions or take in new information. We have found it helpful for patients to tape-record consultations. You will then be able to review your doctor's explanations and recommendations later, when you may be better able to absorb the information.

You may find it helpful to bring the person or persons on whom you will most depend for emotional support with you to the consultation. Family and close friends will be able to be more supportive if they are included from the beginning and understand the intricacies of, and possible side effects from, the tests and treatment you will undergo. They may also assimilate information that you miss, and help you articulate questions and concerns of which they are aware. If those close to you are unable to be present during a consultation, a tape recording will help you share with them what has been discussed.

Chapter 2 on the patient-physician relationship gives more helpful details on this subject.

The Nurse and/or Medical Assistant Physicians choose office nurses and medical assistants carefully, making sure that their attitudes, philosophy and outlook complement the doctor's. The office nurse works with the physician and is responsible for direct delivery of medical care under the doctor's supervision. He or she serves as an important communication link between the patient/family unit and the doctor, and as a key resource in patient education, counseling and coordination of hospital or home care needs.

During your visit, the nurse will update medical records as needed and check your weight, blood pressure and pulse. He or she may also assist with certain types of physical exams. Preparing and administering chemotherapy and immunotherapy are the nurse's job in some offices, as well as reviewing medications, side effects and physician instructions.

Open lines of communication between you, your doctor and your nurse are vital in planning your care. Please feel free to voice your concerns, questions, fears and anxieties. Together your doctor and nurse will assess your individual needs for activity, comfort, diet instruction, elimination aids, equipment, pain relief, safety, skin care and so on. Individual and family needs vary depending on the stage of the disease, the goals of the treatment and the emotional state of the patient and the family.

If you ask, the office nurse will also refer you to community-based services and to rehabilitation and home health agencies for assistance with transportation, escort service, financial aid, social services and locating support groups.

Remember—the office is just a phone call away. If problems arise, the nurse and other office staff can help find solutions.

The Bookkeeper/Accountant Continued visits to a doctor's office, particularly if special tests and lab work are required, are often costly. When you first visit the office, speak to the bookkeeper/accountant about your insurance coverage, and ask any questions you may have about office policy. Many patients have little or no knowledge of what their insurance benefits cover. To help the bookkeeper/accountant with your insurance claims, do the following:

◆ If you have private insurance coverage, give the office the specific form provided by your company, after completing your side, and let the office know where the completed form should be sent.

◆ If you have Blue Shield or Blue Cross POS (point of service) coverage, give the office your card so that they may either make a photocopy of it or write down the necessary identification numbers and coverage. Find out whether your insurance company has a contract with your doctor; if so, you may expect to pay a co-payment amount.

◆ If you are on Medicare, discuss with the bookkeeper how the office handles Medicare claims. Some offices bill the Medicare carrier directly; others ask patients to submit their own bills. When completing a Medicare form, be sure to list, in addition to your name and address, your Medicare number and the nature of your illness in the proper place on the form. You do not need to describe your illness in medical terminology. Put in your own words why you had to see the doctor. If you don't know what to say, ask the nurse or receptionist to help you. Sign the form, attach a copy of the doctor's bill and mail it to the proper address given at the top of the Medicare form. When this information is listed correctly, it will hasten your reimbursement.

◆ If you have a financial problem or are running out of funds and would like some assistance, most cities have social service agencies that help patients who need financial aid. Most doctors' offices are also willing to make financial adjustments when circumstances make it necessary to do so. Contact the bookkeeper to discuss your particular situation.

◆ If you belong to an HMO or a managed-care insurance plan, know what your co-payment is and where your lab work, x-rays and other tests can be done. You usually need a referral from your primary doctor for each specialist visit. The primary doctor's secretary does the referral.

◆ Notify staff of any change in your insurance.

YOUR RESPONSIBILITIES

The Medical Care Plan No matter what illness you are confronted with, you must assume the responsibility of being a partner with your doctor. Your doctor and the nurse will explain why you are being given certain medications and what side effects you can expect, and will give you other instructions concerning diet, exercise, etc., that will hasten your recovery. If your memory is not sharp at that moment, ask your doctor to write everything down so that you won't forget.

Medications

◆ Know the name, dosage and directions of all your medications.

◆ Never stop taking any medication unless given specific orders by your doctor to do so.

◆ A responsible person should handle your medications if you cannot. The visiting nurse will be able to assist you as needed, under your doctor's direction.

◆ Count your pills. When your supply runs low, reorder in time, and on a weekday—not on a weekend.

◆ If you are taking a new medication, the doctor may want you to report to him or her the effects of the drug and whether it was successful before it is reordered.

When you reorder medications from your pharmacy, you should know the following:

1. The pharmacy's name and phone number.
2. The name of the medication, dosage, directions, amount and prescribing physician, all as listed on your cur-

rent bottle. Never expect to order by color! Accurate information will save time and energy. The prescription will state the number of renewals (refills) for your medication, and whether the drug is an over-the-counter item.

◆ The reason for reordering during the doctor's regular office hours is that the pharmacist must call your doctor's office for approval. The pharmacist must do this for every renewal, unless there are refills remaining on the original prescription.

◆ If your doctor cannot be reached for verification and you absolutely need your medication over a weekend, the pharmacist may give you enough to last until Monday, except in the case of drugs for which a special written or triplicate prescription is legally required (such as sleeping pills, narcotics and certain tranquilizers). If you keep proper track of your medications, you won't let them run out.

◆ If you have a language barrier, have a friend serve as your interpreter.

BEING PREPARED FOR EMERGENCIES

List emergency telephone numbers on a card and keep it near the phone. Here is a sample Emergency Phone Numbers Card.

EMERGENCY PHONE NUMBERS	
Police: Tel: ( )	
Fire Department: Tel: ( )	
Physician: Tel:( )	
Pharmacy: Tel: ( )	
Ambulance: Tel: ( )	
Nearest relative or friend: Name	
Relationship	Tel:( )

CONSULTING THE DOCTOR

Write down complex questions or problems before consulting the doctor. Have necessary information available when you call your doctor. For example:

◆ Constipation, diarrhea or bloody stools?
◆ Pulse: regular or irregular (skipping)?
◆ Heart: normal rate, racing beat, thumping?
◆ Nausea or vomiting?
◆ Numbness?
◆ Lightheadedness or dizziness?
◆ Fever? (Take your temperature—own a thermometer and know how to read it. The nurse will teach you, if you are not familiar with it.)
◆ Chills: How long did you shake? What time of day? How often?
◆ Any unusual swelling, redness or evidence of an abscess?
◆ Pain: Where? How long? What intensity? Does it move in different directions? What makes it worse? What seems to alleviate it?

DOCTOR "ON-CALL"

A patient may call the office when another doctor is covering for that patient's regular physician. Your chart is usually available to that doctor so that he or she can make the right decisions about your care. Occasionally the chart is not available because it is on loan to the hospital. To obtain the best help, always call during hours when your doctor's office is open. The office may provide you with a self-care card, which lists valuable information for you to relay in case your doctor is not available and another doctor is taking his or her calls.

SELF-CARE CARD
Name:
Diagnosis:
Treatment:
Drugs:
Allergies:
Name and Telephone Number of Oncologist:
Advance Directives:

28

SOCIAL SERVICES IN THE HOSPITAL, HOME AND OFFICE

Irene Harrison, LCSW, Lee L. Pollak, LCSW, Isadora R. Rosenbaum, MA,
Ernest H. Rosenbaum, MD

───────────◇───────────

This chapter describes the special hospital social services available to cancer patients to supplement medical care and rehabilitation services. Cancer brings with it many practical and emotional problems in addition to medical ones: problems of financial assessment (who will pay or help with hospital or home bills?); transportation (who will bring the patient to the doctor's office or hospital for therapy?); home help (who will plan and carry out medical care and make the practical arrangements?); and emotional crises. The support and guidance of social services can be critical, for finding feasible solutions to acute problems and as a pathway to maximum rehabilitation. (*See also* Chapter 26, "In-Hospital Routines and Health Care Support Teams," and Chapter 27, "In-Home Services and Support Programs.")

THE MEDICAL SOCIAL WORKER

Many hospitals have a Social Services Department with medical social workers available to all patients.

You may never before have needed the services of a social worker. You may even feel that you don't need anyone else to talk with. But cancer brings extraordinary challenges for you and for your family. You will need to marshal all of your emotional energy so that you can participate most effectively in your treatment and rehabilitation. That's why the medical social worker is there: he or she has known many patients who have faced these same emotional and practical problems, and understands what you and your family are going through.

It is the social worker who can best assist with the nonmedical aspects of patient care and support, as well as locating community services to help with home care. Community service agencies can provide professional social services in conjunction with medical teams, adapting services to each patient's situation. They can help solve such typical problems as who will pay or help with mounting bills, work or other activities; how the patient will get to and from medical appointments and treatments; how the practical needs of at-home care will be managed (what might be needed and who will arrange for it); how unexpected crises will be handled; and how the patient and family will handle the intense emotional issues that often arise from a diagnosis of chronic or end-stage disease.

Traditionally, oncology social workers have been found in medical settings, and were available through the hospital social service departments. Today, as medical and inpatient health care are experiencing changes, some services formerly provided within hospital social service departments are being provided by hospital discharge nurses, discharge planners and case managers, and, outside the hospital, by community social service agencies.

Though this may be your first involvement with cancer, the social worker will have worked with many patients and families facing the problems you are now addressing, and will understand what you are all going through. Since you need to marshal your own individual strength to face the challenges ahead, the social worker can provide pertinent information, support and services.

Learning to compensate for and live with disabilities is one of the compromises you must make when you have a chronic illness. The medical social worker can help you adjust while being sensitive to your emotional needs, family obligations and decisions about future goals.

SPECIFIC SUPPORT SERVICES THE SOCIAL WORKER CAN PROVIDE

Initial Diagnosis When they first receive a diagnosis of cancer, many people feel overwhelmed. This may be a time in which you feel least able to reach out for help. Information is coming in too fast to be assimilated. You want to understand your illness, prognosis and treatment choices, yet you don't want to deal with them. During this period, you need to allow yourself time to deal with your illness, your reactions and your understanding at your own pace. Your social worker can be your sounding board and can also help you resolve many practical concerns and determine priorities.

Here are some common practical problems:
◆ What is this going to cost me?
◆ How can I support myself or my family while I am being treated?
◆ How will I manage at home after I leave the hospital?
◆ How can I get back and forth for treatment when I am feeling so weak?
◆ I live out of town, but need to come in to the hospital daily for the next several weeks for treatment; where can I stay?
◆ What do I do about my work?

All of these concerns are real, and the social worker can help with information about insurance coverage; private and government medical and financial benefit programs; and community home health agency, rehabilitation and cancer service programs.

Many cancer patients have difficulty talking about their cancer. Your social worker can help you find ways of talking about it that will put you and others more at ease. Being able to talk with your family about your fears and concerns can result in greater understanding and intimacy and will help you and them to feel less alone. Your friends also need you to be able to talk to them honestly and openly; when they don't know what to say, they may stay away.

The goal for you, with the assistance of your social worker, should be to maintain open communication with all the people on your medical team, as well as with people in your personal and professional life. This will help you feel respected and supported, and will also let you offer respect and support to the people who care about you—who, like you, are undergoing intense responses to your cancer diagnosis.

Social workers on cancer teams have found that one of their most important tasks is to help you deal with some of the myths and misconceptions we all have about cancer, and to help you get past the shock or "not hearing" stage. You may have had some contact with cancer before, either directly in your family or through friends or the media. There is an urge to swap information and compare medical experiences and treatments with others who have cancer, but doing so can result in confusion. There are many different types and stages of cancer: it is not just one disease, but can take many forms. You need all the information you can get about your specific illness.

Cancer does not inevitably lead to death, it is not contagious and it is not a punishment for previous sins. These may seem like strange ideas, but they come up repeatedly among the feelings of people who are beginning to deal with their cancer diagnosis. And all of us have heard about "alternative" cancer treatments, some of which are pure quackery. Discuss any questions you have about these matters with the hospital medical social worker.

Surgery Some treatment options, including surgery, may require hospitalization and outpatient care.

The period while you are waiting for surgery is often one of heightened anxiety. Common concerns include fears about anesthesia, survival, loss of control, pain, mutilation and general effect on lifestyle. These fears are often not discussed with anyone. You will find it helpful to talk to a social worker before surgery to prepare yourself for the operation and its consequences. Talking about your anxieties will help you cope with the actual event. Your social worker can also help you if you need to make practical arrangements before your surgery.

The postsurgical period requires many adaptations, which are often accompanied by mood swings. You may need to mourn something lost or changed. How you react to your surgery will depend on the meaning it has for you. Talking about it can help you understand its unique meaning for you and how you can deal with it.

Postsurgical changes in self-image and fears of rejection may lead to an unnecessarily restricted life. Supportive services can help you adjust; in particular, involvement in programs with other cancer patients will make it easier for you to live a better life with your cancer.

Radiation Therapy The beginning of radiation therapy is another crisis point. Once more, the fear of the unknown has to be confronted. It is frightening to go into the subterranean quarters where most radiation therapy departments are located. Common fears and feelings are:

◆ Will the radiation cause cancer?
◆ Will I be radioactive (overexposed or contaminated)?
◆ I feel alienated and abandoned.
◆ What if the radiation machine fails?
◆ Has the technician forgotten me?
◆ I'm worried about side effects: nausea, vomiting, hair loss, appetite loss.
◆ Will I be able to have children?

As a cancer patient, you have to absorb a great deal of new information. You may misinterpret or distort information that you are not able to assimilate emotionally. To plan realistically for your own care, you need to ask questions repeatedly and learn what you need to know about radiation therapy and about its anticipated side effects, duration and outcome. Hospitals and radiation therapy centers frequently offer group counseling that can help patients share their concerns and cope emotionally with treatment.

Chemotherapy If you are receiving chemotherapy, it is difficult for you to get your mind off your cancer; your life must now accommodate a treatment schedule, and you may often have to deal with uncomfortable side effects, such as hair loss, weight loss and nausea. Feelings of frustration and anger need an outlet. Group therapy programs have proven supportive in helping people participate in their chemotherapy programs; the social worker can advise you about the possibilities.

Recurrences If your cancer recurs, you will be disappointed—and perhaps feel desperate and/or hopeless. You may frantically search for miracles. During this period, you may need special help to mobilize your efforts to participate in further treatment. You may be angry, depressed, weepy or demanding. Individual or group counseling sessions with your social worker can give you a safe and acceptable place to express those feelings.

Remission It is logical to feel joyful when you are in remission. However, many patients find their joy is held in check by the persistent fear that the disease will recur and become uncontrollable. It is common to experience a letdown as it becomes necessary to invest your energy somewhere else besides just dealing with your disease.

Family Support and Counseling

The medical social worker can help your family understand the ramifications of your disease and treatment. Family members often experience crises relating to the changes and concerns brought about by a loved one's illness. Because they are healthy, they may find it particularly difficult to think of their own needs and may need to be encouraged to find an outlet for their feelings.

Common feelings experienced by family members are:
◆ What have I done to make my loved one get cancer?
◆ Why me?
◆ What can I do to make him well? (He doesn't like anything I cook for him.)
◆ I have to devote myself to her needs, and my needs are not important.
◆ I feel so alone, because he doesn't really tell me how he feels.
◆ I am scared that she may die, and I don't know how I will manage without her.
◆ I am worried about expenses.
◆ I am ashamed to take city or state aid (a "handout").
◆ I am ashamed because I feel so angry at her.

All of these feelings are perfectly normal, but they often go unexpressed, either because the relative fears making the person with cancer more ill or because the relative feels ashamed of having such thoughts or concerns.

Your family members need to know that they too are active participants in your treatment program. But they may need help recognizing their own needs as they cope with the changes in family life brought about by your illness. Many hospitals and community agencies have family groups or individual counseling services available to assist family members.

Job-Related Assistance Often patients find it easier if a third party informs their employer that they will not be able to return to work as early as planned or will be unable to return to work for an extended period of time. The medical social worker can help you explain to your employer your present health status and prognosis. If a formal letter is required, that too can be arranged. If you can no longer work at your previous occupation, the medical social worker may also help you learn about vocational transition resources.

Discharge Planning One of the roles of the medical social worker is to help the patient and family with discharge planning. The medical social worker acts as the coordinator of collaborative future health planning, as outlined by the attending physician and other members of the health care team. It is the function of the medical social worker to see that the transition from hospital to other community care facilities is smooth. He or she can arrange for home care, special equipment, meal services, friendly visitors and so on.

Financial Aid You may be unfamiliar with your medical insurance or HMO or PPO managed-care coverage and with the various financial support systems that are available. The social worker is trained to evaluate, investigate and advise you about insurance and financial aid programs.

Transportation Many patients need specialized transportation to the doctor's office, to special therapy centers and to rehabilitation facilities. The medical social worker can provide information or arrange service through the many volunteer organizations in your community.

In certain instances, you may have to travel out of the city or state for consultation or treatment. The medical social worker can arrange for transportation and housing as well as hospitalization.

Support through Crisis Periods Everyone responds differently to cancer. The impact varies with age, sex, personal history and the severity of the illness. But you can expect to encounter at least some changes in how you experience your life; at such times, the social worker can be immensely supportive to you.

The changes aren't necessarily obvious; in fact, they are more likely to involve subtle shifts in your self-image, priorities and attitudes. In some instances, you may experience major disruptions in your lifestyle. These will differ depending on the effect of your illness. Such changes need not be sad, for they can offer new opportunities for you to make changes in your life and to make active choices about how you want to live.

Ironically, it is the points of intense crisis that may offer the greatest opportunities for personal growth and positive changes in your family relationships. During such crossroads periods, cancer patients are often able to make considerable progress in taking control of their situations and in finding new ways to communicate with their loved ones. By acting together in unison, many find tremendous support and connection with important people in their lives. Other cancer patients have identified these same stress periods as times when they felt most insecure and alone and wished they had had professional help for themselves and their families.

Cancer can have its stages of medical necessity, periods of hospitalization and serious outpatient issues. It can also have many long periods of stability. Acute crisis periods force people to face situations as they arise. Dealing with cancer as a chronic illness requires other skills, such as insight, patience and attention to ongoing emotional and practical needs.

Social services can significantly help you to cope with—even grow from—such crossroads and crisis points.

In addition to the social support services and other support services provided by your local hospitals and community agencies, you can obtain information, counseling and practical services from a host of national, regional and local institutions. Your social worker will be your best single resource for information about what is available in your community. The Resources at the end of this book contain the names of some of the organizations that are best known for providing the essential services described in this chapter.

29
HOSPICE CARE

Irene Harrison, LCSW

———◇———

Hospice is derived from the Latin word *hospitium*, "hospitality," an inn for travelers, especially one kept by a religious order. The hospice movement was started by Dr. Cicely Saunders in England in the 1940s, when St. Christopher's Hospice was opened to provide a quiet place where people could die in peace and dignity. It was staffed by nuns who had a sense of commitment to service.

Hospice care was introduced in the United States in 1974 at Yale in New Haven, Connecticut. Since then, the movement has expanded rapidly, with programs based on several organizational models: all-volunteer, hospital-based, integrated with home health agencies or freestanding community hospices. Though diverse, these programs share a philosophy.

PHILOSOPHY

Despite all the advances in diagnosis and treatment, a cure is not always possible. Continued treatment, even if available, may compromise a patient's quality of life. After discussion with the physician and consideration of treatment options and the potential outcomes, it may be appropriate to consider palliative (comfort) care. Some patients and families are frightened by the word hospice, believing that all treatment will be discontinued and the patient is being sent home to die. But many kinds of treatment may be continued to provide comfort and relief of pain.

The hospice philosophy embraces a holistic approach that encompasses physical, emotional and spiritual concerns. The patient and family are seen as the unit of care. Care has to be individualized to meet the patient's and the family's needs, as well as being responsive to differences in lifestyles. The hospice philosophy
- affirms life
- promotes self-determination, as patients and families participate in their plan of care
- provides education to help patients and families provide appropriate care
- promotes understanding and accepting that the journey of life eventually leads to death, and encourages people to view this experience as an opportunity for growth
- emphasizes palliation, which includes physical, psychological and spiritual comfort delivered by a multidisciplinary staff.

WHY CHOOSE A HOSPICE?

When medical treatments have been exhausted or the burden of treatment outweighs the benefits, it may be time to consider hospice care. Most people would like to end their lives surrounded by family and friends. By bringing services into the home, hospices help patients and families provide the necessary care. Patients and families are able to retain a greater sense of control at home than in the hospital. Hospices will also provide services in convalescent homes to ensure pain and symptom management and to provide support to families. The hospice experience can foster spiritual and personal growth as the hospice team empowers patients and families to manage difficult situations.

MEMBERS OF THE HOSPICE TEAM

Medical Director The director is a physician who is committed to the philosophy and goals of hospice care for the terminally ill. She or he attends team meetings and provides consultation to the staff, helps educate other physicians about hospice care and encourage them to make appropriate referrals, and may consult with primary physicians to assist them with pain management.

Nurses Hospice nurses are highly skilled in effective pain management, which is a primary concern to patients and families. Family members are included in education about pain management, since they are the ones providing the daily care at home. Seeing a person in his or her own home is quite different from an office visit. Hospice nurses can thus obtain additional information that lets them collaborate more effectively with the physician.

Medical Social Worker Medical social workers are trained to understand the emotional and social needs of patients and families and how best to help them in this end-of-life stage. They facilitate communication between family members, provide advocacy and teach problem-solving skills. Social workers are aware of cultural diversity and of the belief systems that affect how people respond to hospice services. Social workers link clients to community resources.

Home Health Aides Home health aides are very important members of the team. They provide hands-on care and perform intimate tasks like bathing and grooming. Patients and families may feel more at ease with home health aides than with other personnel and may share their life stories with them. Nurses supervise the home health aides.

Chaplain Since one of the goals of hos-

pice care is to acknowledge a person's spiritual needs, some hospices have a chaplain on their team. Spirituality goes far beyond identifying religious affiliation and where someone worships. It involves the exploration of fears, values and beliefs, especially those relating to what awaits us after death. At this time, many people experience a strong need to review their life and to seek meaning and purpose. Ethnic and religious differences need to be appreciated. Rituals can be helpful in coping with the unknown. Patients may hope for reunification with God or family members, an idea that provides comfort and reduces fear. Even patients who are not affiliated with any specific denomination often wish to get in touch with their spirituality or their existential search for meaning. Life reviews are helpful, and reconciliations help patients "let go" of life. If the team does not have a chaplain, other team members address these issues and also refer the patient to community clerical support.

Volunteers Volunteers are the backbone of many hospice programs. They are trained before they see patients, and supervision continues after their formal training ends. These individuals give willingly of themselves to enhance the quality of life for hospice patients and their families. They may, for example, assist with transportation or stay with patients to give caregivers a break. Sometimes they visit patients in the hospital or nursing home, helping to reduce feelings of loneliness or abandonment. Some volunteers specialize in supporting the bereaved. They make follow-up telephone calls and, if they note any problems, they arrange for a team member to assess the situation. Volunteers are great people with a real commitment to service. They are essential to the success of the hospice program.

Nutritionist A patient's eating habits are

of great concern to the family. Often a patient's appetite and tastes change, and family members may be at their wits' end to find something to prepare. Weight loss affects body image and worries families. The nutritionist can help with information and suggestions that might help to improve appetite. The nutritionist works closely with families and is sensitive to ethnic preferences. Education helps patients and families adjust their usual eating habits. Medications also may affect appetite. Families get particularly upset when their loved ones are no longer able to take food or fluid by mouth, worrying that the patient will die of starvation. Some request tube feedings or intravenous hydration. It is crucial to have a calm discussion with the patient and family to determine the stage of illness and to weigh the advantages and disadvantages of these procedures. Each case needs to be examined individually, keeping in mind that comfort is the goal of hospice care.

Pharmacist Pain control, one of the primary goals of hospice care, is also the patient's main worry. Pharmacists contribute their knowledge of drug potencies and of interactions among drugs to attain maximum pain control and symptom relief.

Physical Therapist Physical therapists help patients maximize their ability to move around and to get in and out of bed, chairs and transportation. The therapist teaches families techniques that will prevent them from injuring themselves while assisting the patient. The therapist will also recommend some exercise to encourage the patient's independence.

Occupational Therapist Occupational therapists help improve the patient's ability to perform the activities of daily living, teaching people how to conserve energy and how to adapt the living environment.

Speech/Language Pathology Services
Speech therapists consult with team members in cases where the patient's ability to speak has been compromised. They help to develop alternative communication systems.

Psychologist Psychologists consult on difficult cases. Depression and pre-existing psychological problems may affect how people cope. Psychologists make recommendations for improving the management of care for patients and families.

HOW ARE HOSPICES FINANCED?
Some hospices are supported by the community with their own fundraising and donations; other programs have a large volunteer component. Hospices may be incorporated with home health agencies or hospitals, or they may receive funds from foundations and grants. Private health insurance and Medicaid are some other forms of reimbursement. In 1982, Medicare began reimbursing certified Medicare hospices, which must adhere to specific guidelines. Part A of Medicare covers most of the costs.

Medicare Hospice Benefit
◆ To qualify for the hospice benefit, patients must be eligible for Medicare.
◆ A physician must certify that the patient has a prognosis of less than six months.
◆ Patients who elect the hospice benefit must waive their rights to traditional benefits.
◆ Patients are entitled to two 90-day periods plus periods of 60-day extensions, which can be extended if the physician certifies the need for further care.
◆ Patients and families receive services from the core hospice staff according to an interdisciplinary team plan.
◆ Patients and families have access to a 24-hour advice line that is answered by a

nurse, who prioritizes problems and arranges for appropriate care.

◆ Equipment for home use is rented, and supplies are furnished.

◆ Medication for symptom management and pain relief is covered.

BEREAVEMENT SERVICES

Hospices are required to provide bereavement services. Some hospices have very comprehensive programs, with staff assigned solely to provide bereavement services; others use their core staff and specially trained bereavement volunteers. Services typically include:

◆ attending funeral services

◆ making home visits

◆ telephoning at regular intervals

◆ contacting the bereaved on birthdays, anniversaries and holidays, which tend to be especially sad times

◆ providing nonthreatening educational programs that offer practical information

◆ hosting social events, often combined with an informative speaker or fundraising component

◆ facilitating bereavement support groups. Such groups are most commonly facilitated by a professional. Bereaved children may need additional intervention. Hospice staff members help teach families how to deal with a child's grief.

Children's groups, such as Good Grief, are a great resource. Referrals to child specialists can be made.

EUTHANASIA OR PHYSICIAN-ASSISTED SUICIDE

To hasten a person's death by active euthanasia is inconsistent with the hospice philosophy of providing quality care at the end of life; but attaining effective pain control may in some cases hasten death. The hospice will focus on helping patients differentiate between giving up and accepting death as a natural progression in life.

MAKING END-OF-LIFE DECISIONS

With the current emphasis on patients' rights, self-determination and informed consent, people are encouraged to make decisions before they become terminally ill. Advance directives are documents that allow individuals to specify their wishes. A person must be mentally competent to complete an advance directive. Chapter 34, "Decisions for Life," provides details on living wills, durable power of attorney for health care and do not resuscitate (DNR) forms.

30
DEALING WITH DEATH IF CANCER BECOMES TERMINAL

Ernest H. Rosenbaum, MD, and Isadora R. Rosenbaum, MA

———◇———

Death is a part of life. We all must die sometime—we don't know when. Yet we persist in thinking of death as something that happens to other people. We do not accept our mortality until a crisis forces us to contemplate nonbeing. Even then, we may fight, bargain and connive to gain more time, but life is elusive as well as precious. It may be snuffed out at a moment's notice or drain away slowly with disease or old age. And although physicians fight to preserve life at almost any cost in time, money or effort, we also know that a day will come when the time is right to let a person die.

In partnership with the physician, cancer patients face many difficult issues. Throughout treatment they share in medical decisions and, if the cancer becomes progressively worse, they will at some point discuss with their physician matters concerning their dying. For example, people often ask that no extraordinary measures be taken to keep them alive when there is no longer any hope of being restored to a good quality of life. Other decisions involve a choice of where to die—home, hospital, nursing home or hospice. Funeral arrangements are also often discussed between patient and physician.

We are all concerned with maintaining dignity in life as well as in dying, and we share certain standards as to what constitutes an acceptable level of dignity. The cancer patient may gradually feel that level recede as he or she experiences diminishing control over personal destiny. A loss of privacy and of the ability to influence one's present or future may become more of a concern than dying. Sometimes people begin to question whether life is worth living under the circumstances, and whether euthanasia might be the best solution. Implementing such a request is neither ethical nor legal, but under the current official guidelines of medical practice, maximum comfort with a minimum of suffering can be promised. A physician can also promise not to interfere with a natural death by keeping a patient alive with special life-sustaining equipment. A patient has a right to die and to direct the physician to see that this wish is honored. (*See* Chapter 34, "Decisions for Life.")

As described in Chapter 29, several forms of hospice units have emerged, helping to ease some of the problems associated with both home and hospital care. In some communities, a hospice unit is a segregated ward in the hospital with an associated staff of physicians, bedside nurses, home-coordinating nurses and social workers managing inpatient care and supporting at-home care by interacting with other community resources. Most units in the United States have developed as out-of-hospital home care agencies, coordinating inpatient services through a loose affiliation with neighboring hospitals.

In some settings, where a separate hospice unit has not been created, a group of hospital-based personnel that includes a physician, a nurse, a social worker and a chaplain is available for consultation and support to patients throughout the institution.

A few freestanding hospices have also been constructed. These low-technology inpatient facilities admit only terminal patients and are often associated with a home care program.

The hospice movement is beginning to fill a void in the medical and psychological care of the terminally ill. But the hospice team should not replace the concerned physician. Patients and families need continuity of care, and physicians should not relinquish their involvement when a patient is admitted to a hospice service. They should remain as physician-of-record, working with the terminal care staff.

COMMUNICATING YOUR WISHES TO YOUR PHYSICIAN

A person can sign a directive to the physician and choose the place where he or she will die. The only thing one cannot dictate is when one will die.

Most people know when they are dying and are sensitive to the suffering of those around them. Yet sometimes when they express a desire for peace, they are made to feel guilty by relatives who prefer to keep them alive under any conditions. To prevent such conflicts, many patients agree in advance with their physician to sign a document, called a living will, that states their request not to be kept alive by artificial means or heroic measures when there is no reasonable expectation of recovery. Living wills can also stipulate other conditions under which the patient wishes either to be freed from life support or to remain on life support.

For some patients, there is a preterminal phase before descending into a coma. At this time, a patient is still alert enough to take comfort in talking with his or her family or with the medical staff. During this phase, anything or anyone especially dear to the patient should be made available. He or she may want to spend time with a particular relative, friend, child or pet.

But we must remember that physicians aren't capable of predicting when a person is going to die. We have only clinical judgment as to the time remaining for any patient. Moreover, no health care professional can prejudge the value of extra days or hours. Some time ago, a patient of mine [Dr. Rosenbaum's] was dying, with marked jaundice, of a massive malignancy that was obstructing his liver. Not wanting him to suffer any longer, I left a spoken order with the interns and the resident that when he died, no efforts at resuscitation should be made. About half an hour later, the patient had a cardiac arrest. Neither the resident nor the interns were in the room, and the nursing staff had changed for the morning shift; the nurse naturally sent for the cardiac resuscitative unit, and the patient was revived. He lived another 48 hours, and during that time several relatives arrived from the Midwest and were able to visit with him. In addition, a brother, from whom he had been estranged for 20 years, flew to San Francisco, and they were reunited. He also had warm, emotionally satisfying talks with his wife and children about their life together.

Such communication is invaluable. It is natural for a dying person to experience a heightened sensitivity to the meaning of life and to want to convey special messages to those close to him or her. But these thoughts are not always expressed, either because of awkwardness at expressing deep feelings or because of a reluctance to talk about death. So survivors are often left without a final message.

PATIENT-FAMILY GOOD-BYES

Saying good-bye before death can be a comfort to everyone concerned—family, friends and patient. We have often participated in such a farewell to life by encouraging patients and key family members to make a tape recording together while the patient is still alert. The recording may include a family history or anecdotes, or it may lead to a philosophical conversation on life and death. A physician or nurse can often be instrumental in helping people to break their silence by initiating similar conversations.

People who find it difficult to speak of their feelings sometimes write a letter expressing their thoughts and love. Such a letter often contains hopes for the future happiness of their loved ones, in effect giving them permission to seek joy and fulfillment in the next phase of their lives.

For example, we recently received a copy of a letter sent by a young woman to her husband several months before she died. She wrote of their life together, her happiness with him and her sadness that it would end soon. She also told him that he would need to return to active living and that he should marry again when he met the right person.

It doesn't matter how eloquently or awkwardly such thoughts are expressed. This conscious, deliberate communication can relieve the stress of silence between two people and bring them closer together. Remorse and guilt may be assuaged in both people. The person who is dying may gain peace of mind, while the survivor experiences a bond that can be a solace during mourning.

Death is never easy to accept, no matter what the cause. Family members need special attention throughout the ordeal, but especially in those final days. Help may come from within the family or from friends; but physicians, nurses, clergy, social workers and hospital volunteers are also available and ready to listen. We always hope that families will find solace in the knowledge that their loved one received good medical care and sensitive emotional support, that he or she lived as long and as well as possible under adverse conditions, and that all possible comfort was provided to ease the process of dying.

31
GRIEF AND RECOVERY

Ernest H. Rosenbaum, MD, Isadora R. Rosenbaum, MA, and Sabrina Selim, BA

The value of life depends on the impact on others.

—*Jackie Robinson*

Grief is a normal, necessary psychological process that helps a person adapt to the loss of a loved one. The survivor is depressed and often withdraws from former interests, activities and even friends. Grief is a very personal experience; even among members of a family who lose the same person, the experience of the loss will be different for each person. The closer the relationship to the deceased, the greater the loss.

For an adult, the psychological work of grief is connected with remembering and reliving the experiences shared with the person who has died. Grief is not a consciously determined task; rather, it is set in motion automatically and proceeds at the rate that is bearable for the individual. Grieving is painful because, as we remember good times as well as bad, the very process of remembering requires a continuing recognition that the person we loved is no longer present.

The outward signs of grief are similar to those of depression and generally include intense mental anguish, remorse and sorrow. But these are mere words, and cannot describe the emotional pain and shock experienced by a person who mourns. He or she has lost love, goals, friendship or security, none of which are immediately replaceable.

The depth of grief is unpredictable because it depends on so many factors, including the availability of support from family, children and friends; one's culture or religion, and the degree of preparation for the event. Although there is no universal approach to the grieving process, many people follow specified religious procedures. Each of the major religions observes a degree of ritual, quite similar in format, when dealing with death.

As health care providers we deal with these problems frequently, and try to prepare a patient's family and friends for an anticipated death. We do this by providing medical information and by holding family conferences on the patient's progress. Yet no matter how thoroughly we prepare them, families still experience shock and momentary disbelief when the death occurs. In addition, questions will be asked and decisions required of them. "Will there be a postmortem?" "What funeral arrangements must be made?" The doctor can be helpful at such a time, because those who were close to the patient are typically not thinking or remembering clearly. If the disease was chronic, funeral arrangements may have already been completed, or at least initiated, by the family.

When the funeral is over, the family, as well as members of the medical team who have been involved with the patient, need time for their sorrow to abate. At this time, we usually write the family a letter expressing both sympathy and hope for the future. A review of the patient's medical problem and the therapy is provided, along with pertinent autopsy information if required. These steps help to clear up any questions or misunderstandings among family members about what actually occurred, especially during the final days, when their comprehension may have been clouded by concern for the patient. We have found this approach very helpful for the grieving process.

During the first few weeks, phone calls, visitors and cards of sympathy distract the attention of the grief-stricken. Often there is a denial of mourning, an attempt to hold back tears and suppress grief. Crying is believed by some people to be a sign of weakness, but it is merely a means of releasing pent-up emotions.

When the attention diminishes and one is left alone with the uncertainty of the future, the feelings of fear and loneliness arise and are natural. However sometimes grief occurs simultaneously with unremitting depression, in which the survivor becomes obsessed with loss. When this happens, feelings of j330

persistent loneliness, helplessness, guilt, shame and anger may lead to a regressed state, and professional help may be required. Grief may seem endless and recovery may seem impossible, but grief must be allowed to run its course.

ONE FAMILY'S STORY

We invited Mary, whose husband had died one year previously, to our monthly conference with the patient service volunteers at Mount Zion Hospital. The topic was grief and recovery. After opening the meeting with remarks on the mechanisms of grief and adaptation to loss, we asked Mary to describe her experiences since Howard's death.

Mary: It's hard to know where to start. During this last year, I have had wildly fluctuating moods and attitudes and have been better or less able to handle what my life is now compared to what it was before. Howard and I were married almost 10 years and had a blessed and easy life. Neither of us, by personality, lived in the future, and so our life together didn't end with many regrets about things we hadn't done or were waiting to do. So I would keep thinking about all the good things that had happened, but each time I did this—and it is still true today—I would have to face the fact that Howard is gone and will not be back. Our children, Noah and Semantha, are now four and six; and the fact that they won't have the influence of this most remarkable man is still, and will probably always be, hard for me to accept.

I feel guilty because I complain. What we had in a relatively short time was probably a whole lot better than many people experience all their lives. It seems ungrateful to complain, but I do. I had thought I would go through a maturing process in my grief and reach a point where I would face the fact of Howard's death and accept it graciously. It is just in the course of the last week, while talking to a friend, that I realize I'm not ever going to accept it. Never, never, never!

The last year has not been a completely sad year for me. I don't feel that my life ended with Howard's death or that good things won't happen, because they have, and I expected they would. Of course, there were the circumstances at the end of his life. All that he was going through, his suffering, was finished, and that was a relief. But, you know, I may live to be 120 years old and have some wild life beyond anything I could imagine in the future—I think that's perfectly possible—but I will never—no matter what happens in the future—be able to accept graciously that Howard died when he did, and the way he did.

In the course of the last year, I have been through different phases of grief. The phases seem to be repetitive and very short. At times, I can be overcome and almost nonfunctional with grief, sad thoughts, resentment and anger. I wonder what I would be like if I didn't have the children to spur me to action and decisions and all the other things.

I might otherwise have apathy or become one of those people who sit in the corner and put the drapes over their head, and everyone would have to work to get me to move. The children saved me from that. They've also had a year of grieving and also have a lot of pleasant memories of Howard. Noah has always been able, without any concerted effort, to talk about Howard or refer to him, because Howard was a big person in our lives and is just naturally a part of our conversations, or record or reference.

Noah will say, "Was that a car like Howard's?" or "Remember when Daddy took us here?" or "That's Howard's book." For me, this has been helpful.

ER: The effect of a parental loss on children is deep. A few months ago, when I said good-bye to Noah after a visit, he replied accusingly, "Ernie, you're not going to come back, just like my daddy."

Mary: One thing I wonder about is my decision that the children should not see Howard after he died. They saw him the morning he died, and he was able to recognize them and talk to them and joke a little. Then they went out of the room, and an hour later Howard died.

I did not have them come back and see Howard, and that is out of my childhood. I went to wakes with open caskets and remember thinking, "That's not what Grandma looked like," and for me that image remained.

I felt this particularly for Noah and Semantha. I did not want that image of Howard to be their most vivid memory of him, and I was concerned that it would be. They had known him such a short time and wouldn't have a store of images to draw on.

They have had a lot of questions since then, and I don't know but what maybe they would have felt better if they had seen him. But I made the decision for them. I still think it was right, but there is one step they can't quite put together. The last time they saw Howard he was alive: and the next time, after I told them he had died, there was the funeral and his body was in a casket.

They have asked me the same questions many times since then. "Was Daddy's whole body in the box? Was he wearing clothes?"

Noah became very angry immediately after Howard's death. He had always been a friendly type, but then he was positively furious. His anger manifested itself with physical displays—throwing things and so forth.

Semantha knew Howard better. She reacted in a more "adult" way. She would be overcome with sobbing and want to talk, but was unable to talk because she just could not get the words out. As the months went by, she became more able to say the words that Howard was dead and that she would never be able to touch him again.

Noah would, on occasion, say things like, "I wish I were dead, because if I were dead then I could see Daddy. Then I would be with Howard." I still don't think the children have accepted it either.

I had a lot of preparation before Howard died, because we knew it was going to happen, and both of us talked about things and did some reading. What I'm trying to say is, I was better able to handle it because of the preparation.

Grieving is a selfish experience but, I guess, a necessary one. Grief is more intense the closer you are to the person who has died. You may have various parts of that relationship filled by other people, so that instead of one person or one source, there are many sources. In that case, the sum of the parts still doesn't equal the whole. Nevertheless, I've had a lot of support, and for that I am very grateful.

The people who have helped me most through the grieving period are those who knew Howard, his complexities and his interests, because they know what he was really like. The support that comes from someone who knew the person—the talk, the conversation, the reminiscing or what-ever—is most helpful. In the grieving thing, it is sort of hard for me to hold myself together. It has been hard some of the time. Right now, I don't think I have a lot left to give to someone else who is grieving.

ER: We all grieve after personal tragedies and losses. We progress from shock to recovery and, with time, move toward a new life. Anger and disbelief subside. Throughout the period of mourn-ing, the concern and support of friends help the bereaved, until a time comes when grief lessens.

A GRANDSON REMEMBERS

Another person wrote the following about the death of his grandfather.

One of the many things that I learned from my grandfather while he was alive was something he taught me in his death from myasthenia gravis.

I had been pretty much living in the intensive care unit with Grandfather for about three weeks. During that time, I spent as much time with him as I could, usually sleeping in a chair in the ICU with him. Throughout the time that he was in the hospital, he had a tube sticking down his throat that made it impossible for him to talk. He was too weak to write, so he couldn't communicate at all. He was also very confused and disoriented. Whenever he was conscious, I would ask him if he knew where he was and why, and he would always shake his head no. I would then explain everything to him as best I could and sit there holding his hand until he went back to sleep. Each time he woke up, the same thing would happen.

All I wanted to be able to do for him was to help him prepare for his death, which (to me) was obviously close at hand. He was frightened, confused and

in a fair amount of physical discomfort. And there was not a damn thing that I could do about it.

After the drugs and treatments had wound their way down and the doctors decided that there was really nothing fur-ther that they could do for him, it was time to allow him to die.

So they took away the medication, and they took him off the breathing machine. I was with him when he began to be aware that it was difficult for him to breathe. He looked into my eyes and mouthed, "Help me, please."

For the entire time that I'd been there, he had been really disoriented because of all the drugs. I'd wanted to talk to him, to help him consciously prepare for his death, but he hadn't been there enough to even start. But this morning there he was, looking right out at me through his eyes and asking me to help him. I started to cry. I held his hand, I looked into his eyes and I told him, "There's nothing else we can do, Grampa. The doctors have tried everything they can, and your lungs just aren't working right."

I sobbed and had difficulty speaking. But for some reason, I suddenly had no difficulty at all in reading his lips. He mouthed, "Does this mean that I am going to die?" He looked right into my eyes. I looked back into his. "Yes, Grampa, you are."

"When is this going to happen?"

"I don't know, Grampa; it could be a few hours, or it could be a few days."

He nodded his head and closed his eyes. He understood. It's a pretty simple matter when you get to the point. There aren't really a whole lot of questions or much to be said.

He squeezed my hand and mouthed, "I want to go outside."

I repeated it back to him in the form of a question: "You want to go outside, Grampa?"

He nodded and mouthed, "Please."

I went to ask the nurse how I could take

him outside, but she said I couldn't. There was no way to take him out in his bed, and there was no way to take him out of his bed without him dying right then and there. And it was snowing and raining and very cold outside, on top of everything else.

I felt trapped. My grandfather made his dying request—something so simple. He just wanted to go outside. But we were stuck in a context of death so complete, a place that kills you so fully that it doesn't even let you die the way you want to.

The rest of the family arrived. He was still fairly alert. Everybody exchanged a lot of love: holding his hand, telling him that everything is okay, that he doesn't have to worry, that he can just rest peacefully. My grandmother asked me why they don't just give him something to knock him out. I explain that I asked them not to unless it seemed like he was really suffering. I asked my grandfather several times during the early part of the day whether he was suffering, whether he wanted some medication to knock him out. He kept shaking his head no.

The day went on. His breathing got shallower. His extremities got colder. His skin got paler. I'd been awake for 30 hours or so, hardly having left his room at all in that time. The family left for the night. It was sort of a shock to me, but at the same time, not too surprising. They all told me that I should call them if anything "happens," but it was clear to me that they didn't want to have to watch him die. It was probably better that way anyway. I was prepared for this. I spoke to him, telling him that I love him, and he squeezed my hand a little bit.

His breathing got shallower and faster. He was breathing 40 breaths a minute, but he couldn't keep that up for long. It slowed down. His oxygen saturation began to drop, and so did his heart rate. The breaths were very shallow then and very slow, but still regular. I held his hand and his head, telling him that it's okay for

him to stop breathing, that he doesn't have to fight anymore, that it's okay to end his association with this body and this world and that his experience will continue in another place.

His breaths were almost nonexistent, and there was a fair amount of time between them. His heart rate went down to about 20. He stopped breathing. He was completely still. I held his head and his hand. His heart continued to beat for a minute, and then he flat-lined. I knew that his brain was still active, so I kept talking to him softly, my lips close to his ear, telling him that it's okay to leave, that he doesn't need to hold on to the body anymore, that he will find people that will help him.

The nurse quickly and carefully helped me disconnect the body from all the machines and turn everything off. I did a little puja [a Hindu prayer] with some incense and asked the nurse to keep anyone from coming into the room for about an hour, and I just sat there in the room with him and meditated.

Aside from the horrible hospital surroundings, it was really an incredibly natural, graceful event. My grandfather lived his life a loving man, and that's the way he died.

The reason that I'm telling you all this is because in his graceful death, my grandfather showed me much "will to live." More, if I'm perfectly honest. Let me explain.

What I kept thinking was how important it is to make the distinction between the "will to live" and the "fear of death." I think that it would be very easy to mistake fear of death, a craven need to hold on to experience in a particular form, for such concepts as "fighting for life." But I think that the true will to live is a matter of love, life and experience in all its forms and transformations. It is an openness to experience of all kinds, a gesture of fullness and love. And death, and whatever lies beyond death, is very much a part of life.

This is no longer a theoretical issue for me. When I sat with my grandfather as he died, the thing that became so perfectly obvious to me was the naturalness of it. Death was very obviously a specific transformation in the course of life, similar to birth. The continuity of consciousness beyond that transition was completely obvious to me. But again, this is a matter of feeling and not intellect. It can be talked about, but not really communicated in words.

THE DURATION OF GRIEF

To the survivor, grief may seem endless and recovery impossible. Nevertheless, a process does begin whereby grief and recovery occur simultaneously in alternating patterns and moods. Of course, nothing is ever quite the same again. The survivor's attitudes may be permanently altered by the long acquaintance with illness, suffering and death; quite likely he or she will emerge from the ordeal a stronger, more mature person.

The means and length of time required for recovery will vary. Those who are alone will have a more difficult time and may need additional and continuing support from clergy, social workers or the medical team to help them through their period of grief.

Slowly a new pattern of life evolves. At first the bereaved may feel guilty when experiencing brief episodes of enjoyment. To feel happiness may seem inappropriate, like being a traitor. Yet it is these interludes of enjoyment that gradually create new hope. As they accumulate, they coalesce into a vision of the future, and the survivor becomes able to acknowledge emotionally what he or she always knew intellectually: that vitality and involvement with others will return.

Little by little, the painful memories of the departed person's suffering and illness become less poignant, and it becomes easier to relive and enjoy thoughts of earlier, happier times. From these cherished memories the bereaved may also derive courage, by identifying with the positive qualities of the person who is gone. At the same time, the survivor begins to recognize with diminishing guilt that his or her own needs continue. This is the turning point.

There is no prescribed time that elapses before a grieving person begins to mobilize his or her interests toward the present and the future. There is no line of demarcation between grief and recovery. Old memories are kept alive while new ones are being created.

ACUTE AND CHRONIC LOSS

The way a person dies can affect how that person's survivors grieve. There is a major difference between grieving an acute loss (a sudden death) and grieving a chronic loss (a death that is expected).

Grief is more acute with a sudden death—for example, than one that results from an auto accident or from an unexpected postsurgical complication. An unexpected death allows no time for planning. On the other hand, when a person has a chronic illness such as cancer, kidney failure or heart disease, people know that death is coming. One is often given support from friends, family and clergy about what to expect where death is concerned.

While someone we care about is dying, we often feel anticipatory grief. We may begin to fear the loss and may go through phases of depression, anger or just difficulty in coping with the situation, knowing that death is near.

This is a time for compassion, where people often put their trust and faith in their belief system or religion. Visits from family, friends and the clergy to offer compassion and support during a chronic illness can prepare the family for death. The family of a patient who enters a hospice program also have time and built-in support; after death, they can get additional counseling.

There is a feeling of sorrow throughout this chronic process; on behalf of the patient who is suffering, we may often wish for mercy—that the process would end. This sometimes leads to feelings of guilt. Accepting that the shortening of life is not fair often results in anger when the impending death occurs.

There are great vicissitudes or changes during the course of illness. With a sudden, unexpected death, there is no time for preparation; suddenly, one experiences a grievous loss. The death of a loved one in war might be expected, yet people on the home front constantly pray and do many acts, often of kindness, aimed psychologically at helping "prevent" that death. When the dreaded telegram arrives, it is therefore such a crushing blow and shock that it totally alters the recovery process. When shootings or assaults result in a sudden death, survivors may suffer psychologically for years. Recovering from an acute death is often difficult and slow.

People try to keep hope alive through the realization that life continues during the many crises one undergoes during a chronic illness—and also in preparing for the eventual death. In Part V, "Planning for the Future," we describe many ways to prepare for death; we also provide forms and sample documents, such as wills and funeral instructions. Having such documents in place can avert suffering and pain, and help family and friends honor the patient's wishes.

We also discuss ethical wills in which people transmit their thoughts either verbally or with an audio or video recording. An ethical will communicates a person's thoughts, love and philosophy to survivors, providing a chance to say good-bye and to leave a legacy of encouragement and support, as well as to give instructions on how the estate and possessions should be distributed.

Frequently, we have participated in conversations where a dying person tries to alleviate feelings of guilt in his or her partner by advising the loved one to become romantically involved again if the opportunity presents itself. We believe grieving can be shortened and eased when the survivors receive explicit permission to continue living, and strong advice that although memories of the deceased will always be alive, life must go on.

The ethical will is a great avenue for recording such thoughts. When curing or controlling a person's cancer is no longer possible or practical, an ethical will can provide the patient with a continuing sense of hope that although he or she may not live longer, he or she will live better. Peace of mind comes with having shared important events in our life and with knowing that we will live what remains of our life without pain and suffering.

The ethical will also allows people to acknowledge that their life has been successful: for example, having raised a family, or leaving a moral or financial inheritance that reflects their values. This often gives a sense not only of the value of life but also of continuing hope for the future—that family and friends will continue to grow, mature and emulate the moral standards and patterns we set. This hope can comfort a dying person, strengthen his or her beliefs and faith, and provide a sense of inner peace despite the most stressful circumstances.

In ethical wills, patients often express hopes that "my family will be all right when I am gone." Some hope for some extra time that has meaning; others, for a peaceful death that will not traumatize their family. Those whose religious faith includes a belief in life after death hope that at some time in the future, they'll be reunited with their loved ones.

Patients have expressed such feelings as "I hope that I die peacefully and painlessly, and that my memory will linger" and "I hope that my life has had meaning that will give strength to my survivors, and that I have served others in a way that has enhanced my feeling of what I term a successful and happy life." Such expressions not only give solace and comfort to the family but are very helpful to remember in the grieving process to come.

Those who have had angry relationships or discord within their family may try to "mend their fences," so that when death does occur, they will have achieved better peace of mind for themselves and their family. People who have not talked to a relative or friend for years—angry because of an incident that occurred a long time ago—have called or met with the other person so that they could make peace. Others have sought forgiveness for deeds they have come to regret. Reaching out in this way can be very helpful for the survivors, softening the grieving process.

Expressions of what a dying person perceives as the meaning of his or her life can also be a touchstone for survivors. Though patients may see no hope for themselves, they may still hope that recalling the events that made their life meaningful will provide their survivors with hope for the future. Often during such a period, religion can play a role through the belief in God who has shown them a path of righteousness and a way of life. They know that when "God takes" them, their family will be comforted by the faith that although their body is no longer present, their spirit will continue and will be remembered.

Some have remarked that their illness has renewed religious feelings, giving them reassurance. This can improve the quality of life for whatever time remains, and can transmit strength to the survivors. The patient and the survivors have put their faith in God's hands for comfort, and know that it is not up to them alone.

We have often heard people say—after either going through a final confession or receiving the sacraments—that they are now at peace and are no longer worried. Receiving absolution helps not only the dying but also the survivors to continue their anticipatory and subsequent grieving process. This often requires an acknowledgment that the dying no longer have control over life or the disease, and that even though they will not attain remission, they are now ready to continue living as best they can.

Those who do not have strong religious convictions can experience similar peace by reaffirming their faith in humanity.

INTIMATE CONVERSATIONS

Saying good-bye may be one of the most difficult aspects of dying for both patient and loved ones.

Discussing and implementing ways to assist survivors, as described in Part V, "Planning for the Future"—by signing living and ethical wills, and by trying to answer difficult questions for relatives, such as "What do you think that cancer has done to you, and how has it affected your life?"—can be very supportive to those around the patient. It can also allow them to interact with one another in loving, supporting ways that can be a touchstone to help in the grieving process. But there are times when such an approach will not work: the dying person may be denying reality, or may not be interested in or able to have such sensitive discussions.

This type of anticipatory grief session or conversation can cause great anxiety as well as sadness, because it accentuates the loss of life that will soon occur. It also means grieving for the time that will never be spent together and the anger at being denied this precious time. Even so, we have found that it gives great strength to the survivors. It can involve admitting some inadequacies—for example, that one has not prepared enough to provide well for one's survivors. It can also involve expressing guilt. But an honest approach to the reality of life can be consoling, and the advice that is given can often be helpful and supportive for family and friends.

There is no "right time" to have such a conversation. Often, though, having it weeks or months before death occurs can help in the anticipatory grief process, as well as lay a foundation for support during the actual after-death grieving. Speaking frankly and setting future standards for one's family's expectations, as well as compassionately discussing and revealing the inadequacies of life, can be very meaningful during this difficult and serious time. Such a somber experience may help renew faith in beliefs and give a sort of breath of life, not only to the dying person (because it may relieve anxieties) but also to his or her survivors (to whom it may give future strength). This is a recognition of the frailty of life and humanity, but it is also an expression of the meaning of one's spirit and philosophy.

Some people hope for a miracle, putting great effort into treatments—whether conventional or alternative—only to experience disappointment and depression when those treatments fail. Talking about one's concerns, one's fears and even one's death can be a strengthening experience that gives people a bridge to the future.

The ability to confide one's thoughts, which may not have been possible for many years, and also the ability to listen nonjudgmentally, can help a dying person acknowledge and reaffirm the feelings of sadness and acceptance, reflecting the resilience of the human spirit and reducing some of the shock, pain and ongoing feelings of loss in the grieving process.

Ways to Help with Grieving
1. Engage in conversations about what

should happen after death. Prepare an ethical will; leave instructions for what kind of funeral you want—for example, who should officiate and whether it should be private. Such information can relieve the guilt that survivors often feel during the crisis that occurs after a loved one's death, when decisions must be made while grief clouds the mind. It can also prevent unnecessary expense, since many people do not wish to have an elaborate funeral. Those who wish to be remembered in a more elaborate way, with a special public memorial, can make this clear.

2. Use a memorial service to try to consolidate the survivors' feelings about the person who has died. This formal means of expressing feelings can initiate and accelerate grieving. Often survivors talk about their feelings and express their love at such a service, which can be a positive, reaffirming experience.

3. During the mourning period, make use of visits from family and friends. Most religions go through rituals and periods of observance that aid in the grieving process. For example, a wake—a party to celebrate a person's life—is a Christian custom. In Judaism, during a week of intense mourning (called shiva, "seven"), mirrors are covered, the immediate family sits on the floor or lower than visitors, and meals are provided by friends and family. After this week, the family gradually progresses back toward living. The setting of the headstone, approximately 11 months later, is supposed to end the period of mourning so that life can go on.

Emotional counseling and support from clergy, family and friends is more available during the first week or two. As time goes on, friends and family return to their homes and their lives. Calls and letters come less frequently, and the grieving person is gradually left more alone to face the finality of the loss. Periodic letters and telephone calls give continued support, but in reality, the grieving person has to take over, regain control of his or her destiny and resume taking care of self, family and friends. Life will go on at its own pace.

We often tell people that this is the time when they need courage and fortitude, and that, in part, they could take such strength from their lost relative or friend, who exemplified strength in going through the illness. The survivors now need to emulate that person, calling on a similar strength to continue living in a way that honors the person's memory.

If grief persists without abating over 6 to 12 months, becoming the dominant force in a survivor's life, spiritual or psychological support becomes essential in order to help the bereaved return to an active and productive life. There is a need for a purpose in life and for setting new goals.

Most terminally ill patients have already thought about these concerns, and the questions they are asked may come as no surprise. Giving the person the chance to express him- or herself, especially in the presence of loved ones, can be a very positive aspect of the coping process.

There are clearly many things on a person's mind during life's final episode. Expressing these concerns can be an effective part of palliative care, improving the quality of the remaining time. It also provides a unique opportunity to help family members bond in a way that fosters both current and future faith and hope, enhancing their courage and giving them strength to face the future.

Love and care begin early in life, and there needs to be some level of satisfaction before death. How a person dies also makes a difference, because survivors will remember many events from the final days, hours and minutes. Compassion shown by the medical team, clergy, psychologists and social workers can reduce the chance that grieving survivors will

feel angry that not everything possible was done. There are always questions along the lines of whether a person could have lived longer had the medical team only kept him or her on the respirator, or the feeling that this death is not fair. Feelings that "my life is now ruined" and "now I have to fend for myself" are normal and natural, but can often be lessened through appropriate guidance during the final episode in life. Attacking the psychosocial as well as the medical issues can reduce or eliminate many of the emotional crises common to grieving.

In facing your own death by taking the steps described in this chapter, you may help your survivors live better and lessen their grief of loss. Not everyone can provide this type of help, though. In part, our resistance to doing so may relate to Freud's suggestion that "the unconscious mind does not recognize its own death, and regards itself as immortal. ... It is indeed impossible to imagine our own death; and whenever we attempt to do so, we can perceive that we are, in fact, still present as spectators."

Often, even near death people act in an unknowing way. A sudden death, which denies the dying person a chance to express helplessness, abandonment or fear of death, presents a more difficult situation. The difficulty, in part, relates to one's ego when the final event is taking place.

In the hospital, the approach of death is often denied until the time it occurs. Media revelations of magical cures and new treatments give false hope. Elisabeth Kübler-Ross reports that only 2 percent of dying patients reject the chance to discuss their dying, but many staff members become so emotionally upset that they cannot participate in helping a dying patient share the experience with staff, family or friends. Such discussions are usually less upsetting to the dying person than to those around him or her. The fear of death can provoke withdrawal, depression or a heroic transcendence into a more giving and gracious attitude. The dying person can provide a touchstone for the survivors and future generations by reflecting on the meaning of life and by giving hope that his or her spirit and thoughts will continue.

The care of the dying provokes a pervasive fear in many people—that they themselves will die and be extinct, helpless, abandoned, lose their self-esteem. People who wallow and struggle in their own mortality during the final episode of the dying process may be detaching themselves from reality. This is one of the normal mechanisms of escape, but such repression of death and anxieties about the future, although normal, can affect not only how the dying person copes but also how the survivors cope.

This leads to what has been termed "appropriate grief," where the mourning resolves around recognizing and integrating each person's feeling of love or hate for the person they are mourning. Our attitudes toward life and death play a role not only in how we live and how we die but also in how we grieve. The process of death and grieving is thus different for each person. Preparing for death through physical means (such as preparing for funerals, buying plots and deciding on code status) and through emotional means (such as making an ethical will) can alter the grieving process.

FINAL THOUGHTS

Courage It takes a lot of courage and compassion to stand and act with others during times of distress. The virtue of courage in approaching reality can be an expression of our inner feelings and philosophy on how to live as well as our emotional capacity to endure difficult crises. This can provide a springboard for thoughts and acts toward relatives and friends, as well as a chance to share strength and support with companions during times of great stress and woe. Benevolent acts, no matter how small, such as doing kind deeds or giving friendship, compassion, and support, can infuse confidence and hope.

The philosopher David Hume stated, "Compassion is a natural feeling which, by moderating the violence of love of self in each individual, contributes to the preservation of the whole species. It is this compassion that hurries us without reflection to the relief of those who are in distress."

By giving compassion, we share our emotions and our philosophy with another, supporting the hope not only that life is worthwhile but also that it will have meaning. This process supports the desire and will to live. Like birth and marriage, death is a turning point for the dying person and for those around him or her. It is only through kindness and giving that one extends oneself.

This is well stated by Emily Dickinson in her poem "If I Can Stop One Heart from Breaking":

> If I can stop one Heart from breaking
> I shall not live in vain
> If I can ease one Life the Aching
> Or cool one Pain
> Or help one fainting Robin
> Unto his Nest again
> I shall not live in vain.

PART V: PLANNING FOR THE FUTURE

32
PAYING FOR CANCER CARE

Joseph S. Bailes, MD, Barbara Quinn, and Malin Dollinger, MD

Newly diagnosed cancer patients are suddenly confronted with critical questions about their insurance coverage. Paying for medical care is complicated. Managed care has introduced new rules and methods of operation. There is a new vocabulary of words and initials that is confusing even to health care workers.

The health insurance industry—both public and private—has its own policies, guidelines and methods of payment specific to cancer care. Each company's rules may be different. It is important for you to understand how your insurance company's payment system works so that you will get the care you need at a cost you should be able to pay. It is especially important to know your policy restrictions.

Group health care plans are often available through employers, labor unions and other associations. As a rule, group plans do not discriminate against pre-existing conditions, including cancer. Individual (nongroup) health insurance plans are also available. In contrast with most group plans, individually purchased plans almost always preclude or at least limit coverage for pre-existing conditions. Some individual plans reject people with serious pre-existing conditions.

As a cancer patient, you are probably uncertain and unclear about the scope of your coverage, as well as about how you can obtain the benefits you are entitled to under your insurance contract. Not being fully informed can put you at great financial risk. You may end up paying for services that should have been covered by your insurance.

TYPES OF HEALTH CARE COVERAGE

There are many types of payment plans, insurance plans and medical groups.

Medicare This government-sponsored health insurance program is for people aged 65 and older. It also covers people who are permanently disabled, provided they have received Social Security disability benefits for at least two years.

Medicare is divided into two parts:
◆ *Part A—Hospital Insurance* This part of the program covers your inpatient hospital stay, limited skilled nursing care, part-time home health care and hospice care for those who are eligible. It is available without payment of a premium, although some services require a deductible or co-payment. Medicare Part A is administered by the Health Care Financing Administration (HCFA) through insurers called intermediaries.
◆ *Part B—Medical Insurance* This part of the program covers physician services and hospital outpatient care, such as blood transfusions, x-rays and lab tests. There is limited coverage for medical equipment such as wheelchairs and walkers. Enrollment is optional, and the payment of a premium is required. Medicare Part B covers 80 percent of allowed charges. You are responsible for the other 20 percent of allowed charges, called co-insurance. You must also meet a yearly deductible (currently $100) before Medicare Part B coverage applies.

Medicare Part B is directed by the federal government through the HCFA and is funded through a monthly premium, which comes out of your Social Security check. It is administered through contracts with insurers (called carriers) throughout the United States.

If you need additional information, as well as a free handbook describing the Medicare program, contact your local Social Security office.

Medigap This insurance is sold by private carriers and traditionally covers the 20 percent co-insurance you are responsible for under Medicare Part B. Federal law stipulates that there be only 10 standard types of Medigap policies available. These policies vary widely in their scope of coverage. You should thoroughly familiarize yourself with the particular Medigap policy you are considering purchasing, so that you will have the coverage appropriate for your situation.

Medicaid This is a joint federal- and state-funded program for low-income individuals. It provides coverage for inpatient care, outpatient services, diagnostic testing, drugs, skilled nursing facility care and home health care. Each state has its own rules about eligibility for the Medicaid program. Your local social service or welfare department is the best place to obtain information about Medicaid.

QMBE This is a program in which the state pays co-insurance and premiums for certain low-income Medicare Part B beneficiaries even if they don't qualify for Medicaid.

Traditional Indemnity Insurance Sometimes called Major Medical Coverage, this type of insurance is sold by numerous private insurance companies. It is the most common type of insurance coverage for people not eligible for Medicare or Medicaid. Such insurance plans typically pay the usual fee for service each time you see your doctor.

There is usually a deductible and/or co-payment associated with traditional indemnity insurance. This means, for example, that you might pay the first $250 or $500 in covered charges each year and/or pay 10 or 20 percent of all fees. There may be limits in the policy (a maximum dollar amount that will be paid); these often apply to hospital room and nursing costs and to treatment for psychological problems. Commonly, reimbursement to a physician is based on the "usual and customary" amount, not on the physician's actual fees.

An employer will often have a plan for general insurance coverage for each employee.

Managed Care Plans Managed care usually requires individuals either to pay a fixed fee for a certain set of services or to see only certain physicians, who have agreed to discount their fees for particular services.

There are many variations of managed care plans (*see also* Chapter 33).

Health Maintenance Organization (HMO) An HMO is a prepaid health plan that requires you to use a specific network or group of provider physicians, hospitals and labs. For a fixed fee each month, HMOs provide care specified by your contract. This care may or may not be all-inclusive, so it is important to read and understand the contract of your particular HMO. For instance, some HMOs have no outpatient prescription drug benefit. In an HMO, you are usually required to select one physician as your primary or family doctor. This individual coordinates all of your care.

Examples of HMOs include Kaiser Permanente, Cigna Health Plans and Blue Cross HMO plans. HMO members aged 65 and older should remember that the HMO plan replaces Medicare coverage, and you must stay within your HMO plan in order for your claims to be paid by Medicare.

Preferred Provider Organization (PPO), Exclusive Provider Organization (EPO) or Independent Practice Association (IPA) Traditionally, PPOs, EPOs and IPAs are groups of physicians and other participating providers who have agreed to offer a discount from their usual fees in order to participate in a particular group. Such groups function as "old-fashioned private practices" in that the physician or other provider receives a fee each time a service is performed or each time you see the physician. There are usually deductibles and/or co-payments for which you are responsible. You do have a choice of using providers or physicians who are not in the plan, but if you do, you will have to pay a larger portion of the cost.

WHAT DOES YOUR PLAN COVER?

Your health benefits manual, insurance representative or the health plan manager at your place of employment should be able to answer the following questions. Because cancer treatment can be quite expensive, it is absolutely essential for a cancer patient to be totally familiar with both the benefits and the restrictions of his or her coverage. Here are some key questions to consider:

◆ What is the effective date of the policy? In other words, when does your coverage begin?

◆ What is your deductible? This is the amount you need to pay before your insurance plan starts paying the rest. Only medical care received as a benefit under your policy is calculated against your deductible. Noncovered services that you pay for do not count toward the deductible.

◆ Do you have a stop loss? This is the annual amount you must pay out of your own pocket before your insurance pays at 100 percent. Stop losses can be very beneficial where diagnosis and treatment are expensive.

◆ What percentage of billed charges is paid by your insurance? Some policies pay 80 percent or 90 percent of some costs but pay only 50 percent of other costs.

◆ Do you have coverage for home care, nursing visits at home, private duty nursing (24-hour care) and care at a skilled nursing facility or convalescent hospital?

◆ Do you have coverage for custodial care? Most insurance companies cover only skilled care. Custodial care—such as housekeeping, bathing, doing laundry and assistance in getting to the bathroom or in preparing meals—is not usually covered.

◆ Does your plan cover hospice care?

◆ Does your insurance provide coverage only if you go to specific providers?

◆ Is a referral or a plan authorization required for doctor's visits, hospital admissions or outpatient testing?

◆ Are there any waivers that would preclude payment for treatment for your condition? This might include prior treatment (within one year, for example) for the same or a similar condition.

◆ What is your lifetime maximum? This is the maximum benefit your insurance will pay in your lifetime. It can be $25,000 or $1 million or more.

◆ How do you get care after hours or in an emergency?

◆ If you have group coverage through your employer, does coverage end if you are fired or laid off? If so, is there a way to continue coverage? (Ask your employer about COBRA, the federal law that requires certain plans to extend your group employer coverage up to 18 months after you are terminated from a job—though you must usually pay the entire premium yourself.)

WHY CLAIMS MAY BE DENIED

Even though your policy may appear comprehensive, denials for medical care claims are common. Sometimes a denial reflects only a practical problem—say, missing information or incorrect documentation. Sometimes the policy does not cover certain types of care. This is often a matter of interpretation. If this is the case, you will need to advocate with your doctor or other health care provider to establish that your care should be covered even though the insurance company's agent interprets the policy as appearing to exclude it. An explanation of common reasons for denial follows, along with recommendations for responding to the denial.

Pre-Existing Condition Your claim may be denied if your medical condition existed before you became eligible for or bought your policy. Be absolutely sure about how your particular plan interprets the term "pre-existing condition."

Noncovered Benefit Most policies have a section that lists illnesses or services that are excluded from coverage. Because of the possibility of noncovered benefits, it is a good idea to check your insurance plan before any treatment or tests are ordered. Some treatments are covered only when given or administered in the hospital, for example.

In such cases, you or your physician's office may be able to make arrangements for outpatient coverage in lieu of hospitalization. Services may actually be cheaper that way.

Not an Authorized Provider Many insurance plans require that you use providers who are part of their network. Seeing a specialist usually requires that you be referred by an authorized provider for a consultation and for all subsequent treatment. Failure to go to contracted providers with a written referral can result in a complete denial of payment for all treatment provided.

Investigational Treatment Virtually all health insurance plans cover standard cancer diagnosis and treatments (e.g., chemotherapy, radiotherapy, surgery), but many insurers will deny claims deemed to be investigational (experimental), unnecessary or inappropriate. Bone marrow transplants and certain other new treatments often fall into this category. While there is no guaranteed way to prevent denial of such a claim, make sure that you attempt to receive pre-approval in writing for the treatment from your insurance carrier. To do this, you should have a "letter of medical necessity" from your physician documenting that the proposed treatment is medically appropriate, along with supporting clinical literature and a full description of the procedure or services to be provided. The anticipated cost and duration of the treatment should also be included.

Off-Label Treatment Your insurer may deny a claim if the drug your doctor has prescribed is used for any reason other than its labeled indication or the use listed on the drug company's package insert. The claim may also be denied if the drug is used in a new dosage or according to a new schedule, given by a different route or combined with other drugs.

You should be aware that fully half of all uses of cancer drugs are not those listed on the official package insert or label. Such uses reflect advances in cancer treatment that occurred after the drug was released onto the market and are in fact the ordinary, proper and accepted uses of such drugs. Not to use certain drugs for established "off-label" uses may be inappropriate.

When your health insurance plan uses "drug use is off-label" to deny a claim, it is very important to appeal this denial to the insurance carrier. Such denials are usually reversed, especially if the use of the drug is standard in the community and is a necessary and effective treatment for your illness. Most pharmaceutical companies will provide clinical literature if needed to help support your claim. In fact, they often provide reimbursement "hotlines" to provide assistance. Your oncologist's insurance or billing staff is usually familiar with ways to help you with this problem should denial occur. In many states, cancer physicians have formed organizations to advise insurance companies about effective new treatments for cancer, especially established drugs in off-label use.

Nonpayment of Premiums It is very difficult to obtain another insurance policy once you have a pre-existing condition. Make sure that premiums for your current policy are kept up to date to ensure that your insurance policy is not canceled.

SUBMITTING CLAIMS

You must bring proper insurance plan identification on your first visit to your oncologist's office. Your insurance provider—whether it is Medicare, Medicaid, a PPO, an HMO or a private indemnity plan—should give you an identification card. This card will have your subscriber identification number (often your social security number), group number, office co-pay amount and the address to which any claims should be submitted. If your insurance does require submission of a claim form, also bring a fully completed and signed claim form to the office.

Always inform your physician's office of any changes in your address, phone number, employment or insurance information. Notifying the office immediately will prevent unnecessary delays in claim submission, avoid the need for re-submission and reduce possible denials of payment. It will also result in quicker payment of claims.

Your physician's office will submit the claim for some plans. This may also be true for hospitals, laboratories and other kinds of service providers.

Most oncology offices have an insurance or finance department. Their patient representatives will explain the billing procedures to you before you begin treatment. Find out whether they will submit your claim or whether you are expected to submit the claim yourself.

Always request a copy of your charges, which should include an itemization of all services and the diagnosis (including its code) for your visit.

Common Terms and Abbreviations To better understand the procedure for submitting and processing claims, you should understand the terms and abbreviations used by most insurance carriers. Here are the most common ones:

◆ *ICD-9 (International Classification of Diseases, 9th Edition) Code* This code identifies your illness. All claims submitted to your insurance carrier will require the correct code. Carriers will not pay your claim if this code is not provided.

◆ *CPT (Current Procedural Terminology) Code* This code identifies the medical, surgical and diagnostic services rendered by your physician. It is used by most insurance carriers to identify what services were performed. Claims are paid using these codes.

◆ *Deductible* This is the amount you have to pay before your insurance starts paying the rest. Only received medical care that is a covered benefit under your policy is counted against your deductible. Noncovered benefits, which you must pay yourself, do not count against your deductible.

◆ *Co-payment* This refers to the amount of your bill that you are responsible for. The co-payment is usually a specific dollar amount rather than a percentage of the bill. Prescription drug programs, for example, often have a co-payment, usually a fixed dollar amount per prescription. Co-payments are generally associated with HMOs.

◆ *Co-insurance* This is the percentage of the bill you are responsible for after you have met your deductible. If your policy has a $100 deductible and a 20 percent co-insurance, for example, you would pay your $100 deductible and 20 percent of all covered expenses. You are also responsible for paying for all services not covered by your policy. Co-insurance provisions are most commonly associated with PPO-type plans.

◆ *EOB (Explanation of Benefits)* This is the statement you will receive from your insurance carrier when your claim has been paid. It will show the provider of services, the place of service and how the benefits were paid. If you have a deductible or co-insurance, this will also be stated on your EOB. If you have a secondary insurance carrier, that company will need a copy of your EOB in order to pay its portion (see "EOMB" below).

◆ *EOMB (Explanation of Medicare Benefits)* This statement, similar to an insurance carrier's EOB, is sent to you as soon as your claim has been paid. It will state the provider of any service, the amount allowed under Medicare's fee schedule, the amount paid and what charges were applied toward your deductible. If your physician is a Medicare provider, the check will be sent directly to his or her office. You will need this explanation of Medicare benefits in order for your secondary insurance company to pay your claim.

◆ *Assignment of Benefits* This is required by most physicians' offices. It means that you give written permission for your insurance company to send payments directly to the service provider. An assignment-of-benefits form is usually provided by the physician's office for you to sign. There is also a place for your assignment-of-benefits signature on your claim form.

◆ *Medicare Assignment* Any physician may accept the fee schedule set by Medicare in an individual case. A participating provider in the Medicare program has agreed to always take the set fee schedule ("assignment").

If your physician takes Medicare assignment (fees), you are then responsible only for noncovered services, for your deductible and for your co-insurance. However, if the physician is not a participating provider in the Medicare program, it is possible for you to end up being responsible for more than the 20 percent co-insurance. If the physician's charge is more than the Medicare allowable charge, for instance, the physician will receive only 80 percent of the Medicare allowable fee, while you will be responsible for the entire rest of the bill. So if you are eligible for Medicare, make sure you ask ahead of time whether your physician participates in the Medicare program and will accept assignment of Medicare benefits for your care.

◆ *UCR (Usual, Customary and Reasonable)* This is the fee determined by your insurance carrier to be the usual fee charged for the same service by the average provider with similar training in your geographic area. This may be different from the fee your physician charges.

◆ *Pre-authorization* This is a requirement by your insurance carrier that certain services be authorized before the services are rendered. If your insurance contains this requirement, make sure your physician's office is aware of it.

◆ *Superbill* This is a standard itemized "checklist of services" in widespread use. It will contain all the required codes (CPT and ICD-9) that will enable you to submit your claim.

◆ *COB (Coordination of Benefits)* When you are enrolled in two separate group insurance plans, those plans will coordinate their benefits so that your claim is paid at no more than 100 percent of the covered benefits. If you have more than one insurance plan, make sure you notify your physician's office so that the office can submit both claims for you.

NEW WAYS OF PAYING FOR MEDICAL CARE

Our society is engaged in a great effort to reform the health care payment system. For example, despite all the numerous types of health insurance and managed care, many Americans have no health coverage.

There used to be only two players in the system: the doctor and the patient. Now there are several others: the health insurance industry, various federal and state regulatory agencies, employers (who often provide employee health care plans) and the federal government. New rules and regulations are being proposed and implemented that will change the basic concepts and practices of health care.

The patient's need for skillful, dedicated and considerate care by the physician has never changed. From the viewpoint of the physician—now called a health care provider—what has changed is that

1. other parties and agencies have taken over some of the decision making that used to belong to the physician alone, and

2. consequently, physicians and hospitals and their staff must now interact continually with these other decision makers. Many decisions now require outside approval. These can include the decision to hospitalize, where to hospitalize, which consultants may be called, what types of treatment may be used and, especially, how health care resources are to be allocated and provided.

Requiring authorization before ordering tests and x-rays is just one example. Many doctors' offices now have more people handling insurance than they have nurses. Physicians will need to be increasingly accountable to outside agencies.

"Managed care" is one common term used to describe a coordinated effort by physicians, hospitals and insurers—also called insurance payers—to create an optimum balance between incredibly sophisticated medical technology on the one hand and our inability as a society to afford paying for every possible treatment and diagnostic test for every person in every situation on the other hand. The practice guidelines now being developed by various insurance carriers will probably become increasingly important in how services are provided and covered.

Because the patterns of delivering and monitoring health care are complex and changing and because new payment systems are being created, it is absolutely essential that you completely understand the provisions of your health insurance plan. With increasingly expensive tests and treatments and more and more controls over payment for medical care, your best insurance is to completely understand the provisions of your own insurance.

In this rapidly changing medical world, there will have to be a greater effort and understanding by all the participants in medical care—the patient, the physician, the health care team and the governmental/insurance payers—to provide cost-effective, state-of-the-art health care.

33

MANAGED CARE AND ONCOLOGY: THE NEW CARE SYSTEMS

Malin Dollinger, MD, and Joel Pollack, CPA

During the past 50 years, there has been a profound shift in patterns of payment for health care. Before World War II, "high-tech" and sophisticated tests and treatment did not yet exist. There were no intensive care units, CT or MRI scans, fancy blood tests or, for that matter, specialists. The cost of medical care was relatively predictable and thrifty, and we simply paid for medical expenses out of pocket.

In 1933 surgeon Dr. Sidney Garfield set up a makeshift hospital in the Mojave Desert to treat workers building the Los Angeles Aqueduct. He provided comprehensive care at a fixed price—a nickel a day—deducted from workers' paychecks. That caught the eye of shipbuilder Henry Kaiser, one of the largest employers in the country. He set up a similar program for workers building the Grand Coulee Dam in Washington State and for workers at shipyards in California, Oregon and Washington. After World War II, Kaiser opened enrollment to the public. Within a year, AFL and CIO members were joining at the rate of 2,000 per month, sparking a revolution in health care.

Kaiser set up an all-inclusive health care system for his employees. For the first time, one plan owned and controlled the hospitals, employed the physicians and other health care providers and managed the whole enterprise, including preventive medicine, under one roof. One monthly payment by the consumer took care of all medical problems, at least as defined by the contract. This became the first and largest health maintenance orga-

nization (HMO) and the first example of "managed care."

Broadly defined, managed care is the application of business principles to the delivery of health care. More specifically, it is a system of health care delivery that provides services at a fair and reasonable price and measures performance outcomes and quality of care. Everyone involved with health care delivery—physicians, hospitals, laboratories—now has to be concerned with efficiency, timeliness, satisfaction, accountability and costs, as well as quality.

HEALTH CARE PAYMENT SYSTEMS

Once the Kaiser model proved successful, other HMOs began to appear. From 1960 to 1980, a number of health care systems existed, offering several combinations and variations. Consumers could choose between systems according to their preferences, tastes and means.

◆ **Direct payment** In this system, the consumer simply pays for health care out of pocket. Even those with insurance plans may need to pay some expenses themselves, such as deductibles, co-payments or extra costs for special and investigational treatments and services that aren't covered.

◆ **Fee-for-service/indemnity insurance** Beginning in the 1960s, this was the most common type of insurance plan through to the 1980s. Health insurance companies issued policies (often, but not always, in association with employers) that allowed the consumers to choose a physician and, indirectly, a hospital. The physician and/or hospital would then bill the insurance company for services rendered.

A primitive form of "quality control" emerged from this process, chiefly related to the concept of "usual and customary fees," which inhibited practitioners from charging, or at least from being paid, excessive fees. Consumers quickly learned to walk away from providers and services that were equivalent in quality but excessive in cost. Competitive market forces began to standardize the costs of hospitalization, laboratory tests, x-ray exams, physical therapy, nursing homes, prescriptions and every other aspect of health care.

◆ **Discounted fee for service** Market forces also began to create discounts for physicians' services. Doctors agreed to accept, for example, a 10 or 20 percent discount in their usual fees. In return, they wanted to be given an "exclusive" for patients of a particular health plan. Physicians' overheads and costs were the same regardless of how many patients were seen. Their margin—the difference between gross income and the cost of doing business—became lower unless they could ensure an adequate number of patients.

◆ **Medicare and Medicaid** In 1965, federal legislation created the Medicare and Medicaid programs. This was a major event in American history. Health care expenditures had been kept under control through prudent spending by physicians and consumers, but federal spending on these new programs unleashed health care expenditures never seen before. Health care turned into a growth industry. Now the consumer had carte blanche for medical care, with the bills paid by Uncle Sam. The impact led health care providers to search for new ways to control costs. They turned to managed care.

MANAGED CARE

In the late 1980s and early 1990s, the gradual evolution of health care payment systems entered a new era. Several forces radically changed our health care payment systems.

◆ Health care more and more came to be delivered by contract between a physician or a group of physicians and the insurance company, which came to be called the payer. New doctors in town not only would announce their names, addresses, specialties and training but, for the first time, needed to indicate which insurance plans they accepted by contract.

◆ Employers began to be primary contractors as well as decision makers for health care. This eventually created the problem of people with chronic and/or pre-existing health problems being unable to change jobs for fear of losing their health insurance and not being able to replace it. On the other hand, a large employer might be able to incorporate people with pre-existing illness (a history of cancer, for example) because of the clout it achieved by having a large number of employees enrolled.

◆ Relationships among health care providers changed dramatically. Physicians were more restricted in their referrals. They could send patients only to physicians and consultants under contract with the same company or plan, unless consumers were willing to pay significantly more for treatment by a physician of their own choice. Each health plan contracted with a certain hospital or hospitals for guaranteed—and often lower—rates. This tended to promote efficiency and drive inefficient or poorly organized hospitals out of business.

◆ The contractual needs linking physicians and health plans made solo or small practices undesirable. Limited groups of physicians could not deliver services to large numbers of potential patients (now called covered lives) or offer the breadth of skills and specialties and geographic availability that came to be standard requirements of health care providers (the new term for doctors). Just as hospitals merged, so did physicians' practices. Small groups became large ones, and solo practitioners became rarities.

COST AND CONTROL

Issues of cost and control became dominant in the 1990s. Each segment of the health care system realized that its piece of the pie was in jeopardy and tried to increase its control. Hospitals either acquired the practices of generalist physicians and internists or formed joint ventures with primary care physicians, thereby capturing their patients and the income derived from their care.

As hospitals and physicians joined forces, practicing medicine became a business as well as a profession. There had always been bills and taxes to pay and records to keep, but in the past doctors had mostly taken care of patients and kept whatever was left over after expenses. Now their livelihood was determined by nonphysicians who controlled which patients they would see, how many patients there would be, which consultants and hospitals could be used and where laboratory tests and x-rays could be done.

In the old days, value was defined as "quality work done by the physician." Now value has another definition, borrowed from business, where value is equal to quality divided by cost. Given equal quality, the one who provides services at a lower cost now provides the greater value.

PATTERNS OF HEALTH CARE DELIVERY

Managed care is becoming the dominant force in the industry and participation is increasing at a rapid rate, especially among Medicare patients. As of 1997, at least half the U.S. population was participating in some system in which the health care providers furnish care based on an integrated economic, contractual, business and professional program, with mutual contracts between all participants, as well as management. California, Florida and Minnesota are leading this trend, but new systems of managed care are quickly gaining predominance in other parts of the country.

There are different patterns of health care delivery under managed care, including Health Maintenance Organizations (HMOs), Preferred Provider Organizations (PPOs), Independent Practice Associations (IPAs), Point of Service (POS) Plans and Independent Physicians Organizations (IPOs).

◆ An HMO integrates under one management system the entire health care program, including physicians, hospitals, outpatient services and other services such as prevention. Physicians are under contract, often on a full-time salaried basis, although the HMO may also contract with PPOs and IPAs to provide contracted physicians' services at standard rates.

◆ PPOs have a list of "approved" providers who agree to provide services at contracted rates. Hospitals usually are also contracted.

◆ An IPA is a group of physicians that contracts with various payer organizations and insurance companies.

THE GATEKEEPER CONCEPT

The dominance of the primary care physician (PCP) is one of the fundamental concepts of HMOs. All members of an HMO managed care plan select or are assigned to a primary care physician, who has complete control of patient care. The PCP determines which doctors the patient will see. If a patient has a lump in her breast, the PCP determines whether she should see an oncologist, usually one within the HMO system. The primary care physician is usually referred to as the "gatekeeper." Some plans specify, however, that a patient may see an eye doctor or skin specialist without asking a PCP for a referral, because everyone agrees such care is appropriate, efficient and cheaper. The expertise is well understood and accepted by all. The cancer specialist is likewise acknowledged as an expert in an area of medicine that requires special training and that many physicians prefer to delegate.

MANAGING RISK

Not only is health care delivery moving toward managed care, but the financial risk of providing health care is being shifted from insurance companies and managed care organizations to the physician. The major types of risk sharing are risk pools, capitation and package-price plans.

Risk Pools Risk pools are common in HMOs. There are several versions. The physician may be paid a salary or a modified salary based on work time and patient allocation. Some of the earnings, however, are placed into a fund that is divided at the end of each year according to a formula based on factors such as productivity and/or saving money by avoiding inappropriate or unnecessary use of services such as laboratory tests, x-ray exams or hospitalization.

Since allocating medical care in HMOs is generally controlled by primary care physicians, the set-aside fund is also used to pay specialists if a member needs specialty care. There is, therefore, an incentive to be thrifty of effort and expense.

The hotly debated question nationally is whether care suffers when such methods of physician reimbursement are used. Federal legislation now requires physicians to disclose valid treatment options not covered by their health plan.

Capitation Under the capitation method, the health care provider is paid a fixed amount each month to take care of anyone in a plan who becomes ill and needs the specified services. There is no further charge for any specific illness or event. The contract provides for taking care of all of the "covered lives" for a certain price per member per month, providing all required (contracted) care that might be needed in the provider's specialty.

An oncology group, for example, might contract on a capitated basis to take care of 100,000 covered lives for a certain sum per member per month. A check for the full amount would arrive each month for any and all care required for those covered persons.

Using various calculations (and not simple ones), the physician group can estimate how many people out of 100,000 would get cancer each month, how much it would cost to see them, what services would be required and how many years of care would be needed. If the estimate proves to be fairly accurate, the physician group might come out okay. If fewer people get cancer that month, money will be left over. If lots of people get cancer, particularly types that are expensive to treat, the physicians will operate at a loss.

In a capitated plan, then, the health care provider takes all the risk. If one person, ten people or a thousand people show up for cancer care, the price is still the same, so enough people have to be covered to make sure that an unusual number of people who need expensive care will not overwhelm the technical and financial ability of the health care provider.

This is analogous to automobile insurance. The insurance company, for a monthly fee, agrees to take care of whatever losses the car owner suffers. The company knows that each month there will be a certain number of car thefts and accidents and is willing to take the risk that the average number will remain roughly the same. The company needs to insure a lot of people to make the risk safer.

Physicians with capitated contracts usually protect themselves by obtaining "reinsurance" ("stop-loss" insurance) to cover any unusual patient or patients who require very expensive care. The reinsurance company needs proof ahead of time that the care given is "standard, reasonable, efficient and cost-effective" to minimize the need to use the reinsurance.

Capitated medical plans are becoming more prevalent, and doctors are finding that they therefore need to understand business principles as much as medical ones. Some physicians choose to concentrate on the business side of things.

Package-Price Plans ("Carve-Outs") In a package-price system, there is a fixed price for a defined "episode" of care. There are already medical plans with a fixed price for certain events that are easy to define from start to finish, such as cataract surgery or coronary artery bypass grafts.

In a "carve-out," the physician and/or organization agrees to provide all the care required for a certain illness, ailment or procedure for a fixed price, which is determined before care is begun. Again, the physician takes all the risk. If it costs less to deliver the care, the physician comes out ahead; if it costs more, he or she loses money.

It's difficult to create such plans in the cancer field because of the complexity and expense of care, the rapid changes in technology and treatments, the length of time that care and follow-up are required (years) and the fact that many facilities and professionals are involved, not just the primary doctor (usually an oncologist). A complex and coordinated effort is required to discover and predict the costs of all the components of care for many different kinds of cancer accurately and reliably, as well as to place under contract (and under risk) the many providers and

health care facilities. The authors of this chapter have created and initiated such plans at the John Wayne Cancer Institute in California. Similar plans exist at the M.D. Anderson Cancer Center in Houston and the Memorial Sloan-Kettering Cancer Center in New York.

One area of uncertainty is how to continue to pay for the vital clinical research trials that test promising new methods of treatment. Insurance companies may not wish to pay for trials of treatments whose role is not yet defined or proven.

MANAGED CARE ISSUES

Before managed care, there was no wish or need for anyone to coordinate the patterns of care or costs in the places where health care was provided—different doctors' offices, hospitals, pharmacies and outpatient care facilities. Inevitably, there was some duplication and excessive use of services, not by intention but because of the way the system developed.

Different physicians might order, for the same patient, the same blood tests or x-rays because the first results were perhaps not available to them. No standard care plan defined which type of physician took care of certain types of problems. It was often unclear which professional was in charge of medical care decisions. A cancer patient, for example, could easily be followed by four physicians: a primary generalist or internist, a surgeon, a radiation oncologist and a medical oncologist. Patients certainly derived a great deal of satisfaction from having all these professionals watching over them, but such a system does produce major increases in the cost of care.

Under managed care guidelines and the gatekeeper concept, a single practitioner determines the location and types of care. While this is often a generalist for most areas of medicine, with referral to specialists as needed, in the cancer field the medical oncologist usually becomes the case manager or "quarterback" who calls on other consultants. The medical oncologist now has to be concerned with cost factors as well as with quality and efficiency.

FEEDBACK

Effective managed care requires attention to several other factors besides quality and cost. There must be feedback to all parties—physician, insurance carrier and payer—about the quality of care, the efficiency of delivery, the results and the satisfaction of patients with the care they receive. Such information must be integrated into the daily care plan and package, often with the aid of computers.

There is also a need for feedback among all participants so that inefficiencies and inappropriate or unnecessary care pathways can be discovered and improved. That is why the package-price plan or "carve-out" has such potential for improving the cancer care system. It puts all the treatment, care management, cost management and communication into one package to achieve the maximum value in quality and cost.

TOTAL HEALTH CARE

For the first time, we need to look at the entire health care picture as a single activity. If a service can be done better or more efficiently or less expensively at a hospital than at a physician's office, that needs to be determined and mandated.

Physician preferences may not determine how things will be done. Only some hospitals will be permitted to perform certain procedures. Laboratory tests, x-rays and other tests and procedures either will be done at a designated facility or will not be paid for or reimbursed. In many managed care markets, the physician already has limited choices in these matters and even now has his or her choice of consultants limited to those on the same plan or contract as the patient.

For the first time in the history of our health care system, the need for total cooperation exceeds the need for autonomy or total control. Doctors, hospitals and other health care suppliers and facilities will need to consider the role of all the other "players" in the system.

Managed care will develop and reward those systems and plans that are able to distill, from the entire spectrum of providers and facilities, an efficient health care package that provides high-quality, cost-effective care. Achieving this goal requires total management of every aspect of care.

Such care packages are being developed at breakneck speed by—and in response to—health care providers, payers and consumers rather than by government. In the cancer field, as in other areas of medicine, we are not sure how the final package will look. But a hint may be found in the not-so-accidental fact that one author of this chapter is a physician and the other is an accountant.

34
DECISIONS FOR LIFE: ADVANCE DIRECTIVES AND LIVING WILLS

Ernest H. Rosenbaum, MD, Isadora R. Rosenbaum, MA, Thomas Addison, MD, Joanna Beam, JD, Meryl Brod, PhD, David Claman, MD, Alan J. Coleman, MD Malin Dollinger, MD, Michael Glover, Nancy Lambert, RN, BSN, Elmo Petterle, Patricia Sparacino, RN, MS, Jeffery Silberman, DMin, Kenneth A. Woeber, MD

With all the changes and advances in medicine, there is more talk about issues concerning life and death.* We all know that we can't get out of this world alive, but at the same time, we Americans avoid as much as possible discussions about life and death.

Although the Patient Self-Determination Act was passed in 1990, less than 10 to 15 percent of our population has prepared advance directives, which are desirable and valuable to patients, families and physicians. Advance directives are legal documents such as Durable Power of Attorney for Health Care, the California Natural Death Act declaration, and the Prehospital Do Not Resuscitate (DNR) form. Why do so few of us complete these important forms? In part, it's a result of the fact that many physicians do not bring up the subject, because they don't want to increase the fear of death in their patients; and in part, it's because the public does not wish to make the kinds of cumbersome decisions required in completing an advance directive.

For many decades, society has avoided discussions about death and dying. Because major advances in medical care can now prolong life, such discussions are becoming vital to improving patient care. One has to assess the medical rationale for performing procedures and interventions, such as cardiopulmonary resuscitation (CPR) or artificial breathing (through use of a ventilator). The patient's quality of life and his or her chances for recovery have to be considered in making such life-and-death decisions.

In our society there is a need to make decisions about how we plan the remaining years of our lives. To aid you in making such decisions, this chapter, along with Chapters 35 ("Your Legacy of Love") and 36 ("Forms and Worksheets for Decision Making"), describes and gives examples of several types of advance directives, as well as worksheets that will help you organize many personal, medical and financial aspects of your life. It is important to work with your physician and to obtain his or her advice on which of the forms is most appropriate for you. Ethical issues and ways to plan in an organized way for your orderly future will also be considered.

Physicians often go to heroic lengths to keep terminal patients alive—often against the patient's wishes. Most people assume that when the time arrives for making life-and-death decisions, their physicians and family will make the choices for them. But the family's and physician's views and decisions may not necessarily agree with the patient's. We should all assess our own values regarding quality of life and make decisions on how we wish to live and the type of care

---

*Reprinted with permission © 1996 the Regents of the University of California

we desire at the end of our life. This can be accomplished through advance directives and/or through filling out other forms that document your wishes about your future.

Chapters 34, 35 and 36 contain the advice of a group of experts who have contributed their thoughts on why and how each person should organize the final details concerning his or her possible illness and death. By completing the forms provided here, you will make life easier for your eventual survivors.

This chapter will help guide you through the maze of issues that are important for you to consider. It will offer suggestions about how decisions can be made before or during a hospitalization. It will also offer a way in which you can help your family and significant others deal with the details if your illness becomes terminal.

These topics may by their very nature be difficult issues for you. However, they represent important factors about how you may want to be treated and how you want your wishes to be carried out if you cannot make decisions for yourself. Some of the necessary documents that will help ensure that your health care wishes are recognized are included.

Here are three case histories for your review and consideration.

Case One

A 24-year-old man has been in an automobile accident resulting in massive injuries. If he is to survive, CPR (cardiopulmonary resuscitation) is needed. Should it be administered?

Yes, you might say: this is an obvious choice. But let's carry the situation a step further. Suppose that the CPR is successful, and the man's life is saved. But due to his injuries and unsuccessful treatment, he goes into a coma from which he is unlikely to recover. He can now be kept alive only by having a tracheal breathing

(windpipe) tube inserted, being connected to a respirator, and by being fed intravenously through a tube. Again, should these measures be taken? Unless the man has made his wishes known, his doctors will keep him alive no matter what the effort, cost or pain.

Most of us would prefer to die peacefully in our sleep rather than to suffer a prolonged, lingering death.

Case Two

A 67-year-old man has a medical history dating back 15 years that includes undergoing lung surgery for low-grade cancer with no recurrence. He also survived a heart attack and a successful heart angioplasty (coronary artery dilation). Recently, this gentleman was admitted to the hospital with severe pneumonia and lung failure. His condition required that he be placed on a respirator in the intensive care unit. As part of his wishes for his emergency health care, he had already signed a Medical Emergency Wallet Card requesting that no CPR be performed on him and that he not be placed on a respirator. However, when advised that a pulmonary respirator might save his life, he verbally canceled his advance directive request that no respirator be used. After 14 days in the ICU, he recovered from the pneumonia. His life and vitality have been restored, and he has returned to work.

Case Three

A 54-year-old woman's health has been failing rapidly. She has advanced metastatic breast cancer and has been admitted to the hospital with acute gastrointestinal bleeding, jaundice and progressive liver metastases. Despite having had many therapies, including a toxic course of chemotherapy, she is dying.

Her physician believes that her condition will not improve and that in her present state of ill health, her quality of life is minimal. He recommends a comfort care program to control pain and suffering and to afford her maximum comfort, rather than continuing active treatment to prolong life with inevitable suffering. She previously signed an advance directive designating her family as her "agent" in her Durable Power of Attorney for Health Care. Now her family is responsible for ensuring that her wishes are carried out.

These are a few examples that illustrate problems faced by patients, families and the medical team. For those you love, a clear advance directive can be a legacy of your thoughts and wishes, and will help alleviate the confusion that often occurs both before and after the death of a loved one. It is your choice: act now or leave these decisions to others later.

PREPARING FOR YOUR DECISIONS

Death is a part of life. We all know that we must die sometime: we just don't know when. Despite this reality, we often think of death as something that happens to other people. Most of us have a difficult time accepting our own mortality, and won't even think about it until a crisis forces us to do so. Even then, we may fight and bargain to gain more time. And accepting death is an issue for doctors as well as for patients. Many doctors fight to preserve life at almost any cost in time, money or effort—but most also know that there are circumstances in which it is right to let a person suffer no longer and die a peaceful death.

FACTORS THAT MAY INFLUENCE YOUR DECISION

How we live our life and how we plan for our death are personal choices. Society also influences us as we observe the attitudes, ceremonies and rituals that surround death and dying in our culture. For guidance in these important decisions, many of us seek religious or spiritual advice. With the technology of medicine forever changing, science may influence our decisions as well.

Since the late 1950s, advances in medical technology and medical practice have changed how patients, lawmakers, physicians, ethicists and society in general think about and define life, death and dying. We may have watched how others have reacted to the death of a loved one. Many of these changes have resulted in serious ethical dilemmas for the medical profession, causing doctors to reassess their role in caring for patients. Patients and their loved ones, faced with the possibility of prolonged suffering and delayed death, have been asking for the power to make their own decisions and to die naturally with dignity. Each person should know about his or her choices for discontinuing aggressive treatment with respect to the newer ethical and professional dilemmas.

Each of us faces serious decisions about how we view the quality of our life in terms of illness and death. Many of us would like to have some control over our medical care toward the end of life. To help us make our decisions known when we're unable to do so, documents called advance directives have been developed. Such documents give us some measure of control over our medical treatment when death threatens our survival. Through them, we can provide clear instructions if we are unable to state our wishes because a serious medical condition impairs our ability to communicate. With such documents we can also ease the burden of responsibility left to our survivors by putting our business, legal and personal affairs in order. In these ways, we can help by making decisions about our death ahead of time and so make things easier for our loved ones.

CHOOSING LIFE: LIVING YOUR LIFE WHILE PLANNING FOR MORTALITY

Despite the inevitability of death and the importance of planning for tomorrow, the purpose of life is to live. The diagnosis of an acute or chronic illness doesn't need to be experienced as an automatic death sentence. A medical diagnosis can be viewed as an important reminder to "live each day as if it were the last."

Not all people are able to cope successfully following the diagnosis of an illness. Some diseases may not respond to treatment, even if the patient has a strong will to live. When this occurs, many find the heartbreak and frustration hard to bear.

Other people say that the uncertainties of living with an illness can make life more meaningful. The smallest pleasures—flowers, the sky, sunshine—are intensified. It is a time to do things you have always wanted to do and to make peace with your family or friends.

Death eventually comes to us all. But we can choose the way we live our life—and, to some extent, the way we die. One remarkable example of a "good" death is that of the national hero Charles Lindbergh, who died in 1974. After being diagnosed with a lymphoma in 1972, he continued to live actively while undergoing radiotherapy and chemotherapy. He hoped that his life and death would reflect his simple birth and that they would serve as a memorial for his children and grandchildren.

When he was informed that he had only a short time to live, he returned to his home on Maui in Hawaii. One of his doctors (Milton M. Howell, MD, in "The Lone Eagle's Last Flight," *Journal of the AMA*, May 1975) noted the following:

In time, he made appropriate legal arrangements for his burial there and selected the site of his grave. Systematically, he arranged his personal affairs, and yet he maintained a sense of the past and an interest in the present. He planned for the next major event in his life, but it did not become an obsession.

He planned ... [the] construction of his grave with a simple coffin. He planned his funeral services along with his family and requested that people attend in their working clothes. There was time for reminiscing, time for discussion and time for laughter. When he lapsed into coma he wanted no respirator, defibrillator (for electric shock) or other complicated paraphernalia. He received excellent, prompt responsive nursing care, oxygen when needed, a minimum of analgesia (for pain), and a great deal of love and consideration from his family and the medical staff (at home).

He stated that he wished his death to be a constructive act in itself. His example of simplicity, his careful planning, his unfailing politeness and consideration for those around him, his public refusal of medical heroics, and his humble funeral are evidence of that wish. Death was another event in his life, as natural as his birth had been in Minnesota more than 72 years before.

MAKING CHOICES ABOUT MEDICAL TREATMENT

Most of us have difficulty coping with the idea of our death and therefore with the preparation that would be best for us and our loved ones. Yet, when we buy life insurance, draw up a will or make a decision about organ donation, we're acknowledging that we will die someday. The decisions you make about your health care, including the use of life-saving treatments and type of code (*see* "Understanding Hospital 'Codes,'" later in this chapter), will protect your wishes as well as ease the burden of difficult decisions for your family.

Today's realities dictate that unless there is an advance directive, your doctors may feel obligated to do whatever is necessary to keep you alive. Sometimes these actions may result in considerable pain and suffering for you as well as emotional suffering for your family and close friends. Other times, these procedures do not prolong meaningful life, but merely delay death.

Decisions about advance directives and when to perform CPR are not simple and may depend on the type of medical condition you have. Many people clearly do not want extraordinary treatment in hopeless situations but may accept such treatment in acute but potentially reversible situations. For instance, using a mechanical breathing machine to treat pneumonia after an operation is usually temporary and may help recovery. The potential risk and benefit of these treatments depend on many factors, including the patient's age, type of illness and other chronic medical problems.

"Standard" advance directives can sometimes cause confusion and need to be discussed with your family and doctor. They should be re-evaluated after each new illness. An acute disease (such as a heart attack) may be reversed by CPR, whereas advanced incurable diseases (such as terminal cancer, severe refractory heart disease, resistant infections, emphysema or kidney failure that can no longer be treated with medical therapy) may instead be best treated with comfort care (care that is aimed at keeping a person comfortable, but does not treat an illness; this may include bathing, nutrition, fluids, massage and pain medications). Different types of general statements are useful with different types of illnesses—especially with regard to the reversibility of a condition. One example might be the following: "I will accept life-supportive treatments for acute potentially reversible conditions that are very likely to be treated successfully and that are like-

ly to result in full recovery and a return to independent life." Here is a more conservative example: "I prefer that all care be directed at comfort and that life-supportive treatments not be used." These directives are often very helpful to physicians and families.

At times, as we saw in Case Two, individuals who have made rational plans when healthy change their minds when faced with a new illness and possible death: they may then change their previous directives to allow for aggressive treatment, including CPR or the use of a respirator.

◆   Any change in one's health can raise new questions.

◆   Talking with your physician and the members of the medical team who are treating your illness will help you make decisions about treatment choices.

◆   A copy of your completed advance directives should be given to your doctor, lawyer, your hospital's Medical Records Department, your family members and any institution where you receive medical treatments.

Note: You, a family member, your guardian or your agent (the authorized person in your Durable Power of Attorney for Health Care) can reverse or cancel your advance directive verbally by telling your doctor that you have changed your mind.

It's important to realize that even if you don't make a decision, that is a decision!

DECIDING ABOUT LIFE-AND-DEATH MEDICAL TREATMENTS

Each of us has the legal right to decide what life-sustaining treatments are acceptable to us. In some circumstances, depending on physical condition, age and personal philosophy, we may choose to refuse certain measures. Part of this decision should be based on whether the illness can be reversed. In the case of a chronic illness, it is vital to consider the pain and suffering, the length of time likely remaining and the likelihood of being able to reverse or improve the disease process or symptoms. To prepare for this kind of serious decision making, it's important to have full medical information, to consider your personal beliefs and to understand what's involved in different types of life-saving measures.

Your decisions about what medical treatment you want may differ depending on the type of medical situation you are considering:

◆ an acute illness that will respond to treatment;

◆ a chronic (incurable) illness that may respond to treatments for a period of time;

◆ an irreversible coma;

◆ an accident resulting in massive irreversible injuries;

◆ a sudden, catastrophic event, such as a heart attack, that cannot be cured by CPR, medicines or an operation; or

◆ progressive failure of body organs (heart, lung, liver, kidney) when transplants are not feasible.

Remember, if no information about your medical treatment decisions is available, your doctors may be obligated to take extraordinary measures to keep you alive. Before you make your decisions, you'll want to discuss all of the potential alternatives and the consequences of those choices with your doctor, agent, lawyer and family, making sure you understand what's involved, so that your doctor and family will understand your wishes.

Here are some of the issues you may want to discuss with your physician:

◆ how many medicines, procedures or other treatments you would want if you were faced with a chronic illness or a potentially fatal illness;

◆ whether you would want to know what "extraordinary" measures to prolong your life could offer you;

◆ whether a cure would be possible;

◆ whether treatment could restore you to a level of activity you could live with or whether it would simply delay death, and

◆ whether, if you had a progressively incurable disease, you would want to reject medical or surgical treatment and simply choose relief of pain and "comfort care"?

TYPES OF LIFE-SAVING MEASURES

There are many life-saving measures that can be used.

Cardiopulmonary Resuscitation (CPR)
When a person's heart stops beating, several kinds of measures may be taken to start it again. These include chest compression (pushing against the breastbone), which in turn compresses the heart so that it will pump blood and thereby maintain circulation; electric shock to keep the heart beating; artificial breathing (see below); and the administration of drugs. The patient's chances for survival depend on what other medical problems are present and on how soon CPR is started. If you are already ill, your chances of recovery may be reduced. When the heart stops beating and the circulation stops, the brain begins to die within four minutes. After 10 minutes, brain damage is usually extensive, even if the person can be revived. If a person's chances of recovery are low, extreme measures are usually not successful.

Artificial Breathing (Use of a Ventilator)
A ventilator is a machine that helps a person breathe. A tube through the person's mouth or nose directs the air from the ventilator into the lungs. Sometimes the tube must go through an opening in the person's neck (a tracheostomy). Breathing with the help of a ventilator is often a temporary situation that can be stopped once other medical treatment reduces or eliminates the breathing problem. A person with severe lung or brain problems may con-

tinue to need the machine to breathe for a long time. You are unable to speak with the tube in place, but you may be able to communicate your wishes. Pneumonia and other infections are possible complications.

Emergency   Surgical   Procedures Emergency surgical procedures include head surgery (craniotomy) for bleeding, spine surgery (laminectomy) to reduce spinal nerve pressure that may cause paralysis, and chest or abdominal surgery for an acute infection (appendicitis) or for acute bleeding. Such procedures can sometimes be life-saving, but at other times may be futile and painful.

Comfort Care Care that helps keep a patient comfortable but does not treat an illness. This can include bathing, nutrition, fluids, massage and pain medications.

Artificial Feeding When you cannot eat or drink enough to keep your body going, food and fluids may need to be given in different ways. A small tube can be inserted through the nose, leading down into the stomach. This may be a temporary measure if your condition improves, or it may be permanent. There is a risk that liquid food, instead of going into the stomach, may enter the lungs by mistake and cause pneumonia. Although this type of pneumonia is usually easy to treat, it can become life threatening. Fluids and liquid feeding solutions can also be given through a tiny plastic tube directly into the veins, using an intravenous (IV) apparatus. Being fed this way is called hyperalimentation. Infection can occur where the tube enters the skin, causing either minor symptoms, such as pain and swelling, or more severe complications, including a blood infection.

Kidney Dialysis (Use of an Artificial Kidney Machine) Dialysis, the treatment used when a person experiences kidney failure, offers a chance to prolong life by clearing waste or toxins from the blood, but does not cure the kidney failure. Transplantation to replace the kidney is the only way to correct irreversible kidney failure.

Chemotherapy (Use of Special Drugs to Fight Cancer) Drugs used in cancer treatment may have many side effects, many of which can be controlled. In some cases, the drugs may actually cure the cancer; in others, they may produce temporary remissions or prolong life.

Pain Medications These medicines are used to control pain and keep patients comfortable.

Antibiotics (Medicines That Fight Infection) Antibiotics are usually, but not always, effective in treating infections. If a serious infection is present and antibiotics are not taken, the patient may die of the infection. Possible side effects of antibiotics include lack of appetite, nausea, diarrhea and allergic reactions.

Diagnostic Tests Diagnostic tests might include such exams as a CT (computerized tomography) scan, MRI (magnetic resonance imaging), x-rays, a spinal tap, a bone marrow aspiration, an endoscopy (the use of a flexible fiber-optic scope to examine the intestines, stomach or colon), or a bronchoscopy (the use of a scope to examine bronchi, the large breathing passages of the lungs). Many of these tests require that a tube be inserted into the patient's body; pain medication is also usually given. Such tests may be necessary to find out what is wrong. The tests may also help the medical team decide whether further medical treatment is appropriate. Each test has risks associated with it, which can be mild to severe.

UNDERSTANDING HOSPITAL "CODES"

An area of information that's important to understand before making your decisions about life-and-death medical treatment is the hospital "codes" that specify what level of resuscitation (CPR) will be provided by your health care team when you are hospitalized.

◆ **Full Code**

A patient with full-code status will receive all of the treatments needed to keep the heart beating and lungs breathing: chest compression, assisted breathing (breathing tubes and respirators), heart electrical shock (defibrillation) and/or special medications.

◆ **Modified Code**

This involves less-aggressive treatment, including a selection of some of the full-code measures listed above. The choice of treatment measures depends on your condition and on your expressed wishes.

◆ **Chemical Code (Pharmacologic Code)**

This restricts treatment to the use of special medicines given into your veins— usually for heart, lung or kidney failure. No aggressive attempts (i.e., CPR) will be made to restart breathing or the heartbeat should they stop.

◆ **No Code (DNR—Do Not Resuscitate)**

This status means that no attempts will made to restart breathing or the heartbeat should they stop. Full efforts for comfort care will be given.

HOW TO SAFEGUARD YOUR DECISIONS

Several kinds of documents can be used to specify your treatment wishes to your doctors and family members. It's important to know that you can change or cancel any of these documents at any time as long as you can communicate your wishes.

Unless you sign (or your surrogate signs) an advance directive stating otherwise, if you have a sudden medical catastrophe, such as a heart attack, you will receive full resuscitative procedures, including cardiac resuscitation, heart electrical shock, assisted breathing (respirator) and drug therapy with life-sustaining drugs given intravenously.

The Medical Emergency Wallet Card (*see* Chapter 36 for an example) is an easy way to specify your decisions in a simple format. It's important to carry information concerning medical treatment and code status requests on a card that you keep with you at all times, preferably near your driver's license. On this card you can indicate which medical directives have been signed and where they can be found.

TYPES OF ADVANCE DIRECTIVES

Several kinds of advance directives can be used to inform care providers of your treatment wishes. The Durable Power of Attorney for Health Care and the California Natural Death Act Declaration are both documents that are legally recognized in California; see Chapter 36 for examples of each document. *The relevant legislation for your state should be available through your local public library or through a lawyer.*

In California, only one of these documents—either the Durable Power of Attorney for Health Care or the California Natural Death Act Declaration—is needed to make your medical treatment desires known to your family, your doctor and your treatment facility. You may, however, use both if you wish. Each of these documents can be revoked or changed as your circumstances change.

After completing your advance directive, remember to give a copy to each of your doctors and to the person you name as your agent (if this is applicable). Also, take a copy with you whenever you go to a hospital or other treatment facility. The advance directive should be on file in the hospital's medical records department.

THE DURABLE POWER OF ATTORNEY FOR HEALTH CARE

The Durable Power of Attorney for Health Care, authorized by California law since 1984, is the most complete and most effective document for ensuring that your desires regarding health care treatment are followed. Your state may have passed similar legislation, available from your local public library or a lawyer.

With this document, you designate someone as your "agent" or "proxy" (attorney-in-fact), authorizing him or her to make decisions about your medical care, including withdrawal of life support, when you are unable to make decisions for yourself. Your agent may make all decisions about your health care, subject to any restrictions on that person's authority that you specify, as well as to any restrictions imposed by law, that are stated within the document.

When naming your agent, consider someone who knows your values, with whom you feel comfortable talking, whom you can trust, who will be there if you become seriously ill and who can carry out the decisions you've made. You will want to discuss your specific wishes with the agent you select. (Even if you do not want to name someone specific to act as your agent, you can still use this document to spell out your intentions.)

You don't need a lawyer to complete this directive. If you are at least 18 years old and of sound mind, you may fill it out. The Durable Power of Attorney for Health Care must be signed by two witnesses other than the person or persons you have designated to act for you, or it must be signed before a notary public. The witnesses cannot be doctors or others involved in your health care, and one of them must be unrelated to you and not an heir to your estate. Your document might include a statement of your specific preferences about treatment (a codicil)

to give to your agent and doctor, or you might want to select one of the general statements below to reflect your wishes:

"I do not want efforts made to prolong my life and I do not want life-sustaining treatment to be provided or continued:

1. if I am in an irreversible coma or persistent vegetative state; or
2. if I am terminally ill and the application of life-sustaining procedures would serve only to artificially delay the moment of my death; or
3. under any circumstances where the burdens of the treatment outweigh the expected benefits. I want my agent to consider the relief of suffering and the quality as well as the extent of the possible extension of my life in making decisions concerning life-sustaining treatments."

(or)

"I want efforts to be made to prolong my life and I want life-sustaining treatment to be provided unless I am in a coma or persistent vegetative state which my doctor reasonably believes to be irreversible. Once my doctor has concluded that I will remain unconscious for the rest of my life, I do not want life-sustaining treatment to be provided or continued."

Durable Power of Attorney for Health Care forms come in different formats. They all contain the same basic information. You can obtain a form from your doctor or hospital. You can also arrange to get one from the California Medical Association and other sources listed in the Resources at the back of this book. Many stationery stores also carry these forms.

To get more information about advance directives, you may call the American Medical Association at 1-800-621-8335 to order the brochure "Advance Medical Directives for Patients," or write to

Pritchett & Hull Associates, Inc. at Suite 110, 3440 Oakcliff Rd NE, Atlanta, GA 30340-3079 to order the book *Decide for Yourself.*

THE CALIFORNIA NATURAL DEATH ACT DECLARATION

This document—provided for by the California Natural Death Act, which became effective January 1, 1992—allows you to instruct your doctor not to use artificial methods to extend the natural process of dying.

The Declaration must be witnessed by two adults, at least one of whom is not mentioned in your will and would have no claim to your estate. You may sign a Declaration if you are at least 18 years old, of sound mind and acting of your own free will. You do not need an attorney.

This document becomes operative when it is communicated to your doctor. Your diagnosis must be certified in writing by both your doctor and a second physician who has personally determined that you are in a terminal condition or a permanent unconscious condition and are no longer able to make decisions regarding the administration of life-sustaining treatment.

The Declaration states:

"If I should have an incurable and irreversible condition that has been diagnosed by two physicians and that will result in my death within a relatively short time without the administration of life-sustaining treatment or that has produced an irreversible coma or persistent vegetative state, and I am no longer able to make decisions regarding my medical treatment, I direct my attending physician, pursuant to the Natural Death Act of California, to withhold or withdraw treatment, including artificially administered nutrition and hydration, that only prolongs the process of dying or the irreversible coma or persistent vegetative state and is not necessary for my comfort or to alleviate pain."

You have the option of deleting the phrase "including artificially administered nutrition and hydration" if you want to continue to receive feeding by means of a tube, even if other treatments are stopped.

Unlike the Durable Power of Attorney for Health Care document, this Declaration does not require you to name an agent to carry out your wishes; however, having an agent is helpful.

A SPECIAL DIRECTIVE— THE PREHOSPITAL DO NOT RESUSCITATE (DNR) FORM FOR CALIFORNIA

This document is for people who are at home, in a health care facility, in a hospice or being transported from one such facility to another. It instructs emergency medical services (EMS) personnel not to resuscitate you. This DNR form is legal in California only for emergency medical services—for instance, when you call 911. The document directs EMS personnel not to perform resuscitation procedures, including chest compression, assisted breathing, cardiac drugs and other extraordinary measures. The document is signed by the patient or an appropriate surrogate (the patient's legal representative—e.g., a Durable Power of Attorney for Health Care agent) and by the patient's physician. Other states may have similar legislation.

Note: To make sure that EMS personnel honor your wishes, you can get a special instructive DNR wallet card and/or a DNR wrist or neck medallion from the Medic Alert Foundation (*see* Medic Alert, p. 374).

If you don't want to draw up a formal document, you can simply inform your doctor of your wishes so that he or she can write them into your medical record, or you can talk with your family and friends. However, a written document signed by you and by the appropriate witnesses, or notarized, is the best way to make sure your intentions are carried out.

Forms for California are found in Chapter 36 of this book and are also avail-able at the UCSF/Mount Zion Hospital Cancer Resource Center, 2356 Sutter Street, 2nd floor, San Francisco, CA 94115 (telephone 415-885-3693).

35
YOUR LEGACY OF LOVE

Ernest H. Rosenbaum, MD, Isadora R. Rosenbaum, MA, Thomas Addison, MD, Joanna Beam, JD, Meryl Brod, PhD, David Claman, MD, Alan J. Coleman, MD Malin Dollinger, MD, Michael Glover, Nancy Lambert, RN, BSN, Elmo Petterle, Patricia Sparacino, RN, MS, Jeffery Silberman, DMin, Kenneth A. Woeber, MD

Life is full of unplanned events. Perhaps the most challenging of these events to cope with is the death of a loved one. It's been estimated that 93 percent of all families are not prepared when a relative dies. Important documents need to be located, funeral arrangements need to be made and vital matters need to be decided.

It's important to realize that death is actually a shared experience. Although each of us must face our own death, our survivors are also affected by and suffer because of our dying. They are left to cope with both the emotional adjustment of losing a loved one and the responsibility of dealing with someone else's affairs.

HOW YOU CAN HELP YOUR SURVIVORS

Your legacy of love for your survivors can, with careful thought and compassion, be one of clear decisions and planned arrangements—a house swept clean of personal, financial and business cobwebs. By sorting out your affairs now, you can spare your survivors an inheritance of scattered papers and countless details to be waded through. Instead, you can bequeath to them the gifts of clear direction, rich memories and unique insights.

The processes of dying and death dictate many decisions that must be carried out by your survivors, typically at a time of great stress. They often have to come up with answers to troubling questions—such as what last-minute medical treatments to accept or reject on your behalf, whom to notify if you die, what arrangements to make to tend to your body and pay tribute to your life, which resources to turn to in order to settle liabilities and disperse assets, and what memories to embrace in order to best remember you.

By taking time and care now to attend to each of the following areas of importance, you'll be providing benefits to yourself and those you love. In the short term, you'll reap the benefit of peace of mind, which comes from organization and control of your affairs, and in the long term, you'll know that what will be done is what you would have wanted.

Before considering the areas listed below, first plan where you are going to store this information file so that those who will need it will know where to find it and will be able to find it easily. Then be sure to tell those who need to know about its location. You might consider putting the most important legal documents in a safe-deposit box, but be sure to tell those who need to know that this box exists, where to find the key and how to gain access to the box. Your legacy of love can best be promoted by completing the forms found in Chapter 36, "Forms and Worksheets for Decision Making."

ADVANCE DIRECTIVES

By completing a Durable Power of Attorney for Health Care form or a Natural Death Act Declaration, you are providing both your family and your health care team with guidance about your decisions. As discussed in Chapter 34, "Decisions for Life," a copy of this directive should be given to a family member and to your doctor for inclusion in your medical record. It should be included in your hospital record if you are hospitalized.

Be sure to include the name, address and phone number of your primary care doctor and any other specialists in this medical information file. (*See* the Medical Emergency Wallet Card in Chapter 36.)

LEGAL WILL

Preparing a will is one of the most important responsibilities you have. Make this a priority. Should you die without a will (called dying intestate) or leave an invalid will, state laws will govern the distribution of your estate. Your estate might wind up being administered by a total stranger appointed by the court. Should both parents of a child or children die without a will, a court-appointed guardian takes custody of any minor children and of the parents' estate.

Preparing a will encourages you to assess your financial situation and to ensure that your property, savings, benefits and assets will be managed according to your wishes. In most cases, you will need a lawyer to guide you and protect your estate. The laws concerning wills are complex and vary by state.

Writing your own will, though, is better than leaving none at all. An entirely handwritten (holographic) will, signed and dated by you, can be binding and enforceable. California accepts holographic wills, but not all states do.

Be sure to review your will periodically to keep your information up to date. If you divorce, separate or remarry or if the status of your named heirs changes, be sure to revise your will appropriately.

In considering your will's contents, be prepared to include information about an executor (the person you name to carry out the terms of your will), your children, anyone you wish to "disinherit," your assets, tax implications, gifts, trusts, revocable living trust (talk to a knowledgeable person about the advantages and disadvantages of this technique to avoid probate), life insurance and charitable contributions.

PERSONS TO NOTIFY

Include the names, addresses and phone numbers of doctors, attorneys, employers, relatives, friends, business associates, the executor or trustee of your estate, religious and social organizations and anyone else who should be notified of your death. (*See* page 375.)

ARRANGEMENTS FOR YOUR BODY

It is important to make decisions regarding organ donation, burial, cremation and donation of your body for scientific research, and then make appropriate plans based on those decisions. You might want to compose your own inscription to appear on a headstone. It is wise to select and designate the plot, location and mortuary of your choice in advance. (*See* pages 376 and 377.)

Note: If you wish to donate your organs, fill out the appropriate places on your driver's license and the Medical Emergency Wallet Card (*see* Chapter 36).

OBITUARY

What would you like your local newspaper to say about you? You can help your family by providing information about your place of birth, career background, education, special achievements, military service, involvement with organizations, hobbies and memorial contribution preferences. (*See* page 377.)

MEMORIAL SERVICE

Your clergy can help provide guidelines regarding mourning or burial rituals. If you know the type of service you want (for instance, public or private), where the service should be held, what music should be played, who should officiate and so on, this is the time to spell out your preferences in writing. Be sure to notify the appropriate family member or friend who would need to know this information. (*See* page 375.)

BENEFIT INFORMATION

Survivors may be entitled to benefits you've earned or provided for. These may include benefits from life insurance, pension and profit-sharing plans, including Keogh plans, IRAs, Social Security, Medicare, supplemental medical insurance, Veterans' benefits or Workers' Compensation benefits. Assemble this information and mark it clearly. Provide account numbers, contact names, and addresses and phone numbers, if possible. (*See* page 371.)

ASSETS AND LIABILITIES

This section of the file should include information about bank and savings and loan accounts (including T-bills and CDs); investments (stocks, bonds and investment funds, including money market accounts, mutual funds, government securities, limited partnerships and annuities); real estate (your home, investment properties, and other assets); notes, first or second mortgages (that you owe or that are owed to you); other liabilities (including home mortgage, investment properties, and business, auto and personal loans); and any recommendations about investments for your survivors.

INSURANCE INFORMATION

Provide information on insurance policies for your home (whether you own or rent it) and auto. (Life insurance is listed above under "Benefit Information.") Record the addresses of all insured properties and the license numbers of all insured cars. Provide the documentation for each insurance policy as well as contact names, addresses and phone numbers. (*See* page 371.)

HOME AND PERSONAL PROPERTY INVENTORY

An inventory is a practical way of listing your belongings, identifying each item, specifying its location, estimating its value and naming the heir to whom you're giving it. (*See* page 372–3.)

Use this opportunity to give away items you're not interested in keeping—donate usable items to charity or have a garage sale. You may want to give away some of your belongings now to your family or friends and take advantage of the opportunity to see them enjoying your former possessions.

YOUR PERSONAL OR "ETHICAL" WILL

This is a rare opportunity to take the time to express your innermost thoughts. You might want to write a personal note to your loved ones or specific personal messages to each of them. You might want to record your thoughts on audiotape or videotape. This is your most meaningful legacy—it expresses who you are, records your autobiography and reflects your life philosophy. The thoughts you share here will provide a lasting and precious memory for your survivors. Include anecdotes, favorite quotations and philosophies. You might also want to include any diaries, pictures or journals you'd like to pass on.

You may wish to make a log booklet or a tape recording of your life history. Talk in depth about your early life experiences, beginning with your youth. Recount memories of parents, grandparents, aunts, uncles, siblings, children, friends, neighbors, colleagues and pets.

Leave a rich family history by providing a family tree. This is also a good time to map out a family medical tree. Write down any medical conditions that you or your relatives may have had—this can be valuable information for your family now and for generations to come.

YOUR PERSONAL OR "ETHICAL" WILL
At this time in my life I wish to share my feelings with you. I would like to tell you of my thoughts, hopes and wishes.

I would like to tell you my life story and what I can remember about my parents, grandparents and family.

Additional personal thoughts for family/friends.

I would like to create a family tree.

| GRANDFATHER | GRANDMOTHER | GRANDFATHER | GRANDMOTHER |

MOTHER   FATHER

CHILDREN

The above diagram is intended as a model only. Please include your Family Tree information with photographs on additional pages as necessary.

36
FORMS AND WORKSHEETS FOR DECISION MAKING

—————◇—————

This chapter contains examples of the various forms described in Chapters 34 and 35, as well as a short glossary of terms that may be helpful when filling out the forms.

CHECKLIST OF FORMS AND WORKSHEETS

Indicate to those who need to know where the following information is being kept. Do not keep this information in a safe-deposit box: give it to your doctor, family, lawyer, agent (as designated in the Durable Power of Attorney for Health Care) and hospital medical records department.

Advance Directives (*See* Chapter 34)
Durable Power of Attorney for Health Care form
California Natural Death Act Declaration (Directive to Physicians)
Prehospital Do Not Resuscitate (DNR) form
Medical Emergency Wallet Card
Your Legacy of Love (*See* Chapter 35)
Legal Will
Persons to Notify
Arrangements for Your Body
Obituary
Memorial Service
Benefit Information
Assets and Liabilities
Insurance Information
Home and Personal Property Inventory
Your Personal or "Ethical" Will

Forms (reprinted later in this chapter)
Additional Considerations for Advance Directives: My Specific Preferences for Life Support (Heroic Measures) form
Family Information form

Location of Records form
Review of Home and Personal Property Assets
Medic Alert form
People to Notify after Death
Instructions to Clergy
Obituary for Newspapers

Many of these documents are available at the UCSF/Mount Zion Cancer Resource Center, 2356 Sutter Street, 2nd floor, San Francisco, CA 94115 (telephone 415-885-3693).

Ninety-three percent of families are said to be unprepared when a death occurs: the time to act is now.

A BRIEF GLOSSARY OF TERMS USED IN THE FORMS THAT FOLLOW

Advance Directives: Advance directives are legal documents, such as the Durable Power of Attorney for Health Care form, the California Natural Death Act Declaration and the Emergency Medical Services Prehospital Do Not Resuscitate (DNR) form. They specify the type of medical care a person wants or does not want.

Cardiopulmonary Resuscitation (CPR): Use of chest compression, drugs and electric shock to restart the heart and/or a breathing tube and ventilator (respirator) to maintain lung function.

Code: Acute heart and/or lung failure requiring cardiopulmonary treatments (CPR) to restart a person's heart or sustain breathing to avoid brain damage.

Comfort Care: Care that helps keep a person comfortable but does not treat an illness. Such measures can include bathing, nutrition, fluids, massage and pain medications (narcotics and sedatives).

Organ Donation: The act of a person who authorizes (by giving his or her signed permission) the giving of one or more of his or her organs (such as a heart, kidney or liver) to another when the organ donor dies.

Persistent Vegetative State: Term used to describe the condition of a person who is in a coma and has no hope of regaining consciousness even with medical treat-ment. The person may move and respond to pain, but cannot think.

FORMS AND WORKSHEETS
Getting Your Affairs in Order: Practical Financial, Retirement and Estate-Planning Worksheets, by Elmo Petterle.

Filling in the forms on the pages that follow will help you ensure that your loved ones are cared for after your death.

TO SEAL YOUR CARD AT HOME —WRAP IN SCOTCH TAPE

MEDICAL EMERGENCY WALLET CARD©

NAME   SS NO.

    DOB   /   /

ADDRESS

    TEL.   /

NEAREST RELATIVE   TEL.   /   CITY

PHYSICIAN   TEL.   /   CITY

CLERGY   TEL.   /   CITY

DIAGNOSIS

MEDICATIONS

LEGAL WILL   YES☐ / NO☐   LOCATION OF DOCUMENTS

Advance Directives Location _____

Durable Power of Attorney for Health Care   YES☐ NO☐

Desig. Agent   Tel.   /   City

California Natural Death Act (Declaration to Physician)   YES☐ NO☐

Prehospital Do Not Resuscitate (DNR) (Declaration to Physician) YES☐ NO☐

Resuscitation:

	Chest Compression	Mechanical Ventilation	Drugs Therapy
Acute (Reversible)	YES☐ NO☐	YES☐ NO☐	YES☐ NO☐
Chronic (incurable)	YES☐ NO☐	YES☐ NO☐	YES☐ NO☐

Organ Donation: Cornea Y☐ N☐   Liver Y☐ N☐   Bones Y☐ N☐
      Heart Y☐ N☐   Skin Y☐ N☐
      Kidney Y☐ N☐   Middle Ear Y☐ N☐

Signature   Date   /   /

Witness   Relationship

ADDITIONAL CONSIDERATIONS FOR THE ADVANCE DIRECTIVES
MY SPECIFIC PREFERENCES FOR LIFE SUPPORT (HEROIC MEASURES)

People's preferences for use or non-use of life sustaining measures may vary depending upon the specific life sustaining measure being considered. In addition, preferences are influenced by different health conditions. Below are several health situations you may encounter. Please check which life sustaining measures you want, do not want, or are undecided about for each of these different situations. In situation 5, you may put your own situation if it has not been covered. If you would like a limited trial only, place a T in the "I want" column.

If you would like, you may attach this form to your Durable Power of Attorney for Health Care or your California Natural Death Act form. If it is attached, signed and witnessed, it will be considered a legally binding preference for your physician or designated surrogate decision maker.

NAME

DATE

WITNESS

WITNESS

(Please use the same witnesses as on Durable Powers Form)

LIFE SUSTAINING MEASURES	Situation 1 — I do not have a terminal illness and I can care for myself. However, everything takes much effort and I am in constant pain (as in arthritis). If I suddenly require medical help (as in a heart attack or pneumonia), treatment for this emergency can return me to my usual level of functioning. If not treated, I will most likely die. In such a case, my preferences are:			Situation 2 — I have a chronic and terminal disease. I cannot accomplish my own self-care such as eating, toileting, dressing, walking, but I do recognize everyone around me. (This could be the case in advanced cancer, lung disease, paralysis from stroke.) If an emergency arises, my preferences are:			Situation 3 — I have a disease from which I will become progressively confused and incapacitated, such as in Alzheimer's Disease. I may not always be able to take care of myself or recognize people. In an emergency occurs my preferences are:			Situation 4 — I am in a persistent state of vegetation (coma). I cannot eat, dress, toilet myself or recognize people. (This could occur in the stages of Alzheimer's disease or severe stroke.) If an emergency occurs, my preferences are:			Situation 5 — Please write in any other scenario which is important to you:		
	I WANT	I DO NOT WANT	UNDECIDED	I WANT	I DO NOT WANT	UNDECIDED	I WANT	I DO NOT WANT	UNDECIDED	I WANT	I DO NOT WANT	UNDECIDED	I WANT	I DO NOT WANT	UNDECIDED
1. Cardiopulmonary Resuscitation															
2. Mechanical Breathing															
3. Artificial Food & Fluids															
4. Painful or Potentially Harmful Diagnostic Tests															
5. Antibotics															
6. Include here any other directives important to you															

FAMILY INFORMATION	
Name	
Residence	
Telephone	
Birthdate and Place	
Social Security Number	
Military Service Serial Number	
Spouse or Next of Kin	
Children	Telephone
Special plans for children in event of parent's death	
Designated Guardian	
Mother	Telephone
Father	Telephone
Maternal Grandparents	
Paternal Grandparents	
Grandchildren	
Blood/Genetic Information	
VA Claim Number	
Date and Place of Discharge	
Significant Other Person	Telephone
Special plans for pets (name/type of/who will adopt)	
Additional significant information	
Signature	Date
Spouse/Partner	Date

LOCATION OF RECORDS

ITEM	LOCATION	
Wills	Legal Will	Living Trust
Durable Power of Attorney		
Calif. Natural Death Act		
Pre-nuptial Agreement		
Financial	Who has access	
Safe-deposit box	Key	Number
Banks/Account Nos:	Savings	Money Market Funds
	Checking	
*Stocks and Bonds		
*Deeds of Trust		
Loans	Loan Accounts	
Loans Owed to Us		
*T-bills, Cert. of Deposit		
Trusts	Attorney	
Address		
Business Records	Briefcase combination	
Limited Partnerships		
Real Estate Records		
Mortgage Documents		
Miscellaneous Contracts		
Pensions	IRA	Keough
Work/Company Pension Plan		
Workers Comp. Records		
Social Security Records		
Tax I.D. Number(s)		
Veterans Records		
*Insurance Policies		
*Auto Ownership Certificates		
Credit Cards		
Installment Payments		
Warranties		
Personal		
Passports		
*Birth Certificates		
Ministorage or Warehouse	Key/combination	
Charitable Gifts		
Church		
Individuals		
Organizations		

Signature _____ Date _____

Spouse/Partner _____ Date _____

*Recommend keeping in safe-deposit box

REVIEW OF HOME AND PERSONAL PROPERTY ASSETS
(Brief Review — To Be Expanded As Needed)

1. Stocks and Bonds (Broker)   Location—To be given to

2. Properties (Name, Mortgage)   Location—To be given to

3. Bank Accounts (Account Numbers)   Location—To be given to

   Business

   Checking

4. Insurance Policies (Agent)   Location—To be given to

5. Cars

6. Current Liabilities and Loans   Document Location

   Home Mortgage   = $

   Business Loans   = $

   Automobile Loans = $

   Personal Loans   = $

   IRS Income Tax   = $

   Credit Union   = $

7. Home Assets Inventory

   Living Room   Designated Recipient

    Furniture

    Paintings

    Rugs

    Piano

   Dining Room

Furniture

Dishes

Miscellaneous

Silver

Crystal

Miscellaneous (Mirrors, lamps)

Antiques

Jewelry

Appliances

Televisions

Audio Equipment

Records/Audio- and Videotapes

Refrigerator/Stove

Washer/Dryer

Bedrooms

Stamp collection

Coin collection

Miscellaneous
It is worth making a home inventory list with an appraisal and designating the person(s) to whom you wish to will items. Dividing and distributing family pictures, heirlooms and special items can make decisions easier for those you love and can make a willed gift more appreciated.

Signature   Date

Spouse/Partner   Date

MEDIC ALERT® SERVICE FORM

TO ENROLL BY PHONE Call 1-800-432-5378 anytime. Have the following information ready: 1) Credit card number and expiration date; 2) Medical information; 3) Name, telephone number and address of persons and physician(s) to contact in an emergency; 4) Bracelet size (when ordering bracelet)

TO ENROLL BY MAIL Complete form and mail with payment to Medic Alert®, 2323 Colorado Ave, Turlock, CA 95382 Please photocopy form for other enrollees.

1. **ARE YOU OR HAVE YOU BEEN A MEDIC ALERT MEMBER?**   Yes ☐   No ☐   If yes, Enter Member Number

2. **PERSONAL INFORMATION:** Print or type clearly.   Sex   Social Security Number

Last name	First	Middle

Date of Birth
Mo.   Day   Year

Mailing address	Phone Area Code ( )

City	State	Zip

EMERGENCY CONTACTS: As a free service, Medic Alert will advise your physician of your enrollment, and emergency information.

Person 1	Phone ( )	Person 2	Phone ( )
Physician 1	Phone ( )	Physician 2	Phone ( )
Address		Address	

3. **MEDICAL INFORMATION TO BE ENGRAVED ON EMBLEM:** (will also appear on computer record and wallet card). Dosage data not needed. Engraving space is limited. Small bracelet emblem: limit: 60 spaces. Large bracelet emblem and necklace emblems: limit 90 spaces. Allow one space between words.

4. **OTHER EMERGENCY MEDICAL INFORMATION:** For your computer record and wallet card. Dosage data not needed.

5. **STYLE AND SIZE OF EMBLEM:** *Select your emblem below by checking box:*

Metal Type	Necklace	Large Bracelet	Small Bracelet	Fee**
Stainless Steel	☐	☐	☐	$35
Sterling Silver (Raised)	☐	☐	☐	$50
Gold Filled (Raised design, 10 KT)	☐	☐	☐	$75
Designer Silver (Recessed Design)		☐	☐	$115

(Fees & Terms as of 10/93, subject to change without notice.)

*Bracelet Size: ☐   ☐   ☐   ☐   ☐   ☐   ☐
6"   6½"   7"   7½"   8"   8½"   9"

6. **PAYMENT CALCULATION**

REGISTRATION FEE:.................................. $_____
(Tax deductible medical expense.) Includes issuance of ID number, wallet card and one custom engraved emblem with chain.

ANNUAL MEMBERSHIP FEE: $15 (first year free)............. $_____
Covers 24 hour year round emergency hot line service and free updating of your computer record.

CONTRIBUTION: (tax deductible)................................. $_____
Medic Alert, a non profit foundation, is partly supported by contributions for professional and public education programs.

TOTAL AMOUNT ENCLOSED:...................................... $_____

7. **METHOD OF PAYMENT:**
☐ Check ☐ MasterCard ☐ VISA ☐ Discover
☐ Money Order   *(no other cards accepted.)*

No CODs. Payment must accompany order. Send to:
Medic Alert, 2323 Colorado Ave., Turlock, CA 95382

Card Number
Expiration Date   ____   ____

LEGAL STATEMENT: IMPORTANT: The member agrees not to wear the emblem or carry the wallet card until the emergency record has been carefully checked by the member for correctness, and agrees to inform Medic Alert in writing of any error found. The member authorizes Medic Alert to relay information in response to emergency telephone calls. The member agrees to immediately notify Medic Alert Whenever his/her medical condition or address changes.

8. **I understand and accept the legal statement printed above.**

1643

PEOPLE TO NOTIFY AFTER DEATH

Directory of Officials, Relatives and Friends
Clergy
Telephone
Office Staff
Telephone Number(s)
Funeral Director
Telephone
For Organ Donation
Contact
Telephone
Attorney
Telephone
Accountant
Telephone
Executor/Executrix of Will
Telephone Number(s)
Life Insurance Agent
Telephone
Bank Trust Officer
Telephone
Social Security Admin
Veterans Administrator

ALSO NOTIFY

Other Relatives and Close Friends	Telephone Number(s)

Signature	Date
Spouse/Partner	Date

INSTRUCTIONS TO CLERGY
Type of burial memorial
☐ Cremation   ☐ Casket
In church/temple
At funeral home
Open or closed casket
At the gravesite
The Committal should be   ☐ public   ☐ private
If cremation, instruction for ashes
Specific desires for the service, i.e., suggested readings/music
Viewing
Grave marker (tombstone)
Decoration
Flowers
Inscription
Casket: ☐ wood   ☐ metal
Burial: ☐ shroud   ☐ street clothes
Gravesite
Family plot located
Previously purchased gravesite location
Memorial gifts/donations to agencies or foundations
Other comments, instructions or wishes

Signature	Date
Spouse/Partner	Date

OBITUARY FOR NEWSPAPERS

Name

Notes about life and achievements

Birthplace

Career

Hobbies

Organizations

Names of Relatives

Achievements

College   Degree(s)

Military Service

Memorial Donations

Preferred Funeral Arrangements

Place of Funeral Service   Time

Additional Information or Instructions

Signature   Date

Spouse/Partner   Date

CONCLUSION: CHOOSING LIFE

Ernest H. Rosenbaum, MD, and Isadora R. Rosenbaum, MA

Look to this day, for it is life, ...
For yesterday is but a dream,
And tomorrow is only a vision.
But today, well lived,
Makes every yesterday a dream of happiness,
And every tomorrow a vision of hope.

—Sanskrit Proverb

———————⬦———————

TO THE PATIENT

This guide has presented concepts, information and methods that can help give direction to your desire to rehabilitate yourself. Our concept of rehabilitation is one that requires a total approach to the person with cancer—one that includes the mind and body with exercise, nutrition, sexuality and supportive care, as well as the efforts of your health care team.

Only by acquiring specific knowledge can we begin to conceive possible solutions to our complex health problems. To achieve any level of success, you, the patient, must accept responsibility for the role you can play in your medical care. Having made the critical decision that you want to get well, you must believe that it is worth the effort and be willing to make sacrifices and give sufficient attention to the task.

Frequently, coping requires a compromise—to accept what cannot be changed and to proceed from there. A patient who copes can set new, realistic goals. He or she must leave anger and bitterness behind and free up energies to live in the present.

To live in the present a patient must have hope, because hope is an essential part of the will to live. Hope can come from many sources: from the doctor who shares his or her therapeutic plans with the patient, or from the family members and friends who seek to help. But primarily, hope will come from the patient who is willing to help him- or herself.

THE MIND

By knowing yourself, your goals in life, your limits and capacities and how to compensate for the stresses and trials of daily life, you can accelerate your rehabilitation. Knowing how to keep your "cool," how to keep your frustration level low and how to make appropriate use of support systems can make the difference between success and failure in treatment. Psychological and spiritual aids can help control the disturbances of external mental pressures.

THE BODY

When you have a disease, there is an accompanying chronic feeling of tiredness, often so subtle that it may not be recognized for what it really is.

376

Expending energy appropriately is paramount, lest the tiredness be compounded and come to characterize daily life. An energy deficit manifests itself in how we feel, emotionally and physically. It can mean the difference between health or illness, misery or happiness. Fortunately, we have an energy reserve upon which to draw. Energy needs may be constant and predictable, yet vary in the ways they are met. The better our mental and physical state, the greater our vitality and energy reserves. The concepts and methods discussed in this book are designed to help you achieve the highest level of functioning possible within the limits of your disease.

GUIDELINES TO KEEP IN MIND

Adequate Sleep Your need for sleep will vary, depending in part on your activities and habits (not all people require eight hours of sleep nightly). Prolonged lack of sleep reduces efficiency and the ability to function. How you sleep is important too. A good night's sleep is "as good as gold. " If sleeping pills or tranquilizers are helpful in obtaining an adequate night's rest, they should be used. Resolving any perplexing and annoying emotional problems helps immeasurably. The use of relaxing techniques, meditation and biofeedback is often invaluable.

Nutrition Fad nutritional notions and diets should be avoided. Eating balanced meals, with adequate protein and calories, is vital in helping you to tolerate therapy, to fight disease and to gain the strength to return to active life.

Physical Exercise An active and organized exercise program—with appropriate rest periods—is absolutely essential in maintaining good physical status. Exercise provides a feeling of well-being, reduces stress, aids relaxation, increases reserve strength and promotes better sleep. Graduated levels of exercise that add increasing variations as you improve will prevent fatigue and frustration. Nothing is more reassuring than to see and feel self-improvement. Concurrent use of an occupational physical therapy program will help accelerate your recovery.

Sexuality Your sexuality is still a part of your total being when you have a chronic illness, and it is an area of concern that should not be ignored. If adjustments in your patterns of sexual expression are necessary, communication between you and your partner may enable you to work these out alone. For those who need help, counseling is available.

Relaxation Time Periods of "trained relaxation" two to three times a day will help make life more enjoyable. We go through so many changes daily—from hectic stress periods to periods of diversion and relaxation—that we need a tool to help us cope with them. Meditation, biofeedback and other techniques can relax the mind and reduce stress. Outlets such as hobbies, sports and various types of mental or physical games help maintain energy resources. Allot specific time to "be good to yourself." These times should be private, personal and inviolate. Don't use your relaxation time as a work period! To do so will only increase mental tension and physical exhaustion.

In short, a person needs to restructure his or her life to succeed in obtaining as full a rehabilitation as possible, no matter what the problem. A person cannot change completely, but daily habit patterns, even some of life-long duration, can be adjusted and altered by setting reasonable goals and personal priorities, so that time is used both efficiently and constructively. The self-help/self-support programs described in this guide are designed to help you formulate a better recovery program.

TO THE FAMILY AND FRIENDS

There are many resources for patients with cancer, but probably the greatest allies to the physician are you, the close family and friends who are available for help when the need arises; you offer a reserve that cannot be found in any other resource. Your continued love and compassion give hope and courage to the patient.

We all need love. The person who is ill is particularly vulnerable to the feelings of being alone and abandoned. Thus, the importance of the family's and friends' understanding of the patient cannot be overestimated. Without your support, the patient's recovery process may be prolonged.

Illness, incapacity and the threat of death are difficult subjects for a patient and his or her family and friends to discuss together. You may want to talk to each other but be hindered in your desires because you want to protect one another or because you do not wish to face the truth yourselves. The inability to communicate can occur with all people at any time, but it is usually heightened under conditions of stress.

Families and friends faced with the life-threatening illness of a loved one have the dual problem of trying to control their own fears and anxieties while giving encouragement and support to the patient. They may spend their time wondering how to ease the patient's emotional suffering, while the patient is busy worrying about the despair of those he or she loves. Each is searching for the most tactful way to deal with the other.

Our experience with patients has shown, however, that a deliberate policy of candor and openness will create an atmosphere that is beneficial to all concerned. It can remove the burden of secrecy and open the door for the alleviation of apprehensions. Candor may not be easily achieved, for often people are not in the habit of speaking about their deepest concerns. Even those who have established close relationships may become faint-hearted in the presence of cancer and the threat of death. To achieve openness and to maintain it under stress is part of the challenge of living with cancer—for both the patient and the patient's family and friends.

Hearing what the other is experiencing is never as devastating as what the imagination can conjure up. Fears and frustrations should be talked about as they arise rather than being left to fester until they become too frightening to mention, or until a habit of withholding evolves into inevitable isolation. Confronting each other's fears therefore becomes a means of keeping those fears under control. Candor will allow relationships to operate in a new realm, in which despair can be minimized or set aside and enjoyment and pleasure can resume their rightful places.

Candor between a patient and his or her family and friends includes recognizing one another's needs as well as one another's fears. Family and friends need to give, to feel they are doing something practical to hasten the patient's recovery, whether at home or in the hospital.

The separation caused by hospitalization is particularly traumatic to the family. They leave the hospital each evening and worry about whether their loved one will ever again lead a normal life, or whether he or she will even leave the hospital. Feeling impotent, they need to give of themselves. Fortunately there are many practical services a patient's family and friends can perform while the patient is in the hospital—services such as feeding, walking, turning, massaging. These, along with the offer of special foods, a favorite pillow or a comforting hand, become the routine of the daily hospital visit, giving solace to the family and friends as well as to the patient.

When the patient is critically ill, it is not unusual for at least one family member to be in attendance around the clock. This may mean sleeping in a chair beside the patient's bed. To obtain up-to-date information on the patient's condition, relatives may rearrange their schedules so as to be present when the doctor makes rounds or a particularly helpful nurse is on duty.

When the patient is at home, functioning well, there are still many opportunities for family and friends to give emotional and practical support. One need only consider what the cancer patient must sometimes be feeling: anxiety about a visit to the doctor, wondering whether a new problem will be discovered or a new treatment recommended, dreading the side effects from the day's treatment, concern about lack of transportation to and from the doctor's office. A family member or friend can offer a ride or go with the patient on the bus. If everyone is working and cannot be with the patient during the day, there is still the evening, when the side effects of therapy may have to be endured. Patient, family and friends benefit from any means by which love and encouragement can be expressed.

To be realistic, however, not everyone is able to be open, loving or intelligently supportive in crisis. Even stable relationships may be severely threatened by the pressures of long-term illness. Latent problems may emerge, and anger or guilt may surface in sudden attacks or recrim-

inations, or in indifferent or overly solicitous behavior. The exhaustion and frustration of constant worry and care may break the most loyal supporter. Family and friends must be reminded that they need time to themselves and moments of rest if they are to keep emotionally and physically fit. Calling on other friends or relatives for assistance can provide a respite from the responsibilities and worries of constant caring.

Children of cancer patients often need special understanding. Absence of a parent during hospitalization and the parent's fatigue following treatment may cause children to feel neglected and lost. Children may also feel they caused the illness; this misconception must be corrected quickly. Reassurance from other family members is important for children to realize they are still loved. Adolescents are particularly vulnerable to stress, as they may be asked to assume a supportive role, to approximate an adult partner or spouse. If this responsibility is beyond the adolescent's capabilities, he or she may rebel by not making hospital visits or by excessive drinking or drug use. Adolescents are adults—up to a point— but they still require the reassurance and comfort routinely given to younger children.

Lengthy illness can also break the most courageous of patients. When a person has fought long and hard against cancer, losing and regaining hope many times, and then realizes that the battle is not to be won, he or she may at times experience rage or depression that will focus on the nearest available person—the patient's spouse or significant other, child, parent or friend, or the nurse on duty. This anger usually manifests itself as irritation over trivial matters that normally would not even concern the patient. The person under attack needs to understand that this is not a rejection, but a cry of anguish.

In addition to anger and depression, a patient must also endure the endless boredom of being ill, as well as the fear of being a burden when he or she really wants and needs special attention. Ironically, the people from whom this attention is demanded may be suffering from the same tedium or from feelings of inadequacy and guilt for being unable to relieve the suffering. They may not be able to cope with the reality in which the patient is imprisoned. The result may be a gradual diminishing of attention and care by the family, and increased bitterness and fear of isolation for the patient.

No one should be blamed for the ways he or she responds to the crisis of a long-term illness or the threat of change and loss. Some people and some relationships grow stronger, experiencing new depths of love, respect and understanding; some waver, yet hold together; and some collapse.

The most important thing that family and friends can do for a patient is to be supportive and to give encouragement in doing everything possible to promote his or her recovery. However, it is vital that they do not err on the side of being overly solicitous, because this deprives the patient of the accomplishments that can give a sense of independence, purpose and self-esteem, and concrete proof of progress in returning to a normal life.

The purpose of life is to live. The goal of the physician who treats cancer patients is not only to administer medical therapy but also to help them live as normally as possible while undergoing treatment.

There is a widespread belief that a diagnosis of cancer is an automatic death sentence. This is not true. Today 50 percent of all cancer patients are cured; the majority of those who are not cured are leading active, productive lives with the same odds and life expectancy as people who live with other chronic diseases.

Of course, a cure for cancer is not just around the corner. No single breakthrough will produce all the answers; the answers will come one by one, just as they have until now. Nevertheless, as of 1996, more than 14 types of cancer were curable when diagnosed at an advanced stage. New forms of cancer will continue to be added to this list, because new discoveries are constantly being made and known techniques perfected. New methods of giving radiation therapy, new chemotherapeutic drugs and combinations of drugs, the use of adjuvant chemotherapy, hormonal therapy and experimental therapies—such as immunotherapy and hyperthermia—all give hope for the future.

In spite of the promise of these medical advances, though, living with cancer is an anxious, fearful time. Undergoing therapy and experiencing the side effects of treatment involve compromise. This compromise consists in accepting what has happened and at the same time being willing to fight for your life. But no matter how well informed you become about current therapies and available treatment alternatives, you will still feel a loss of control over your fate because you must trust the judgment of cancer specialists and pray for good luck. One day you are hopeful, the next day full of gloom.

Sometimes we are able to survive a current crisis because of the way we coped with a crisis in the past. We acquire resilience; we learn how tough we really are and develop confidence in our ability to endure. By turning to these inner resources and to the resources offered by members of the medical team, a cancer patient will give him- or herself the best chance of maintaining a good quality of life while living with cancer. Attention to nutrition and muscle strength can have marked physical and emotional benefits for the patient. Knowledgeable, sensitive nurses and physicians can assuage fear and offer reassurance as well as good medical care. Medical social workers can help with insurance problems, or arrange for home care or participation in a discussion group. Every patient should be aware of these services.

Thus help is available from people in many professions who understand your needs. These needs can also be met by other cancer patients who have formed support groups. We are here to help each other. How you live with cancer is your choice.

All cancer patients must live with their disease. The decision on how to approach the problem is theirs. With the proper support from family, friends and the medical team, and with their own inner resources of courage and hope, they can continue to live a meaningful life.

Choose life—only that and always, and at whatever risk. To let life leak out, to let it wear away by the mere passage of time, to withhold giving it and spreading it, is to choose nothing.

—Sister Helen Kelley

APPENDIX

THE PATIENT'S BILL OF RIGHTS

In recognition of patients' human dignity, their legal rights and their rights to information concerning medical care, the American Hospital Association has developed the following Patient's Bill of Rights, which has been approved by more than 75 percent of American hospitals.

The American Hospital Association presents a Patient's Bill of Rights with the expectation that observance of these rights will contribute to more effective patient care and greater satisfaction for the patient, physician and the hospital organization. Further, the association presents these rights in the expectation that they will be supported by the hospital on behalf of its patients, as an integral part of the healing process. It is recognized that a personal relationship between the physician and the patient is essential for the provision of proper medical care. The traditional physician-patient relationship takes on a new dimension when care is rendered within an organizational structure. Legal precedent has established that the institution itself also has a responsibility to the patient. It is in recognition of these factors that these rights are affirmed.

PATIENT'S RIGHTS

a) Hospitals and medical staffs shall adopt a written policy on patients' rights.
b) A list of these patients' rights shall be posted in both Spanish and English in appropriate places within the hospital so that such rights may be read by patients. This list shall include but not be limited to the patients' rights to:

1. Exercise these rights without regard to sex or cultural, economic, educational or religious background or the source of payment for care.
2. Considerate and respectful care.
3. Knowledge of the name of the physician who has primary responsibility for coordinating the care and the names and professional relationship of other physicians and nonphysicians who will see the patient.
4. Receive information about the illness, the course of treatment, and prospects for recovery in terms that the patient can understand.
5. Receive as much information about any proposed treatment or procedure as the patient may need in order to give informed consent or to refuse this course of treatment. Except in emergencies, this information shall include a description of the procedure or treatment, the medically significant risks involved in this treatment, alternate courses of treatment or nontreatment and the risks involved in each and to know the name of the person who will carry out the procedure or treatment.
6. Participate actively in decisions regarding medical care. To the extent permitted by law, this includes the right to refuse treatment.
7. Full consideration of privacy concerning the medical care program. Case discussion, consultation, examination and treatment are confidential and should be conducted discreetly. The patient has the right to be advised as to the reason for the presence of any individual.

8. Confidential treatment of all communications and records pertaining to the care and the stay in the hospital. Written permission shall be obtained before the medical records can be made available to anyone not directly concerned in the care.
9. Reasonable responses to any reasonable requests made for service.
10. Leave the hospital even against the advice of physicians.
11. Reasonable continuity of care and to know in advance the time and location of appointment as well as the identity of persons providing the care.
12. Be advised if hospital/personal physician proposes to engage in or perform human experimentation affecting care or treatment. The patient has the right to refuse to participate in such research projects.
13. Be informed of continuing health care requirements following discharge from the hospital.
14. Examine and receive an explanation of the bill regardless of source of payment.
15. Know which hospital rules and policies apply to the patient's conduct while a patient.
16. Have all patients' rights apply to the person who may have legal responsibility to make decisions regarding medical care on behalf of the patient.

c) A procedure shall be established whereby patient complaints are forwarded to the hospital administration for appropriate response.

d) All hospital personnel shall observe these patients' rights.

Note: Authority cited: Section 208(a) and 1275. Health and Safety Code. Reference: Section 1276, Health and Safety Code. Source. Amendment of subsection (b) filed 3-13-80, effective thirtieth day thereafter (Register 80, No. 11).

PART VI:
RESOURCES

THE NATIONAL CANCER INSTITUTE: A RELIABLE SOURCE OF CURRENT AND COMPREHENSIVE CANCER INFORMATION

Susan Molloy Hubbard, BS, RN, MPA

◇

Information is a critical component of shared decision making for any patient with a diagnosis of cancer and any individual known to be at high risk of developing cancer. The challenge facing patients, families and individuals at risk is finding readily available, authoritative and current information from a trustworthy source. The World Wide Web, a worldwide network of computers on the Internet, now provides a readily accessible, inexpensive and popular source of almost any type of information imaginable. The National Cancer Institute (NCI), the major source of federal funding for cancer research, has developed a computerized information system called PDQ (Physician Data Query) to make the most current information on the treatment of cancer, cancer screening and prevention and approaches to the management of disease and treatment-related complications more widely known. Information in the PDQ system is based on careful and ongoing reviews of the medical literature by cancer experts. PDQ also contains up-to-date information on clinical trials that are being conducted to evaluate new approaches to cancer treatment in patients with cancer and new approaches to cancer screening, and prevention in those at risk of developing cancer; a directory of physicians who care for cancer patients and individuals with significant risk factors, and a directory of facilities that have accredited cancer screening and/or cancer care programs.

NCI staff also developed, maintain and update CancerNet, a World Wide Web site that features information from PDQ and CANCERLIT, a bibliographic database of published cancer literature, educational resources produced by other NCI divisions and offices, a glossary of medical terms and links to complementary web sites with supplemental cancer information. The address is: http://cancernet.nci.nih.gov.

PDQ and CancerNet are reliable resources that cancer patients, those at significant risk of developing cancer and their loved ones can use to find up-to-date information to enable them to discuss management options with medical experts as well as prevention and screening options that may be appropriate for family members and actively participate in the decision-making process.

PDQ AND CANCERNET CONTENT

Cancer Information The cancer information developed for the PDQ system and CancerNet contains treatment summaries for adult and pediatric cancers, supportive care information on common complications of cancer or its treatment, and statements on approaches to cancer prevention and screening. The summaries feature information on:
- the prognosis (chance of recovery)
- staging (extent of spread)
- histopathology (tumor cell type)

◆ state-of-the-art (effective or standard) treatment options

◆ promising clinical research (research studies, protocols or clinical trials)

◆ the management of complications (supportive care)

◆ the early detection of cancer (screening)

◆ approaches in use to prevent cancer development (cancer prevention).

Treatment The treatment summaries in PDQ and CancerNet are written by cancer specialists with input from experts around the country and are available in both English and Spanish. Treatment options are provided for more than 90 different types of cancer, and information on rare cancers is being added over time. They are provided in two formats:

◆ Statements for health care professionals written in highly technical medical terminology that contain references to medical literature containing information that supports the use of the treatment options discussed; and

◆ Complementary summaries written for patients and the public that contain references to additional, less-technical educational resources written for cancer patients, their families and the public. These summaries are designed to complement discussions with a health care professional and to be shared with patients when prognosis and treatment options are discussed rather than to serve as a primary and free-standing source of treatment advice.

Because treatments that are appropriate for patients with cancers that are very localized (have not spread from the site of origin) are often markedly different from those that can be offered to a patient whose tumor has spread to other organs (metastasized), PDQ and CancerNet generally present treatment options by stage of disease (extent of spread). In certain types of cancer, other considerations, such as the anatomic location of the tumor or the type of cells that have become can-

cerous, can be more important in the selection of treatment. In such situations, these features govern the discussion of treatment options. When there is no effective therapy, PDQ and CancerNet recommend that patients consider participation in clinical trials that are evaluating new approaches to treatment.

Supportive Care and Survivorship Issues PDQ and CancerNet provide information on support that can ease the physical and psychosocial adverse effects of cancer or its treatment, such as pain, digestive problems, nausea and vomiting, fever, itching, fatigue, depression and grief and loss. These statements are also available in both English and Spanish.

Cancer survivors serve on the Editorial Boards that develop these summaries and participate in the refinement of existing summaries. Survivors are also setting priorities for the development of new topics.

Screening and Prevention Information on screening for cancers of the breast, cervix, colon and rectum, stomach, oral cavity, ovaries, prostate, neuroblastoma, endometrium, skin and testes is also summarized in PDQ and CancerNet. Each summary provides information on the strength of the evidence supporting the use of the technique (1) to detect cancer in asymptomatic individuals and (2) to reduce cancer mortality. Evidence-based statements on the prevention of cancers of the lung, breast, cervix, colon and rectum, ovaries and skin are also available. These summaries provide information on matters that increase or decrease cancer risk and information on current approaches to cancer prevention.

Information on Cancer in Racial and Ethnic Minorities In the near future, users will be able to search CancerNet for information on the incidence, mortality, screening, prevention and treatment of cancer in racial and ethnic groups. The resource features data from an NCI monograph on racial and ethnic patterns of cancer and prompts that point the user to the PDQ screening, prevention, treatment statements and clinical trials that may be appropriate for patients and individuals at high risk of developing certain cancers. A fully functional resource for both health professionals and patients on cancer in African-Americans was implemented on CancerNet in 1997. This prototype is the model for a similar resource for Alaskan Natives, Asian Americans, Hispanic Americans, Native Americans, Native Hawaiian/Pacific Islanders and white non-Hispanics.

Keeping PDQ and CancerNet Information Current All of the treatment, supportive care and screening and prevention summaries in PDQ and CancerNet are regularly updated by the members of four Editorial Boards. These boards are composed of more than 60 prominent physicians, nurses, psychiatrists, pharmacists, statisticians and social workers with expertise in the care of cancer patients. The Editorial Board that reviews information on the treatment of cancers that occur in adults and the Supportive Care and Survivorship Board each meet nine times a year; the boards that review information on pediatric cancers and on Cancer Screening and Prevention each meet five times a year. At each board meeting, members review and discuss information from recently published medical and scientific articles to update existing statements and develop new ones. An International Advisory Board of Editors comprising more than 100 specialists with expertise in cancer treatment, supportive care, screening and prevention complements and extends the expertise of these four core Editorial Boards.

INFORMATION ON CLINICAL TRIALS IN PDQ AND CANCERNET

New methods of cancer screening, pre-vention and treatment must be proved safe and effective before they can become standards of care and made widely available to individuals at risk and cancer patients. PDQ and CancerNet contain summaries of interventions under evaluation in patients that are designed to identify new and better ways to help cancer patients. These organized research programs are called research studies, clinical trials or protocols.

PDQ and CancerNet provide two overviews on the design and conduct of clinical trials: one written for health professionals and one for patients and their families. These summaries describe what protocols or clinical trials are, what their objectives are, the types of research questions they attempt to answer, and how the trials are conducted. These summaries also discuss the many biomedical, ethical and practical concerns that pertain to participation in cancer clinical trials.

There are many types of clinical trials. They range from studies of new methods to prevent, detect, diagnose, control and treat cancer to studies of new measures to enhance comfort and quality of life or measure the psychological impact of cancer on individuals. On average, about 1,500 clinical trials that actively seek patient participation are summarized in PDQ and CancerNet. All of the clinical trials supported by the NCI are listed in PDQ and CancerNet. NCI also invites physicians conducting clinical trials that are being supported by other sources to submit them to PDQ and CancerNet. These clinical trials are listed following review and approval by a board of cancer specialists that ensures that each trial is appropriate for use in the patient population that is to be studied.

The review evaluates whether the clinical trial adequately meets the following basic criteria:
◆ Is the study reasonable in design?
◆ Is it based on rational scientific information?

◆ Is it likely to yield some useful information?

◆ Is it unduly risky to patients?

◆ Are the entry criteria clear and complete?

◆ Is the statistical section clear and complete?

If the board decides that the trial does not meet one or more of the criteria, the chairperson sends a letter explaining the board's concerns to the principal investigator, who is invited to modify the protocol document to respond to their concerns or to clarify information in the protocol document. Once the principal investigator responds, the protocol is re-reviewed and a decision is made. More than 93 percent of the non–NCI sponsored trials submitted for review are included in PDQ.

How to Find a Clinical Trial New treatments often employ new methods of surgery, radiation therapy, chemotherapy and / or biological therapy. New treatments may be given alone or in combination with one another. Clinical trials in PDQ and CancerNet are classified by:

◆ the research goal (prevention, screening, treatment or management of complications)

◆ the primary tumor type (colon or breast cancer, for example)

◆ specific drugs or biologic substances

◆ the modality, or type, of treatment (surgery, radiotherapy, chemotherapy, biological therapy, screening, chemoprevention or supportive care)

◆ accrual status (open, closed, approved but not yet active, or investigational)

◆ the study phase (Phase I, II, III or adjuvant trial)

◆ sponsorship (NCI-sponsored, pharmaceutical or other organizational support)

Information on clinical trials is provided in two formats: physician-oriented and consumer-oriented summaries. The physician-oriented summaries provide technical details on the objectives of the study, the patient entry criteria (medical requirements) and the regimen, including drug dosages and schedules. In addition, each clinical trial includes the names, addresses and phone numbers of the physicians conducting the study. Information on clinical trials in PDQ and CancerNet is updated monthly. It's easy to search PDQ and CancerNet to identify clinical trials for a specific type and stage of cancer as well as a specific location (one or more cities, states, countries or ZIP codes) in the United States, Canada, Europe, Asia and several other locations.

Concise, consumer-oriented summaries were created for all active breast cancer clinical trials in PDQ and CancerNet in 1996. These single-paragraph summaries describe the rationale, purpose, entry criteria and regimen so patients can understand the basic design of the trials and find those for which they might be eligible. Special links in the text of the summary enable patients searching CancerNet to click on words that are hyperlinked to a glossary containing the definitions of medical terms used in the trial summaries. Each summary also provides the names and phone numbers of a physician conducting the study and a link to the longer and more technical summary written for physicians. NCI staff evaluated and refined the breast cancer prototype in collaboration with the patient advocate community and has offered to help advocates distribute consumer-oriented summaries for all types of trials on patient advocate web sites and newsletters. These short summaries are now integrated into the online PDQ system as well.

The Phases of a Clinical Trial Clinical trials are designed to demonstrate whether a therapy is effective and / or if it is more effective than another treatment. They are designed to take advantage of what has worked in the past and to improve on this foundation. For example, a clinical trial may compare the best-known surgical treatment with a newer operation to see if one produces more cures and/or causes fewer side effects than the other.

Clinical trials are carried out in stages called phases of investigation. Each phase is designed to discover different types of information. Each phase depends on, and builds on, information from an earlier phase. Patients may be eligible for studies in different phases, depending on their general condition and the type and stage of their cancer.

Most of the treatments we now consider standard therapies were first shown to be effective in clinical trials.

◆ *Phase I trials* The purpose of a Phase I study is to find the best way to give a new treatment and, if it is a new drug or biologic substance, how much of it can be given safely. Important findings of Phase I trials include the documentation of anticancer activity and any adverse effects associated with the treatment. Each new treatment (or new dose level) is given to a small number of patients under the careful eye of health professionals who evaluate each individual for any harmful side effects. Each patient is carefully assessed for anticancer effects via the measurement of tumor masses that are present at the beginning of the treatment. If any or all of the masses shrink appreciably, the patient is said to have responded to the treatment. Although each treatment has been thoroughly tested in laboratory animal studies, side effects in humans are not always predictable. For this reason, Phase I studies may involve significant risks and are offered only to patients whose cancers have spread and who are not likely to be helped by other known treatments.

◆ *Phase II trials* Once a safe dose and schedule for the treatment are established in Phase I trials, it can be advanced to a Phase II study, where investigators try to determine how effective it is against dif-

ferent types of cancer. Usually, 30 to 40 patients with a specific type and stage of cancer receive a Phase II treatment. Anticancer activity and adverse effects are assessed and a tentative response rate to the new therapy is established. If at least one out of five patients (20 percent) responds, the treatment is judged active against their tumor type. A treatment that shows this level of activity will move to Phase III. Since more patients receive the new treatment in Phase II trials, each patient is carefully assessed for new or unusual side effects.

◆ *Phase III trials* Phase III trials are comparative studies that require large numbers of patients, sometimes many thousands, to determine the superiority of one treatment over others in a special type of clinical trial. In Phase III trials, patients are assigned to a treatment group in a random (by chance) manner to avoid any bias in the selection of treatment for any patient. One group of patients receives the standard care for that type and stage of cancer (the "control" group). The other group receives the new treatment. At the end of the study, treatment outcomes are compared. All patients are monitored closely for anticancer and adverse effects. A Phase III trial is conducted under strict rules that terminate the study if outcomes show that one treatment is significantly superior to the other or if the treatments appear equal in efficacy but the side effects of one treatment are significantly more severe than the other.

◆ *Adjuvant trials* Adjuvant trials are conducted to determine if the administration of a supplemental form of therapy (the adjuvant therapy) can improve the chance of a cure in patients with localized cancer who are known to have a significant risk of recurrence after surgery or radiation therapy. Adjuvant trials of chemotherapy that compared surgery alone against surgery plus chemotherapy in women with breast cancer showed that the combination of surgery and chemotherapy led to fewer recurrences than the use of surgery alone. As a result of these studies, surgery and chemotherapy has become the standard therapy for many women with localized breast cancer who are at significant risk of recurrence.

Taking Part in a Clinical Trial Clinical trials offer patients the most up-to-date care available. Patients who take part in clinical trials have the first opportunity to benefit from new research and can make a very important contribution to medicine and science. The medical requirements for participating in a clinical trial depend on many factors. Patients who want to know more about clinical trials should review the summary on the design of clinical trials in PDQ and CancerNet and talk with their physicians about their options.

Patients should learn as much as they can about the trials before making up their minds. A cancer specialist is often the best person to counsel a patient about the selection of a standard option or a clinical trial. Patients should ask questions about the clinical trials that are available before deciding whether to participate in one. Some of the right questions to ask include:

◆ What is the purpose of the study?
◆ What are other choices and their advantages and disadvantages? Are there standard treatments for my case and how does the study compare with them?
◆ What does the study involve? What kinds of tests and treatments are done and how are they done?
◆ What is likely to happen in my case with or without this new research treatment?
◆ How could the study affect my daily life?
◆ What side effects could I expect from the study?

◆ How long will the study last? Will it require an extra time commitment on my part?
◆ Will I have to be hospitalized? If so, how often and for how long?
◆ Will the treatment be free? Will I incur any costs? If so, what are they?
◆ If I am harmed as a result of the research, what treatment would I be entitled to?
◆ What type of long-term follow-up care is part of the study?

THE PDQ AND CANCERNET DIRECTORIES

Physician Directory This directory contains the names, addresses, telephone numbers and medical specialties of more than 24,000 physicians who spend the majority of their time managing cancer patients or individuals at significant risk of developing cancer. These names have been compiled from the membership directories of 17 medical specialty organizations. All of the physicians conducting clinical trials listed in the PDQ and CancerNet are in the directory file.

Genetic Counseling Directory Since 1997, CancerNet users can search for genetic counselors by name, city, state and by the professional services required. Genetics counselors submitting applications for inclusion in the CancerNet database must have (1) a professional degree in genetics counseling or (2) a professional license or national certification, and (3) a membership in an approved national oncology or genetics society.

Organization Directory PDQ and CancerNet list more than 2,500 health care organizations that have certified programs of cancer care.

Note: The inclusion of individual doctors, counselors and organizations in the directory file does not imply endorsement by the NCI.

ACCESS TO PDQ AND CANCERNET INFORMATION

Cancer Information Service Patients and others who want to know more about cancer and how it may be screened for, prevented and treated can also obtain information from PDQ and CancerNet by contacting the NCI's Cancer Information Service (CIS). The CIS is staffed by trained information specialists who provide up-to-date information and answer questions from the public, cancer patients and their families, health care professionals and the media about cancer and cancer-related issues. Counselors who speak Spanish are available. Individuals with questions can call a toll-free number, 1-800-4-CANCER (1-800-422-6237), TTY 1-800-332-8615, to be connected to the CIS office serving their area. The counselors at the CIS use PDQ to obtain information about cancer screening, prevention, treatment, supportive care and clinical trials.

Patients and the public can access the PDQ database directly in several different ways. The PDQ system can be searched interactively over the Internet via the NCI's Information Associates Program, the National Library of Medicine's (NLM) MEDLARS system or through commercial and nonprofit information providers who have licensed PDQ as an online or CD-ROM service. A user needs a computer, a modem and telecommunications software to link over a standard telephone line to a remote computer containing the PDQ system. Those using a CD-ROM product need a CD-ROM reader. Although not essential, it is also highly desirable to have a printer so that the information seen on the screen can be produced for review. Information on vendors can be obtained from the International Cancer Information Center by contacting the Licensing Coordinator at 301-496-4907 or by looking for "PDQ Distributors" on CancerFax, CancerMail or CancerNet.

CancerFax The NCI disseminates PDQ data in English and Spanish through its CancerFax service, which enables people to obtain access to cancer treatment information via a facsimile machine. Users dial the CancerFax telephone number (301-402-5874) from the telephone handset on their fax machine, request a contents list, enter a code number from the CancerFax contents list for the desired information and follow the voice prompts to receive a faxed image of any of the information that is available through the CancerNet Mail Service. The service is available 24 hours a day and there is no cost to the user other than the telephone call. In addition, CancerFax provides current information on the NCI's scientific journals, its patient education materials and commercial vendors that distribute PDQ.

CancerMail Another source of PDQ information is CancerMail, an electronic mail service. An e-mail user simply submits an electronic message (e-mail) to the ICIC's mail server (cancermail@icic.nci.nih.gov) with the word "help" in the body of the message to get a table of contents and instructions for requesting information. Almost all of the information on CancerFax can be found on CancerMail. (Graphics cannot be transmitted on CancerMail.) Like PDQ, CancerMail and CancerFax are updated each month.

CancerNet As has been discussed, users can also get information from CancerNet, the ICIC's web site located at http://cancernet.nci.nih.gov. Users need a computer equipped with a modem and telecommunications software and Internet browsing software. Almost all of the information from PDQ is available in CancerNet, including all of the cancer information summaries for health professionals and patients, in English and Spanish, and the abstracts for all 1,500 or so ongoing clinical trials. In addition, CancerNet contains more than 80 topic-specific citations and abstract "digests" derived from the monthly updates to CANCERLIT, a bibliographic database of more than 1.2 million citations, also produced by the ICIC. CancerNet includes nearly 20 different CANCERLIT topic searches in the field of genetics, NCI news articles, educational booklets and bulletins, a variety of scientific and science policy publications and information produced by NCI researchers. The ease of updating a web site makes it a particularly suitable medium for transmitting time-sensitive material, including late-breaking news from the NCI and the National Institutes of Health (NIH).

Both CancerNet and the CancerNet Mail Service have greatly improved foreign access to PDQ information. One-third of the users on the Internet are accessing these services from foreign countries. By June of 1998, CancerNet was accessed more than 3.2 million times a month, and a growing number of medical facilities, cancer centers, community health information networks and health-oriented web sites link to CancerNet.

CancerNet Links Along with the wide range of information contained in CancerNet, ICIC provides hyperlinks to other web sites that offer valuable information. In keeping with the ICIC's goal of offering current, reliable information, each site is reviewed by an editorial board comprising health professionals, health educators and patient advocates before a link is established. Each review is designed to determine if the site meets the following criteria:

◆ Is the information related to the ICIC's mission of information dissemination?

◆ Is the information something that the ICIC does not already provide that would be useful to users?

◆ Is the information accurate and up-to-date?

◆ Is there an acceptable review process

in place to maintain the quality and currency of the material on the site?

Review board members also consider the following characteristics in their review of each site:

◆ Information on which users would base important health care decisions: reviewers are asked to carefully review any information in this category that may be incorrect or misleading,

◆ Inaccuracies that compromise meaning (missing text, misaligned tables): whether or not to link to a site with problems of this nature is decided by assessing the importance of information and the extent to which the information is likely to be misinterpreted, and

◆ Organizational and cosmetic flaws: whether or not to link to a site with these problems will be decided by assessing the importance of information versus the difficulty of locating specific details, and the unprofessional appearance of the information.

Once a link has been established, each site is reviewed at least twice a year. These criteria and information on how to request a link from CancerNet can be found on CancerNet's global resources page.

ACKNOWLEDGMENT

The information in PDQ is developed, maintained and disseminated by the staff at the International Cancer Information Center. The staff includes content and technical specialists whose goal is to ensure that PDQ is of high quality and easily accessible to health professionals, patients and the public. The author gratefully acknowledges their work and the many contributions of the patients who have advanced our knowledge on cancer screening, prevention, treatment and support.

THE CANCER RESOURCE CENTER

Keren Stronach, MPH

A cancer resource center, usually found in a cancer treatment center, can empower patients to become active and informed participants in health care decisions, improve the quality of their lives by fostering coping skills, link patients to community-wide resources and promote a sense of community among people affected by cancer. Its functions include providing medical information and listing support groups, classes and lectures on topics of interest as well as spiritual support services. By addressing the multiple needs of patients, the resource center can play an integrative role, bringing together the disparate aspects of patient care.

MEDICAL INFORMATION

One of the primary purposes of a resource center is to provide people with cancer with information about their condition and treatment options, as well as about nutrition, exercise and other lifestyle factors that can have an impact on their health.

It is one of the few forums where time is not a factor and patients can pursue their questions at leisure, either alone or with the help of a health care professional. By providing access to the Internet and health information search engines, the resource center can tailor information to patients' specific needs. Newly diagnosed patients who are unfamiliar with medical terminology can pick up pamphlets about their condition or electronically explore sources of health information in lay terms. Patients who are more comfortable with medical terminology or are interested in cutting-edge research can do Medline searches, obtain printouts of medical journal articles or explore medical textbooks.

The resource center is also an ideal forum in which to give individualized lessons on searching the Internet and using Medline, thus providing tools to explore questions that arise during the course of treatment. By furnishing patients with disease-specific Internet sites and listserves where patients who share the same condition can interact with each other, the resource center provides a launching pad for patients to explore the myriad psychological, emotional and medical issues that emerge with any diagnosis.

EMOTIONAL AND SPIRITUAL SUPPORT

Another important goal of a resource center is to address the emotional and spiritual needs of people with cancer. Patients can learn about support groups and counseling options for themselves and their families. Within the intimate environment of a support group, patients and their families can share their feelings and experiences, form ties with others in similar situations and learn important coping skills through the experiences and suggestions of others.

If they prefer one-on-one counseling, the resource center can direct them to a variety of individual counseling options that are available and have a sliding scale of payment.

Another potential function of a resource center is to link newly diagnosed patients with veteran patients who are familiar with the ins and outs of the medical system. Veteran patients can serve as an important source of support and information during the initial period of diagnosis when new patients are often overwhelmed. Even simple information, such as the whereabouts of a good restaurant near the hospital or whom to call for certain information, can be helpful. More important, however, linking new and veteran patients helps reduce the isolation that newly diagnosed patients often feel. At the same time, veteran patients can use their knowledge and experience in a meaningful way, thus imparting significance to their own experience.

The resource center can also fulfill its support function by supplying a rich collection of books, videotapes and audiotapes on relaxation techniques. These resources can be used by patients and their families to learn more about visualization, meditation and self-hypnosis to reduce stress, manage pain and cope during the period of treatment. Books about the experiences of others with cancer can also often serve as a source of inspiration and can give validation to many of the feelings that arise with a cancer diagnosis.

OTHER PROGRAMS AND CLASSES

Another role of a resource center is to develop programs and classes that encourage patients to live healthier lifestyles. Examples of such programs include nutrition and cooking classes to encourage healthy eating. Weekly exercise classes can provide patients with the opportunity to tone up their bodies, strengthen their muscles and improve physical functioning. Patients who exercise are able to maintain their health better than patients who do not exercise and are also likely to experience less fatigue and improved mental well-being. Other possibilities include programs such as art and dance therapy that provide avenues for artistic expression, and for sharing and interaction among patients.

COMMUNITY RESOURCES

The resource center can identify and locate support services for patients and their families. During the period of diagnosis and treatment, when patient and families often face financial and emotional difficulties, a comprehensive listing of resources can be invaluable in linking patient and families to important sources of support.

RESOURCES ON THE INTERNET

Achoo
http://www.achoo.com
Internet Health Care Directory.

American Cancer Society
http://www.cancer.org
Information on support sources, statistics on cancer.

American Institute for Cancer Research
http://www.aicr.org
AICR provides updates on nutrition and cancer research plus general information on better health and lower cancer risk.

Ask Noah About: Cancer
http://www.noah.cuny.edu/cancer/cancer.html

Cap Cure
http://www.capcure.org/
Good source of current research and articles.

Cancer Facts
e-mail to: listserv@sjuvm.stjohns.edu
message: afd ada cancer faq

Cancer List
e-mail to: listserv@wvnvm.edu
message: subscribe cancer-L (your name)

CancerNet (NCI)
http://www.icic.nci.nih.gov
e-mail to: CancerNet@icic.nci.nih.gov
message: help
CancerNet is a comprehensive and up-to-date source of information about cancer maintained by the National Cancer Institute.

800 Numbers
http://nysernet.org/bcic/numbers/eight.html

Food and Drug Administration
http://www.fda.gov
The FDA provides a variety of health information.

Grateful Med
http://igm.nlm.nih.gov/
Available via the Internet or via modem access from PCs or Macs. A one-time fee of $29.95 gives individuals a user ID and a password, as well as yearly software updates. Individual searches of MEDLINE and CANCERLIT are very inexpensive; access to AIDSLINE, AIDS DRUGS and AIDS TRIALS is free.

Guide to Internet Resources on Cancer
http://www.ncl.ac.uk/~nchwww/guides/clinks1.htm
Index list of linked sites with general and disease-specific treatment information about cancers, resources listed by country, clinical trial information and discussion lists and groups.

Healthfinder
http://www.healthfinder.gov
A gateway site to help consumers find health and human services information quickly. The site offers an alphabetical list of resources, toll-free numbers by health topic and clinical and nonclinical subject areas.

Healthgate
http://www.healthgate.com/
Search MEDLINE, CANCERLIT and MDX Family Health Library without charge. Also good information about herbs, roots and supplements. Fees for access to specific databases and medical and drug information resources.

Healthweb: Oncology
http://www.medlib.iupui.edu/hw/onco/home.html
Oncology-related treatment statements, clinical trials information, list servers and newsgroups listings, and links to oncology-related sites.

International Cancer Information Center
http://www.icic.nci.nih.gov
Sponsored by the National Cancer Institute.

The Med Help International
http://medhlp.netusa.net/
Has a large consumer health library, a place to post questions to health care professionals and a place to interact with patients.

Medicine On-Line
http://www.meds.com
Information on leukemia and cancer of the colon and lung. Provides information about list servers.

Medinfo.Org Oncology Resources
http://www.medinfo.org/
Oncology-related mailing lists, links to CancerNet, archived oncology-related articles from medical journals.

MEDLINE
http://www.nlm.nih.gov
The world's most extensive collection of published medical information, coordinated by the National Library of Medicine. Originally designed primarily for health professionals and researchers, MEDLINE is also valuable for people seeking specific information about health conditions, research and treatment. Free.

Memorial Sloan-Kettering Cancer Center
http://www.mskcc.org

NCCS Guide to Cancer Resources: Cansearch
http://www.access.digex.net/~mkragen/cansearch.html
Information on different types of cancer, newsgroups, lists and frequently asked questions (FAQs).

National Health Care Center
http://nhic-nt.health.org
A referral service sponsored by the Department of Health and Human Services. Will put you in touch with organizations best able to provide health answers.

NIH Health Information Page
http://www.nih.gov/health/
Provides a single access point to the consumer health information resources of the National Institutes of Health.

Northern California Cancer Information Service Regional Bulletin
http://www.nccc.org

Oncolink
http://oncolink.upenn.edu
Excellent oncology resource from the University of Pennsylvania. Includes a keyword search engine, psychosocial support, chemotherapy education materials for patients, clinical trials, anticancer drug regimens, publications, large collection of peer-reviewed information, descriptions of oncology-related mailing lists and newsgroups, and frequently asked questions.

PDQ
http://www.cancernet.nci.nih.gov/pdq.htm
Comprehensive cancer information database of the NCI; contains the most current available information on screening, detection and treatment of cancers, including investigational drugs.

Partners Against Pain
http://www.partnersagainstpain.com/
Information geared to professionals and patients; pain management guidelines.

Patient Education Materials
http://www/aetnaushc.com/topics/index

Quick Information about Cancer for Patients and Their Families
http://asa.ugl.lib.umich.edu/chdocs/cancer/cancerguide.html
Description of cancer, possible causes, treatment and support information.

Pubmed
http://www.ncbi.nlm.nih.gov/Pubmed/

Statistics
http://www.census.gov/stat_abstract/

University of Texas M. D. Anderson Cancer Center Home Page
http:utmdacc.mda.uth.tmc.edu/
Directory of information concerning M. D. Anderson's programs, services, departments and research. Includes links to other cancer-related sites.

ALTERNATIVE TREATMENTS

Alternative Medicine Home Page
http://www.pitt.edu/~cbw/altm.html

Commonweal Home Page
http://www.commonwealhealth.org

National Institutes of Health — Office of Alternative Medicine
http://altmed.od.nih.gov/

BONE MARROW TRANSPLANTS

Blood and Marrow Transplant Newsletter
http://www.bmtnews.org

BMT-Talk
To subscribe send an e-mail message to bmt-talk-request@ai.mit.edu. Put only

the word "subscribe" in the body of the message. To send mail to people on the bmt-talk list, address your e-mail to bmttalk@ai.mit.edu.

BREAST CANCER

Breast Cancer List
To subscribe send an e-mail message to listserver@morgan.ucs.mun.ca. In the body of the message put "subscribe breast-cancer." To send a message to people on the breast-cancer list, send e-mail to Breast-cancer@morgan.ucs.mun.ca.

Breast Cancer Information Clearinghouse
http://nysernet.org/

National Alliance of Breast Cancer Organizations (NABCO)
http://www.nabco.org
Central resource for information and network of 370 organizations; has resource list and newsletter.

CLINICAL TRIALS

Breast Cancer Clinical Trial Directory
http://www.nabco.org/directory.html

Centerwatch
http://www.centerwatch.com
Lists ongoing cancer research trials.

National Cancer Institute
http://cancernet.nci.nih.gov/trials/h_clinic.htm
or
http://cancernet.nci.nih.gov/prot/protsrch.html
Includes international trials.

DRUGS

Drug Infonet
http://www.druginfonet.com/
Drug and disease information, health care news and links to medical reference sources and medical sites.

Healthgate
http://www.healthgate.com/
Search MEDLINE, CANCERLIT and MDX Family Health Library for free. Also good information about herbs, roots and supplements. Fees for access to specific databases and medical and drug information resources.

Pharmaceutical Information Network
http://pharminfo.com/

RXList
http://www.rxlist.com/
Searchable database of prescription and over-the-counter drug information and interactions; some oncology drugs.

DYING, DEATH AND BEREAVEMENT

Bereavement and Hospice Support Netline
http://ube.ubalt.edu/www/bereavement/
Resource directory providing a national listing of free or very low cost bereavement support groups, services, newsletters and professional organizations and associations.

Griefnet
http://griefnet.org/index.html
Comprehensive, interactive site offering support groups, a library, links to emergency services and much more.

Hospice Hands
http://hospicecares.com/welcome.html
Hospice information, links to hospice organizations and sites, reference materials for patients and families, articles on pain and pain management, and discussion groups.

GYNECOLOGIC CANCERS

Gynecologic Oncology
http://www.oncolink.upenn.edu/specialty/gyn_onc/

Oncolink Ovarian Cancer
oncolink.upenn.edu/specialty/gyn_onc/ovarian

Ovarian
http://gynoncology.obgyn.washington.edu/Tutorials/OvarianCancer.html

Ovarian Cancer Discussion List
send e-mail to:
Listserv@sjuvm.stjohns.edu

NUTRITION

American Cancer Society
http://www.cancer.org/
Includes FAQs and guidelines for diet, nutrition and cancer prevention.

The American Dietetic Association Home Page
http://www.eatright.org!
Includes nutrition resources, FAQs and fact sheets.

Center for Nutrition Policy and Promotion
http://www.usda.gov/fcs/cnpp.htm
Links resources with USDA for dietary guidelines, nutrition educators services, food consumer services and many more.

Healthtouch
http://www.healthtouch.com/
Includes links to Food and Drug Administration, National Diabetes Information Clearinghouse and Weight Control Information Network.

Wellness Web
http://www.wellweb.com/
Includes a nutrition index and alternative/complementary section for information on herbs, vitamins and minerals.

PROSTATE CANCER

American Foundation for Urologic Disease
http://www.access.digex.net/~afud

American Prostate Society
http://www.ameripros.org/
Web link where cancer information can be requested by e-mail.

Doctor's Guide to Prostate Cancer
http://www.pslgroup.com/
PROSTCANCER.HTM
An excellent source of prostate cancer news and information for anyone.

Enter the Circle
http://rattler.cameron.edu/circle/

Mediconsult
http://www.mediconsult.com/prostate

**National Prostate Cancer Coalition —
Mailing Lists**
http://rattler.cameron.edu/mlist/mlist.html

Prostate Cancer Discussion
send e-mail to:
Listserv@sjuvm.stjohns.edu
To subscribe put only the word "subscribe" in your message and leave your name and e-mail address.

The Prostate Cancer Infolink
http://www.comed.com/Prostate/

Prostate Pointers
http://rattler.cameron.edu/prostate/
#lay
Lots of information about prostate cancer.

**University of Michigan Prostate
Cancer Home Page**
http://www.cancer.med.umich.edu/prostcan/prostcan.html

Urology Information Site
http://www.wwilkins.com/urology/
Has a list of journal articles with abstracts.

Us-Too, International, Inc.
http://www.ustoo.com
Provides medical information as well as lists of patients who have had prostate

cancer and are willing to be contacted.

Virgil's Prostate Online
http://www.prostate-online.com

OTHER CANCERS

Hematology/Oncology List
listserv@sjuvm.stjohns.edu
To subscribe put only the word "subscribe" and your name in the body of the message.

Hodgkin's and Non-Hodgkin's
http://www.avonlink.co.uk/amanda/index.html

International Myeloma Foundation
http://myeloma.org/IMF

**Lymphoma Research Foundation of
America**
http://www.lymphoma.org

**The Malignant Melanoma Research
Page**
http://users.aol.com/private/mel.html

Mark's Melanoma Hotlist
http://www.geocities.com/HotSprings
/1704/marksmel.htm

Melanoma Patients' Information Page
http://www.sonic.net/~jpat/getwell/getwell.html

SPANISH LANGUAGES

**National Cancer Institute (NCI)
CancerNet Database**
http://imsdd.meb.uni-bonn.de/
cancernet/cancernet.html

WWW Cancer
http://www.arc.com/cancernet/cancernet.html

ORGANIZATIONS AND SUPPORT GROUPS

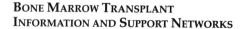

BONE MARROW TRANSPLANT INFORMATION AND SUPPORT NETWORKS

American Bone Marrow Donor Registry
c/o The Caitlin Raymond International Registry
University of Massachusetts Medical Center
Worcester, MA 01655
800-7-A-MATCH if you need a bone marrow donor
800-7-DONATE if you wish to become a donor
508-756-6444
fax: 508-752-1496

BMT Family Support Network
P.O. Box 845
Avon, CT 06001
800-826-9376

The HLA Registry Foundation
(New Jersey, New York, Pennsylvania, Massachusetts)
70 Grand Ave.
River Edge, NJ 07661-1935
800-336-3363
201-487-0883

International Bone Marrow Transplant Registry (IBMTR)
Medical College of Wisconsin
P.O. Box 26509
Milwaukee, WI 53226
414-257-8325

National Bone Marrow Transplant Link
29209 Northwestern Hwy. #624
Southfield, MI 48034
800-LINK-BMT
fax: 810-932-8483

National Marrow Donor Program (NMDP)
3433 Broadway Street N.E., Suite 400
Minneapolis, MN 55413
800-MARROW-2 (or 800-627-7692)
or 612-627-5844
fax: 612-627-5877 or 612-627-5877
Office of Patient Advocacy 800-526-7809

The Oncology Nursing Society
(publishes a directory of major BMT centers in the U.S.)
BMT Special Interest Group
501 Holiday Drive
Pittsburgh, PA 15220-2749
412-921-7373

CANCER SUPPORT AND INFORMATION

American Cancer Society (ACS)
1599 Clifton Road N.E.
Atlanta, GA 30329
404-320-3333
800-ACS-2345 (hotline)

American Red Cross
431 18th Street N.W.
Washington, DC 20006
202-737-8300

Cancer Care, Inc.
1180 Avenue of the Americas
New York, NY 10036
212-302-2400
800-813-HOPE (4673)
Provides supportive services for people with cancer and families, one-page information sheets free to callers to 800 number, one-to-one telephone counseling and referrals to local resources.

Cancer Information Service
National Cancer Institute
Bldg. 31, Room 10A07
9000 Rockville Pike

Bethesda, MD 20892
800-4-CANCER (800-422-6237)

Cancer Support Network
802 E. Jefferson
Bloomington, IL 61701
309-829-2273
Provides support groups, lending library, wig bank.

Candlelighter's Childhood Cancer Foundation
7910 Woodmount Ave., Suite 460
Bethesda, MD 20814
800-366-CCCF
301-657-8401

CanSurmount
(contact a local ACS office)
An ACS program that provides information and support for cancer survivors, family members and health professionals.

Center for Attitudinal Healing
33 Buchanan Drive
Sausalito, CA 94965
415-331-6161
fax: 415-331-4545
Provides support for patients with life-threatening illnesses.

Choice in Dying, Inc.
200 Varick Street
New York, NY 10014
212-366-5540
Distributes state-specific information on living wills, health care proxies, etc.

ENCORE
Contact your local YWCA or write:
600 Lexington Ave.
New York, NY 10022
Provides support and rehabilitation for postmastectomy patients.

Foundation for Hospice and Homecare
513 C Street N.E.
Washington, DC 20002
202-547-6586
fax: 202-546-8968

Helps people set up quality home care, including hospice, as an alternative to institutional care. Pamphlets and agency names available on request.

Friend's Health Connection
908-483-7436
Connects people with same health problems for purpose of mutual support.

Hospice Education Institute Hospicelink
190 Westbrook Road
Essex, CT 06426
800-331-1620
203-767-1620
Provides information on hospices and palliative care, and referrals to local hospices, palliative care units and bereavement support services.

I Can Cope
(contact a local ACS office)
An ACS program that provides information on treatment for cancer patients and family members.

International Association of Laryngectomees
(contact a local ACS office)
An ACS program that provides information and services for laryngectomy patients.

International Myeloma Foundation
2120 Stanley Hills Drive
Los Angeles, CA 90046
800-452-CURE (800-452-2873)

International Pain Foundation
909 N.E. 43rd Street, Suite 306
Seattle, WA 98105
206-547-2157
Provides information about pain control.

Leukemia Society of America, Inc.
600 Third Ave.
New York, NY 10016
212-573-8484
800-955-4572 (information hotline)

Provides information, referrals, support and financial aid for patients with leukemia, Hodgkin's disease and lymphoma.

Look Good ... Feel Better
800-558-5005
(contact a local ACS office)
An ACS program that teaches makeup techniques to women patients.

National Childhood Cancer Foundation
440 East Huntington Drive
P.O. Box 60012
Arcadia, CA 91066-6012
818-447-1674
fax: 818-447-6359
http://www.ncf.org/

National Children's Cancer Society
1015 Locust #1040
St. Louis, MO 63101
800-5-FAMILY
314-241-1600

National Coalition for Cancer Survivorship
1010 Wayne Ave., 5th Floor
Silver Spring, MD 20910
301-650-8868

National Council Against Health Fraud
Resource Center
3521 Broadway
Kansas City, MO 64111
800-821-6671
Provides information on questionable health practices and health organizations.

National Council Against Health Fraud
P.O. Box 1276
Loma Linda, CA 92354

National Hospice Organization
1901 N. Moore Street, Suite 901
Arlington, VA 22209
800-658-8898
Provides information, referrals and support.

National Women's Health Network
1325 G Street N.W.
Washington, DC 20005
202-347-1140
Provides information on women's cancers and other issues related to women's health.

Ostomy Rehabilitation Program
(contact a local ACS office)
An ACS program that provides information and services for ostomy patients.

Reach to Recovery
Contact a local ACS office or write:
Reach to Recovery, American Cancer Society
777 Third Ave.
New York, NY 10017
An ACS program that provides information and services for patients with breast cancer.

United Ostomy Association, Inc.
1111 Wilshire Blvd.
Los Angeles, CA 90017
213-481-2811

Vital Options
4419 Coldwater Canyon Ave., Suite A-C
Studio City, CA 91604
818-508-5657
Provides information and support for young adults with cancer.

Well Spouse Foundation
610 Lexington Ave., Suite 814
New York, NY 10022-6005
800-838-0879
212-644-1241

Women's Cancer Resource Center
3023 Shattuck Ave.
Berkeley, CA 94705
510-548-9272

FERTILITY

American Society for Reproductive Medicine
1209 Montgomery Hwy.
Birmingham, AL 35216
205-978-5000

Genetics and Invitro Fertilization Institute (ovary freezing)
3020 Javier Road
Fairfax, VA 22031
800-552-4363
703-698-7355

Resolve Inc.
1310 Broadway
Somerville, MA 02144-1731
Help line: 617-623-0744
http://www.ihr.com/resolve/

FINANCIAL ASSISTANCE, FUNDRAISING AND INSURANCE INFORMATION

Health Care Financing Administration, Medicare Issues
U.S. Department of Health and Human Services
7500 Security Blvd.
Baltimore, MD 21244-1850
800-638-6833
800-772-1212
Focuses on consumer education and assistance. Provides information on Medicare coverage and related topics.

Health Insurance Association of America
1025 Connecticut Ave. N.W., Suite 1200
Washington, DC 20036
202-223-7780

Indigent Drug Program
United States Senate, Department of Aging
202-224-5364, 202-224-1467

Provides a list of drug companies and drugs that are provided free under the indigent drug program.

LIFE-CORE (Oregon and neighboring states)
P.O. Box 291
Bend, OR 97709
503-385-9125

National Association of Hospital Hospitality Houses
800-542-9730

Provides information on hospitality programs that provide lodging and supportive services in a caring environment for families receiving medical care away from home.

The National Children's Cancer Society
800-5-FAMILY
Provides financial aid to children who need a bone marrow transplant, as well as fundraising advice.

National Insurance Consumer Helpline
1001 Pennsylvania Ave. N.W.
Washington, DC 20004
800-942-4242
Aids consumers in finding insurance companies that fit their needs, including handling inquiries about insurance issues, consumer complaints and where to find insurance. Also provides information on coping with treatment, pain, disabilities, doctors and hospitals.

VOICE (Victims of Insurance Company Error)
533 N. Pacific Coast Hwy., Box 278
Redondo Beach, CA 90277
310-372-7439

DIAGNOSIS/DISEASE-RELATED INFORMATION

ANEMIA

Aplastic Anemia Foundation of America (also serving MDS patients)
P.O. Box 22689
Baltimore, MD 21203
800-747-2820

Myeloproliferative Disease Research Center
950 Park Ave.
New York, NY 10028-0320
800-HELP-MPD
212-535-8181
fax: 212-535-7744

BRAIN TUMOR

American Brain Tumor Association
2720 River Road, Suite 146
Des Plains, IL 60018
800-886-2282
708-827-9910

National Brain Tumor Foundation
785 Market Street, Suite 1600
San Francisco, CA 94103
800-934-CURE
800-934-2873

BREAST CANCER

National Alliance of Breast Cancer Organizations (NABCO)
9 E. 37th Street, 10th Floor
New York, NY 10016
212-719-0154
fax: 212-719-0263
http://www.nabco.org

Susan G. Koman Breast Cancer Foundation
5005 L.B.J. Freeway, Ste 370
Dallas, TX 75244
972-855-1600
fax: 972-855-1605

The New York Statewide Breast Cancer Hotline
Adelphi University
Breast Cancer Support Program
Box 703
Garden City, NY 11530
800-877-8077 (from within New York state)
516-877-4444 (outside New York state)

Y-Me National Breast Cancer Organization
212 W. Van Buren
Chicago, IL 60607-3908
800-221-2141 (24-hour hotline)
fax: 312-294-8598
http://www.y-me.org

IMMUNE DEFICIENCY DISORDERS

Immune Deficiency Foundation
25 W. Chesapeake Ave., Suite 206
Towson, MD 21204
800-296-4433
410-321-6647

National Organization for Rare Disorders (NORD)
P.O. Box 8923
New Fairfield, CT 06812-8923
800-999-NORD or 800-999-6673

LEUKEMIA

Children's Leukemia Foundation of Michigan (serving adults and children in Michigan)
29777 Telegraph Road, Suite 1651
Southfield, MI 48034
800-825-2536
fax: 810-353-0157

Leukemia Research Foundation
(Illinois/Indiana residents within a 100-mile radius of Chicago)
4761 W. Touhy Ave., #211
Lincolnwood, IL 60646
708-982-1480

Leukemia Society of America
600 Third Ave.
New York, NY 10016
800-456-5413
Public Information Resource Line 800-955-4LSA (4572)

National Leukemia Association
585 Stewart Ave., Suite 536
Garden City, NY 11503
516-222-1944

Wellness Community National Headquarters
2200 Colorado Ave.
Santa Monica, CA 90404
310-453-2300
Provides support; helps patients to improve their quality of life.

TRANSPORTATION SUPPORT

Mercy Medical Airlift
P.O.Box 1940
Manassas, VA 20108-0804
To find charitable, long-distance medical air transportation dial the National Patient Air Transport Helpline 800-296-1217. This hotline, operated by Mercy Medical Airlift, has the latest information on all known air medical charity programs in the U.S. Here you can find information for 35 public benefit flying charities. Web site for the National Patient Air Transport Helpline (NPATH) is at www.npath.org. Within that web site you can read information about the whole of the National Charitable Patient Air Transportation System, and the NPATH 800 number is the "door" to all of that help.

ACTIVITIES OF DAILY LIVING

The following self-help companies deal directly with the consumer and provide catalogs of their products.

Cleo Living Aids
3957 Mayfield Road
Cleveland, OH 44121

Fred Sammons, Inc.
Be O/K Sales Company
Box 32
Brookfield, IL 60513

Medi-Gym
Ernest H. Rosenbaum, MD
Mount Zion Hospital and Medical Center
P.O. Box 7921
San Francisco, CA 94120

PLANNING FOR THE FUTURE

Willmaker 5.0 for Windows
by Nolo Press
For wills, living wills and final arrangements.

Do-It-Yourself Kit "Living Will"
E-Z Legal Forms

Family Tree Maker Deluxe CD-ROM Edition
by Banner Blue Software

To receive advance directive forms and information regarding these documents:

American Association of Retired Persons
202-434-2277

American Medical Association
800-621-8335

California Health Decisions
714-647-4920

California Medical Association
415-882-5175

Choice In Dying
212-366-5540

National Hospice Organization
800-658-8898

Self-Determination Directory and Resource Guide
National Heath Lawyers' Association
202-833-1100

BOOKS, CD-ROMS, NEWSLETTERS

◇

Alternative Treatments

Cassileth, Barrie R., PhD. *The Alternative Medicine Handbook*. New York: WW Norton, 1998.

Hsu, Hong-Yen. *Treating Cancer with Chinese Herbs*. Los Angeles: Oriental Healing Arts Institute, 1982.

Kaptchuk, Ted J. *Web That Has No Weaver: Understanding Chinese Medicine*. New York: Congdon & Weed, 1983.

Lerner, Michael. *Choices in Healing: Integrating the Best of Conventional and Complementary Approaches to Cancer*. Cambridge, MA: MIT Press, 1994. An excellent and nonjudgmental review of conventional and alternative treatments to cancer therapy and provides valuable information on coping and living fully with cancer, choosing a physician and conventional therapies and selecting suitable alternative therapies.

Pelton, Ross R., PhD. *Alternatives in Cancer Therapy*. New York: Fireside, 1994.

Randall, R. C., ed. *Cancer Treatment and Marijuana Therapy: Marijuana's Use in the Reduction of Nausea and Vomiting and for Appetite Stimulation in Cancer Patients*. Washington, DC: Galen Press, 1990. Testimony from historic federal hearings on marijuana's medical use.

Breast Cancer

Bruning, Nancy. *Breast Implants: Everything You Need to Know*, 2nd rev. ed. Alameda, CA: Hunter House, 1995.

Hirshaut, Yashar, MD, FACP, and Peter Pressman, MD, FACS. *Breast Cancer: The Complete Guide*. New York: Bantam Books, 1992.

Kelly, Patricia T. *Understanding Breast Cancer Risk*. Philadelphia: Temple University Press, 1991.

Love, Susan, MD, with Karen Lindsey. *Dr. Susan Love's Breast Book*, 2nd ed. Reading, MA: Addison-Wesley, 1995.

Ploski, Cynthia. *Conversations with My Healers: My Journey to Wellness from Breast Cancer*. Tulsa, OK: Council Oak Books, 1995.

Coping/Support

Benjamin, Harold, PhD. *From Victim to Victor: The Wellness Community Guide to Fighting for Recovery for Cancer Patients and Their Families*. Los Angeles: Jeremy Tarcher, 1987.

Bloch, R., and A. Bloch. *Cancer — There's Hope*. Kansas City: R. A. Bloch Cancer Foundation, 1981. Advice for cancer patients, their family and friends about what is involved in diagnosis, decision making and treatment.

Cousins, Norman. *Anatomy of an Illness as Perceived by a Patient.* New York: Bantam Books, 1981. Patient story discussing the effects of positive emotions and relationships on the natural healing process.

————. *Head First: The Biology of Hope.* New York: Dutton, 1989. Explores the connection between personal beliefs and the body's healing resources.

Frank, Arthur. *At the Will of the Body.* Boston: Houghton Mifflin, *1991.*

LeShan, Lawrence L. *Cancer as a Turning Point: A Handbook for People with Cancer, Their Families and Health Professionals.* New York: Dutton, 1989. A research and clinical psychologist discusses taking control of one's life and developing a lifestyle suited to new needs.

Moyer, B. *Healing and the Mind.* New York: Doubleday, 1993. Explores the connection between mind and body, focusing on cancer and treatments.

Rosenblum, Daniel, MD. *A Time to Hear, a Time to Help: Learning to Listen to People with Cancer.* New York: Maxwell Macmillan International, 1993.

Siegel, Bernie, MD. *Love, Medicine and Miracles: Lessons Learned about Self-Healing from a Surgeon's Experience with Exceptional Patients.* New York: Harper & Row, 1986. Healing viewed as a process of exploring the meaning of illness in one's life.

————. *Peace, Love and Healing: Body-Mind Communication and the Path to Self-Healing: An Exploration.* New York: Harper & Row, 1989. Encourages taking responsibility for one's health and emotions.

Smith, Gregory White and Steven Naifeh. *Making Miracles Happen.* Boston: Little, Brown and Company, 1997.

Spiegel, David, MD. *Living Beyond Limits: New Hope for Facing Life-Threatening Illness.* New York: Time Books, 1993.

Dying, Death and Bereavement Resources

Akner, L. F. *How to Survive the Loss of a Parent: A Guide for Adults.* New York: William Morrow, 1993.

Colgrove, M., H. H. Bloomfield, and P. McWilliams. *How to Survive the Loss of a Love.* Los Angeles: Prelude Press, 1991.

Dossey, Larry, MD. *Dr. Larry Dossey's Healing Words.* San Francisco: HarperCollins, 1993.

Ellis, A., and M. Abrams. *How to Cope with a Fatal Illness: The Rational Management of Death and Dying.* New York: Barricade Books, 1994.

Groopman, Jerome, MD. *The Measure of Our Days.* New York: Viking Press, 1997.

Humphry, Derek. *Final Exit: The Practicalities of Self-Deliverance and Assisted Suicide for the Dying,* 2nd ed. New York: Dell, 1996.

Kübler-Ross, E. *On Death and Dying.* New York: Macmillan, 1969.

Kushner, H. S. *When Bad Things Happen to Good People.* New York: Avon, 1983. Discussion of guilt, blame and other reactions by family members and cancer survivors. Countless patients have drawn inspiration and solace from this compassionate reflection on "Why me?"

Meyer, C. *Surviving Death: A Practical Guide to Caring for the Dying and Bereaved.* Mystic, CT: Twenty-Third Publications, 1991.

Middlebrook, C. *Seeing the Crab: A Memoir of Dying.* New York: Basic Books, 1996.

Miller, J. E. *How Can I Help? 12 Things to Do When Someone You Know Suffers a Loss and What Will Help Me? 12 Things to Remember When You Have Suffered a Loss.* Fort Wayne, IN: Willowgreen Publishing, 1994.

Nuland, Sherwin. *How We Die: Reflections on Life's Final Chapter.* New York: Vintage Books, 1995.

Paget, M. A. *A Complex Sorrow: Reflections on Cancer and an Abbreviated Life.* Philadelphia: Temple University Press, 1993.

Rinpoche, Sogyal. *The Tibetan Book of Living and Dying.* San Francisco: Harper Books, 1993. Lucidly presents the teachings of Tibetan Buddhism on the meaning of life and death, and introduces the practices and philosophy of Buddhist spirituality.

Smith, Rodney. *Lessons from the Dying.* Seattle: Wisdom Publications, 1998.

Tatelbaum, J. *The Courage to Grieve: Creative Living, Recovery and Growth through Grief.* New York: Harper & Row, 1980.

Nutrition

Aker, S. *A Guide to Good Nutrition During and After Chemotherapy and Radiation.* Seattle: Fred Hutchinson, 1988. To order, call 206-467-4834.

Barrett, S., and V. Herbert. *The Vitamin Pushers.* Amherst, NY: Prometheus, 1994.

Bender, David A. *Nutrition: A Reference Handbook.* New York: Oxford University Press, 1997.

Black, A. S. *Nutrition Management of the Cancer Patient.* Sapen, 1990.

Block, Gladys, PhD. *Nutrition DISCovery,* CD-ROM, University of California — Berkeley. Features a unique interactive program where audio, music and video enhancements make nutrition learning easy and fun. The process begins with a personal dietary assessment. It also considers the effects that diet and lifestyle habits — such as smoking, dieting for weight loss, cooking with fat, frequency of dining out and vitamin/mineral supplement usage — may have on nutritional status.

Bohannon, R. *Food for Life: The Cancer Prevention Cookbook.* Chicago: Contemporary Books, 1987. More than 300 recipes.

Brody, J. *Nutrition Book.* New York: Bantam Books, 1987.

Coppers, K. H. MD. *Antioxidant Revolution.* Nashville: Thomas Nelson, 1994.

Claiborne, Craig, Timothy Ryan, and Mary Deidre Donovan. *Techniques of Healthy Cooking.* New York: Van Nostrand Reinhold, 1997.

Franz, M. J., D. D. Etzwiler, J. O. Joynes, and P. M. Hollander. *Learning to Live with Diabetes.* Minneapolis: DCI Publishing, 1991.

Hailer J. *What to Eat When You Don't Feel Like Eating.* Hantsport, Nova Scotia: Lancelot Press, 1994.

Jones, J. *Eating Smart*. New York: Macmillan, 1992.

Lindsay, Anne, in consultation with Diane J. Fink. *American Cancer Society Cookbook: A Menu for Good Health*, rev. ed. New York: Hearst Books, 1988.

National Cancer Institute. *Action Guide for Health Eating*. Washington, DC: NCI, 1995 (95-3877). USDA dietary guidelines for healthy eating and lowering cancer risk.

————— . *Eating Hints for Cancer Patients*. Washington, DC: NCI, 1995 (95-2079). Includes dietary needs, suggested menus, recipes, resources and a glossary.

Newell, Guy R., and Neil M. Ellison, eds. *Nutrition and Cancer: Etiology and Treatment*. New York: Raven Press, 1981.

Nixon, Daniel W., MD, with Jane A. Zanca. *The Cancer Recovery Eating Plan: The Right Foods to Help Fuel Your Recovery*. New York: Times Books, 1996.

Pennington, Jean A. T. *Bowes & Church's Food Values of Portions Commonly Used*, 16th ed. Philadelphia: Lippincott, 1994.

Piscatella, J. C. *What to Eat If You Have Cancer*. Chicago: Contemporary Books, 1991.

Raichlen, Steven. *Controlling Your Fat Tooth*. New York: Workman Publishing, 1995.

————— . *High-Flavor, Low-Fat Vegetarian Cooking*. New York: Viking Penguin, 1997.

Ramstack, J. L., and E. H. Rosenbaum. *Nutrition for the Chemotherapy Patient*. Palo Alto, CA: Bull Publishing, 1990.

Robertson, Laurel, Carol Flinders, and Brian Ruppenthal. *The New Laurel's Kitchen: A Handbook for Vegetarian Cooking and Nutrition*. Berkeley, CA: Ten Speed Press, 1986. The Blue Mountain Center of Meditation, Inc., Berkeley CA 94707.

Rosenbaum, Ernest H., MD, et al. *Recipes for the Chemotherapy Patient*. Palo Alto, CA: Bull Publishing, 1992.

Rosenfeld, I., MD. *Doctor, What Should I Eat?* New York: Random House, 1995.

Ross Laboratories. *Nutrition: An Ally in Cancer Therapy*. Columbus, OH: Ross Laboratories, 1989. Describes ways to use nutrition supplements.

Rosso, Julie, and Sheila Lukins. *The New Basics Cookbook*. New York: Workman Publishing, 1989.

Simone, C., MD. *Cancer and Nutrition*. New York: Avery Publishing Group, 1994.

Simopoulos, A. P., V. Herbert, and B. Jacobson. *The Healing Diet*. New York: Macmillan, 1995.

Spear, R. *Low Fat and Loving It*. New York: Warner Books, 1990. More than 200 recipes, information on diet and cancer, fat and cholesterol and an easy-to-follow diet plan. Written by a breast cancer survivor.

U.S. Department of Health and Human Services. *Recipes and Hints for Better Nutrition During Cancer Treatment*. Washington, DC: National Cancer Institute, 1992.

Watson, R. R., and I. M. Siraj. *Nutrition and Cancer Prevention*. New York: CRC Press, 1996.

Protein and Calorie Contents of Diet Supplements

Ross Laboratories
Columbus, OH 43215
800-544-7495

Mead-Johnson and Company
Evansville, IN 947721

General Cancer Information

The Alpha Institute. *Alpha Book on Cancer and Living: For Patients, Family and Friends.* Alameda, CA: The Alpha Institute, 1993.

Griffith, H. Winter, MD. *Complete Guide to Prescription and Non-Prescription Drugs.* Berkeley, CA: The Body Press, Perigee Books, 1994.

Morra, Marion, and Eve Potts. *Realistic Alternatives in Cancer Treatment.* New York: Avon Books, 1994.

Stronach, Keren. *Survivors' Guide to A Bone Marrow Transplant.* Southfield, MI: National Bone Marrow Translant Link, 1997.

Reference Books

Altman, R., and M. J. Sarg. *The Cancer Dictionary.* New York: Facts on File, 1992.

Bennett, J. C., and F. Plum, eds. *Cecil Textbook of Medicine.* Philadelphia: Saunders, 1996. Considered an authoritative source in internal medicine.

Clayman, C. B., ed. *The American Medical Association Family Medical Guide.* New York: Random House, 1994.

Conn, R. B., ed. *Current Diagnosis.* Philadelphia: Saunders, 1991.

Cooper, Geoffrey M. *The Cancer Book: A Guide to Understanding the Causes, Prevention and Treatment of Cancer.* Boston: Jones and Bartlett Publishers, 1993.

DeVita, V. T., S. Hellman, and S. Rosenberg, eds. *Cancer: Principles and Practice of Oncology.* Philadelphia: Lippincott-Raven, 1997.

Dollinger, M., MD, E. H. Rosenbaum, MD, and G. Cable. *Everyone's Guide to Cancer Therapy: How Cancer Is Diagnosed, Treated, and Managed Day to Day,* 3rd ed. Kansas City, MO: Andrews and McMeel, 1997.

Frank, Arthur W. *The Wounded Storyteller: Body, Illness, and Ethics.* Chicago: The University of Chicago Press, 1995.

Fischbach, F. T. *Quick Reference re Common Laboratory and Diagnostic Tests.* Philadelphia: Lippincott, 1995.

Holland, J. F., et al., eds. *Cancer Medicine,* 4th ed. Baltimore: Williams & Wilkins, 1997.

Isselbacher, K. J., et al., eds. *Principles of Internal Medicine.* New York: McGraw-Hill, 1994. Considered an authoritative source in internal medicine.

Larson, D. E., ed. *Mayo Clinic Family Health Book.* New York: William Morrow, 1990.

Love, Susan, MD, with Karen Lindsey. *Dr. Susan Love's Hormone Book.* New York: Random House, 1997.

McAllister, R. M., S. T. Horowitz, and R. V. Gilden. *Cancer.* New York: Basic Books, 1993.

Morra, M., and E. Potts. *Choices.* New York: Avon Books, 1994.

Pazdur, P., ed. *Medical Oncology: A Comprehensive Review.* Huntington, NY: PRR, 1995.

Pazdur, P., et al., eds. *Cancer Management: A Multidisciplinary Approach, Medical, Surgical and Radiation Oncology.* Huntington, NY: PRR, 1996.

Rakel, R. E., ed. *Conn's Current Therapy.* Philadelphia: Saunders, 1996.

Shaw, M., ed. *Everything You Need to Know about Medical Tests.* Springhouse, PA: Springhouse, 1996.

Tierney, L. M., S. J. McPhee, and M. A. Papadakis, eds. *Current Medical Diagnosis and Treatment.* Stamford, CT: Appleton & Lange, 1996.

Tilkian, S. M., M. B. Conover, and A. G. Tilkian, eds. *Clinical Nursing Implications of Laboratory Tests.* St. Louis: Mosby, 1995.

Walsh, Patrick C. MD, and Janet Farrar Worthington. *The Prostrate: A Guide for Men & the Women Who Love Them.* Baltimore: The John Hopkins University Press, 1995.

Mind, Body, Spirit

Achterberg, J. *Imagery in Healing: Shamanism and Modern Medicine.* Boston: New Science Library, Shambhala Publications, 1985.

Ader, R., D. L. Felten, and N. Cohen, eds. *Psychoneuroimmunology,* 2nd ed. San Diego: Academic Press, 1991.

Burish, T. G. "Behavioral Relaxation Techniques in Reducing Stress from Cancer." *Oncology Nursing Forum,* 1993, 10:32-35.

Elliott, William. *Tying Rocks to Clouds: Meetings and Conversations with Wise and Spiritual People.* Wheaton, IL: Quest Books, 1995. Interviews with religious and spiritual teachers from a wide range of traditions and perspectives who address questions about life's purpose, the nature of God or an ultimate reality, and the meaning of suffering.

Ferguson, Tom, MD. *Health Online: How to Find Health Information, Support Groups and Self-Help.* Reading, MA: Addison-Wesley, 1996. Information about how to get on line as well as numerous online addresses.

Gawain, S. *Creative Visualization.* New York: Bantam, 1978. How-to book on visualization, affirmations and meditation in healthful living.

Krippner, S. "The Role of Imagery in Health and Healing: A Review." *Saybrook Review,* vol. 5, no. 1 (1985):32–41.

Lutheran General Health Care System. *Health and Medicine in the "Religious" Tradition.* New York: Crossroad Publishing. A series of scholarly books that explore the ways religious traditions understand medicine and health. The volumes cover several traditions, including Methodist, Anglican, Jewish, Lutheran and Reformed.

Remen, Rachel Naomi. *Kitchen Table Wisdom: Stories That Heal.* New York: Riverhead Books, 1996. A collection of inspirational stories told by people with life-threatening illness.

Rossman, M. L. *Healing Yourself: A Step-by-Step Program for Better Health Through Imagery.* New York: Walker and Company, 1987.

Simonton, O. C., S. Matthews-Simonton, and J. Creighton. *Getting Well Again: A Step-by-Step Guide for Overcoming Cancer for Patients and Their Families.* New York: Bantam Books, 1978.

Stress

Biofeedback and Self-Control: An Aldine Annual on the Regulation of Bodily Processes and Consciousness. Chicago: Aldine. Published annually. Highlights of scientific research in the field of self-regulation.

Borysenko, J. *Minding the Body: Minding the Mind*. Menlo Park, CA: Addison-Wesley, 1987. How to manage stress and anxiety and how to reframe life.

Cannon, Walter B. *The Wisdom of the Body*. New York: Norton, 1963. Original description of the "emergency" or "fight or flight" response and its relation to health and body functioning.

Chopra, Deepak. *Quantum Healing: Exploring the Frontiers of Mind-Body Medicine*. New York: Bantam Books, 1989. Explores the inner dimensions of healing using Eastern and Western thought patterns.

LeShan, Lawrence L. *You Can Fight for Your Life*. New York: Harcourt Brace Jovanovich, 1978. Describes psychotherapeutic experiences with cancer patients and how attitude appears related to outcome, both positively and negatively.

Pelletier, Kenneth. *Mind as Healer, Mind as Slayer*. New York: Delacorte Press, 1977. Summary of scientific research on stress and major illness, and description of treatment modes available.

Selye, Hans. *The Stress of Life*. New York: McGraw-Hill, 1978. Original work by the leading figure in the field of stress. Discusses the biochemical impact of stress upon the body.

Simonton, Carl and Stephanie. *Getting Well Again*. Los Angeles: J. P. Tarcher, 1978. Discussion of scientific basis for comprehensive cancer treatment and for encouraging and developing "the will to live."

Pain Control

Carlson, Richard, PhD, and Benjamin Shield, eds. *Healers on Healing*. Los Angeles: Jeremy P. Tarcher, 1989. In 37 original essays, many of the world's leaders in healing explore the complex nature of healing and the underlying principles on which healing rests.

Catalano, Ellen, MA, and Kimeron Hardin, PhD. *The Chronic Pain Control Workbook*, 2nd ed. Oakland, CA: New Harbinger Publications, 1997. This book offers practical self-help instructions for managing pain, and includes breathing and stretching exercises, stress management techniques and self-hypnosis.

Caudill, Margaret A., MD. *Managing Pain Before It Manages You*. New York: Guilford Publications, 1995.

Freese, Arthur S. *Pain*. New York: Penguin, 1975. Summary of all aspects of the pain problem — disorders, causes and treatment.

Kabbat-Zinn, Jon. *Full Catastrophe Living: Using the Wisdom of Your Body and Mind to Face Stress, Pain and Illness*. New York: Dell, 1990. Provides information on stress and illness, health and healing as well as step-by-step instructions on how to meditate.

———— . *Wherever You Go There You Are*. New York: Hyperion, 1994. Provides easy access to the essence of mindfulness medication and its applications, for people whose lives may or may not be dominated by immediate problems of stress, pain and illness.

Exercise, Massage and the Activities of Daily Living

Downing, George. *Massage Book*. New York: Random House, 1972. Discusses and illustrates massage techniques.

Hofer, Jack. *Total Massage*. New York: Grosset & Dunlap, 1976. Describes and illustrates massage techniques.

Khor, Senior Master Gary E. A. *Tai Chi Gigong For Stress Control and Relaxation.* San Francisco: Heian International, 1993.

Klinger, Judith Lannefeld, OT, ed. *Mealtime Manual for People with Disabilities and the Aging,* rev. ed. New York: The Institute of Rehabilitation Medicine, New York University Medical Center and the Campbell Soup Co., 1997. (Available from: Mealtime Manual, Box 38, Ronks, PA 17572, for $3.25 including postage.) Offers descriptions of and sources for assistive kitchen devices. Gives meal planning tips and recipes.

Winningham, M.L. "Walking Program for People with Cancer. Getting Started." *Cancer Nursing,* vol. 14, no. 5 (1991): 270–276.

Planning for the Future

Blum, Laurie. *Free Money for Heart Disease and Cancer Care.* New York: Simon & Schuster, 1992.

Clifford, D. *Who Will Handle Your Finances If You Can't?* Berkeley, CA: Nolo Press, 1992. Information and forms for creating power of attorney for financial affairs.

Colen, B. *The Essential Guide to a Living Will: How to Protect Your Right to Refuse Medical Treatment.* New York: Prentice-Hall, 1991. Explains the living will laws, why you may want a living will, what can happen if you don't; provides forms for the states that have living will laws.

Dollinger, Malin, MD, Ernest Rosenbaum, MD, and Greg Cable. *Everyone's Guide to Cancer Therapy,* 3rd ed. Chapter 16, "Living with Cancer," by Ernest Rosenbaum, MD, Malin Dollinger, MD, and Isadora Rosenbaum, MA, and Chapter 29, "Living with Mortality," by Malin Dollinger, MD, and Bernard Dubrow. Kansas City, MO: Andrews and McMeel, 1997.

Hastings Center. *Guidelines on the Termination of Life-Sustaining Treatment and the Care of the Dying.* Briarcliff Manor, NY: Hastings Center Report, 1987.

Knox, Lucinda P. and Michael D. *Last Wishes: A Handbook to Guide Your Survivors.* Ulysses Press, 1994.

Petterle, Elmo A. *Starting to Plan for Lifetime Financial Independence: A Book for Immediate and Ongoing Use.* Glendale, CA: Griffin Publishing, 1993.

Petterle, Elmo A., with contributing editors Robert C. Kahn and Marianne Rogoff. *Getting Your Affairs in Order: Make Life Easier for Those You Leave Behind.* Bolinas, CA: Shelter Publications, 1993.

"Practicing the Patient Self-Determination Act," Hastings Center Report Special Supplement, vol. 21, no. 5 (1991):S1–16.

Rosenbaum, Ernest, MD. *Living with Cancer.* New York: New American Library, 1982.

———, and Jay S. Luxenberg, MD. *You Can't Live Forever: You Can Live 10 Years Longer with Better Health.* San Francisco: Better Health Foundation, 1993.

Sexuality

Barbach, Lonnie G. *For Yourself: The Fulfillment of Female Sexuality.* New York: Doubleday, 1976. A classic that empowers women to enjoy their own sexuality, with suggestions for women who want to learn to become orgasmic.

Boston Women's Health Book Collective. *The New Our Bodies, Ourselves.* New York: Touchstone, 1992. An excellent book by and about women, their health and sexuality.

Butler, Robert, and M. I. Lewis. *Love and Sex After 60,* rev. ed. New York: Ballantine, 1993. Compassionate and helpful book for men and women who want to continue to enjoy their sexuality into their elder years.

Dackman, Linda. *Up Front: Sex and the Post-Mastectomy Woman.* New York: Viking, 1990. Moving and insightful account of one woman's experiences.

Mullen, Barbara Dorr, and Kerry Anne McGinn. *The Ostomy Book: Living Comfortably with Colostomies, Ileostomies, and Urostomies,* 2nd ed. Palo Alto, CA: Bull Publishing, 1992. An accurate and lively account of why colostomies, ileostomies and urostomies are necessary, and how to live with them.

Schover, Leslie R. *Prime Time: Sexual Health for Men over Fifty.* New York: Holt, Rinehart and Winston, 1984. Provides validation and useful suggestions for men and their partners.

———. "Sexuality and Cancer: For the Man Who Has Cancer, and His Partner."

———. "Sexuality and Cancer: For the Woman Who Has Cancer, and Her Partner." New York: American Cancer Society, 1988. Excellent comprehensive booklets outlining effects of cancer and treatment on sexuality, with suggestions for staying sexually healthy.

———. *Sexuality and Fertility after Cancer.* New York: John Wiley & Sons, 1997.

Zilbergeld, Bernie. *The New Male Sexuality.* Boston: Bantam, 1992. A commonsense, practical antidote to media pressures on males to be sexual superstars. Excellent discussion of the fantasy model of sex and myths of male sexuality, the importance of an individual's conditions for good sex, and specific self-help chapters dealing with common male sexual problems.

Survivorship Issues

Card, I. "What Cancer Survivors Need to Know about Health Insurance." Silver Spring, MD: National Coalition for Cancer Survivorship, 1993. An overview of health insurance.

Coleman, B. "A Consumer Guide to Home Health Care." Washington, DC: National Consumers League, 1985. (National Consumers League, 815 15th Street N.W., Washington, DC 20005, 202-639-8140.) Describes basic facts of home health care.

Nessim, Susan, and Judith Ellis. *Cancervive: The Challenge of Life After Cancer.* Boston: Houghton Mifflin, 1991.

The Will to Live

Benson, Herbert, MD. *The Relaxation Response.* New York: Avon, 1975.

Borysenko, Joan, PhD. *Minding the Body, Mending the Mind.* New York: Bantam, 1987.

Coleman, Daniel, and Joel Gurin, eds. *Mind Body Medicine: How to Use Your Mind for Better Health.* Yonkers, NY: Consumer Reports Books, 1993.

Fiore, Neil A., PhD. *The Road Back to Health: Coping with the Emotional Aspects of Cancer.* New York: Bantam, 1984.

Johnson, Judi, and Linda Klein. *I Can Cope: Staying Healthy with Cancer,* 2nd ed. Chronimed Publishing, 1994.

Pollin, Irene, MSW, and Susan K. Golant. *Taking Charge: Overcoming the Challenges of Long-Term Illness.* New York: Times Books, 1994.

Rosenbaum, Ernest and Isadora. *Inner Fire, Your Will To Live.* Austin, TX: Plexus Press, 1998.

Newsletters

BMT Newsletter
c/o Susan Stewart
1985 Spruce Ave.
Highland Park, IL 60035
847-831-1913

Coping
2019 N. Carothers
Franklin, TN 37064
615-790-2400
This quarterly carries articles on subjects of interest to cancer patients and on developments in cancer treatment and research.

Surviving!
Stanford University Medical Center
Patient Research Center, Room H0103
Division of Radiation Oncology
300 Pasteur Drive
Stanford, CA 94305
415-723-7881
This patient newsletter provides information on Hodgkin's disease, plus stories, essays and artwork by Hodgkin's survivors.

Y-Me Hotline
18220 Harwood Ave.
Homewood, IL 60430
708-799-8338
708-799-8228 (24-hour hotline)
800-221-2141
A newsletter for women who are coping with breast cancer.

Consumer Reports Health Letter
P.O. Box 52145
Boulder, CO 80321-2148

GLOSSARY OF MEDICAL TERMS

Malin Dollinger, MD

◇

A

Absolute neutrophil count (ANC)

The actual count of the white blood cells (also called polys or granulocytes) that engulf and destroy bacteria. There is some concern about infection if the count is less than 1,000.

Acupressure

The use of finger pressure over various points on the body (the same points used in acupuncture) to treat symptoms or disease.

Adjuvant chemotherapy

Chemotherapy used along with surgery or radiation therapy. It is usually given after all visible and known cancer has been removed by surgery or radiotherapy, but is sometimes given before surgery (neoadjuvant chemotherapy). Adjuvant chemotherapy is usually used in cases where there is a high risk of hidden cancer cells remaining and may increase the likelihood of cure by destroying small amounts of undetectable cancer.

Advance Directives

Legal documents that specify the type of medical care a person wants or doesn't want in certain circumstances.

Allogeneic transplant

A form of transplantation or transfer of a tissue—bone marrow, for example—from one individual to another. It is preferable that the tissue types match, but this is not always possible.

Amenorrhea

The temporary or permanent lack of menstrual periods. This may be a normal part of the menopause or is sometimes brought on by severe physical or emotional stresses. Some anticancer drugs can produce amenorrhea, especially if the woman is near the age when menopause would normally occur.

Amino acids

The building blocks of proteins, analogous to the freight cars making up a train.

Analgesic

A drug that relieves pain. Analgesics may be mild (aspirin or acetaminophen), stronger (codeine) or very strong (morphine). There are also a large number of mild, moderate or strong synthetic analgesics.

Anemia

Having less than the normal amount of hemoglobin or red cells in the blood. This may be due to bleeding, lack of blood production by the bone marrow or to the brief survival of blood already manufactured. Symptoms include tiredness, shortness of breath and weakness.

Antibody

A protein (gamma globulin) made by the body in response to a specific foreign protein, or antigen. The antigen may result from an infection, a cancer or some other source. If the same alien substance attacks again, the white blood cells are able to recognize it and reproduce the specific antibody to fight it.

Antigens

Substances that cause activation of the immune system.

Aspiration

Removal of fluid or tissue, usually with a needle or tube, from a specific area of the body. This procedure may be done to obtain a diagnosis or to relieve symptoms.

Atrophy
A withering or reduction in size of a tissue or a part of the body. This may result from lack of use during immobilization or prolonged bedrest or from pressure from an adjacent tumor.

Autologous transplant
Removal of a patient's own tissue, especially bone marrow, and its return to the same patient after chemotherapy. This might more correctly be called bone marrow reinfusion, or protection, rather than transplantation.

B

Biologic modifiers
Substances and agents that may have a direct antitumor effect, and also affect tumors indirectly by stimulating or triggering the immune system to fight cancer. Examples include interferon, IL-2 and LAK cells.

Biological therapy
Certain complex substances produced within the body regulate cell growth and immunity. Biological therapy, which includes immunotherapy, is the use of these same substances to treat cancer. They may be produced in the laboratory or a production facility, or the person with cancer may be given drugs that stimulate the production of these substances.

Biopsy
The surgical removal of a small portion of tissue for diagnosis. In almost all cases a biopsy diagnosis of cancer is required before appropriate and correct treatment planning can take place. In some cases a needle biopsy may be enough for diagnosis, but in others the removal of a pea-sized wedge of tissue is needed. In many cases, the biopsy may be the first step of the definitive surgical procedure that not only proves the diagnosis but attempts to cure the cancer by completely removing the tumor.

Blood cells
The red cells, white cells and platelets that make up the blood. They are made in the bone marrow.

Blood chemistry panel
Multiple chemical analyses prepared by an automatic apparatus from a single blood sample. These panels often include measurements of electrolytes (minerals) and proteins as well as tests of liver, kidney and thyroid function. The advantages of panels include less cost and greater accuracy and speed, with results often available the same or the following day.

Bone marrow
A soft substance found within bone cavities. Marrow is composed of developing red cells, white cells, platelets and fat. Some forms of cancer can be diagnosed by examining bone marrow.

Bypass
A surgical procedure to "go around" an organ or area affected by cancer and allow normal flow or drainage to continue. In cancer of the pancreas, for example, the bile ducts may be blocked. A bypass procedure will allow the bile to drain into the small bowel, as it should.

C

Calcium
An important body mineral that is a vital component of bone. The calcium level may be elevated if tumors involve bone.

Carcinoma
A form of cancer that develops in the tissues covering or lining organs of the body such as the skin, uterus, lung or breast (epithelial tissues). Eighty to 90 percent of all cancers are carcinomas.

Cardiopulmonary Resuscitation (CPR)
Use of chest compression, drugs and electric shock to restart the heart and/or a breathing tube and ventilator to maintain lung function.

Caregiver
The common term for a family member or friend who provides emotional and physical support. If you are admitted to hospital, it may be possible for you to have one caregiver stay with you.

CAT scan
See CT scan

Catheter
A tube made of rubber, plastic or metal that can be inserted into a body cavity such as the bladder to drain fluid or to deliver fluids or medication.

CEA (carcinoembryonic antigen)
A "tumor marker" in the blood that may indicate the presence of cancer. It may be elevated in some cancers, especially of the breast, bowel and lung. By monitoring the amount of CEA, doctors can detect the presence of these cancers and assess the progress of treatment.

Cell-cycle-specific
Chemotherapeutic drugs that kill only cells that are dividing rather than resting.

Cells
The fundamental unit, or building blocks, of human tissues.

Cervix
The lower portion of the uterus, which protrudes into the vagina and forms a portion of the birth canal during delivery. The Pap smear test is designed to check this area for cancer.

Chemotherapy
The treatment of cancer by chemicals (drugs) designed to kill cancer cells or stop them from growing.

Choriocarcinoma
A carcinoma composed of cells arising in the placenta or the testes.

Chromosomes
The fundamental strands of genetic material (DNA) that carry all our genes. There are 23 pairs in each cell. Tumor cells some-

times have more or fewer than 23 pairs.

Clinical
Refers to the treatment of humans, as opposed to animals or laboratory studies. Also refers to the general use of a treatment by a practicing physician, as opposed to research done in cancer research centers ("preclinical").

Clinical trials
The procedure in which new cancer treatments are tested in humans. Clinical trials are conducted after experiments in animals and preliminary studies in humans have shown that a new treatment method might be effective.

Clone
A strain of cells—whether normal or malignant—derived from a single original cell.

Cobalt; cobalt treatment
A radiotherapy machine using gamma rays generated from the radioisotope cobalt 60.

Comfort Care
Care that helps keep a person comfortable but does not treat an illness. Such measures may include bathing, nutrition, fluids, massage and pain medications.

Computerized tomography
See CT scan

Congestive heart failure
Weakness of the heart muscle usually due to heart disease, but sometimes due to other causes, causing a buildup of fluid in body tissues.

Cortisone
A natural hormone produced by the adrenal glands. The term is also loosely used to designate synthetic forms of the hormone (such as prednisone) that are used to treat inflammatory conditions and diseases, including certain cancers.

CT scan
A CT (computerized tomography) scan

creates cross-section images of the body, which may show cancer or metastases earlier and more accurately than other imaging methods. This type of x-ray machine has revolutionized the diagnosis of cancer and other diseases.

Cytokine
A substance secreted by immune system cells, usually to send "messages" to other immune cells.

D
Diuretics
Drugs that increase the elimination of water and salts in the urine.

DNA (deoxyribonucleic acid)
The building block of our genetic material. DNA is responsible for passing on hereditary characteristics and information on cell growth, division and function.

Drug resistance
The development of resistance in cancer cells to a specific drug or drugs. If resistance develops, a patient in remission from chemotherapy may relapse despite continued administration of anticancer drugs.

E
Electrolytes
Certain chemicals—including sodium, potassium, chloride and bicarbonate—found in the tissues and blood. They are often measured as an aid to patient care.

Enteral nutrition
Administration of liquid food (nutrients) through a tube inserted into the stomach or intestine.

Enzymes
Proteins that play a part in specific chemical reactions. The level of enzymes in the blood is often measured because abnormal levels may be a sign of various diseases.

Epstein-Barr (EB) virus
A virus known to cause infectious mononucleosis and associated with Burkitt's lymphoma and certain cancers of the head and neck.

Estrogen
The female sex hormone produced by the ovaries. Estrogen controls the development of physical sexual characteristics, menstruation and pregnancy. Synthetic forms are used in oral contraceptives and in various therapies.

Excision
Surgical removal of tissue.

F
Familial polyposis
A hereditary condition in which members of the same family develop intestinal polyps. Also called Gardner's syndrome, it is considered a risk factor for colorectal cancer.

Frozen section
A procedure done by the pathologist during surgery to give the surgeon an immediate answer as to whether a tissue is benign or malignant. Tissue is removed by biopsy, frozen, cut into thin slices, stained and examined under a microscope. This information is vital in helping the surgeon decide the most appropriate course of action.

G
Gamma rays
The form of electromagnetic radiation produced by certain radioactive sources. They are similar to x-rays but have a shorter wave-length.

Gene
A biological unit of DNA capable of transmitting a single characteristic from parent to offspring.

Grade of tumor
A way of describing tumors by their appearance under a microscope. Low-grade tumors are slow to grow and spread, whereas high-grade tumors grow and spread rapidly.

Graft-versus-host (GVH) disease
After bone marrow transplantation, immune cells in the donated (grafted) material may identify the patient's tissues (the host) as foreign and try to destroy them. This can be a serious problem, and drugs are available to combat it. However, in some cases, a GVH reaction actually helps control the cancer.

Granulocyte
The most common type of white blood cell. Its function is to kill bacteria (also called neutrophil, poly, PMN).

H
Hematology
The study of the blood and blood disorders.

Hemoglobin
A way of measuring the red cell content of the blood. The normal value in men is about 13 to 15 grams, in women from 12.5 to 14 grams.

Hepatic
Pertaining to the liver.

Hormonal anticancer therapy
A form of therapy that takes advantage of the tendency of some cancers—especially breast and prostate cancers—to stabilize or shrink if certain hormones are administered.

Hormones
Naturally occurring substances that are released by the endocrine organs and circulate in the blood. Hormones control growth, metabolism, reproduction and other functions, and can stimulate or turn off the growth or activity of specific target cells. Some hormones are used after surgery to treat breast, ovarian, prostate, uterine and other cancers.

Hospice
A facility and a philosophy of care that stress comfort, peace of mind and the control of symptoms. Hospice care, provided on either an outpatient or inpatient basis, is generally invoked when no further anticancer therapy is available and life expectancy is very short. Hospice also helps family and friends to care for and cope with the loss of a dying loved one.

I
IL-2
See Interleukins

Ileostomy
An artificial opening in the skin of the abdomen, leading to the small bowel (ileum). (See Ostomy)

Immune; immunity
A state of adequate defense against infections or foreign substances. Some cancers are believed to produce immune responses.

Immune system
The body mechanisms that resist and fight disease. The main defenders are white blood cells and antibodies, which, along with other specialized defenders, react to the presence of foreign substances in the body and try to destroy them.

Immunosuppression
The state of having decreased immunity and thus being less able to fight infections and disease.

Immunosuppressive drug
A drug that modifies the natural immune response so that it will not react to foreign substances. This type of drug is most commonly given after organ transplants so that the new organ will not be rejected.

Immunotherapy
A method of cancer therapy that stimulates the body's defense mechanism to attack cancer cells or combat a specific disease.

Inflammation
The triggering of local body defenses causing defensive white blood cells (leukocytes) to pour into the tissues from the circulatory system. It is characterized by redness, heat, pain and swelling.

Informed consent
A legal standard defining how much a patient must know about the potential benefits and risks of therapy before agreeing to receive it.

Infusion
Administration of fluids and / or medications into a vein or artery over a period of time.

Interferons
Natural substances produced in response to infections. They have been created artificially by recombinant DNA technology in an attempt to control cancer.

Interleukins
A group of cytokines produced by body cells that convey molecular messages between cells of the immune system. Interleukin-2 (IL-2), the best known of these, acts primarily on T lymphocytes; it is being used in the treatment of cancer.

Intramuscular (IM)
The injection of a drug into a muscle; from there it is absorbed into the circulation.

Intravenous (IV)
Administration of drugs or fluids directly into a vein.

Invasive cancer
Cancer that spreads to the healthy tissue surrounding the original tumor site. This contrasts with in situ cancer, which has not yet begun to spread.

Isotope
A radioactive substance used for diagnosis (tracer dose used for scans) or treatment (therapeutic dose).

K
Kidney failure
Malfunction of the kidneys due to disease or the toxic effects of drugs or chemicals. Urine volume may or may not be diminished.

L
Linear accelerator
A radiation therapy machine that produces a high energy beam.

Localized
A cancer confined to the site of origin without evidence of spread.

Low-Residue Diet
The indigestible material in food, sometimes called fiber. A low-residue diet minimizes stool output, thereby reducing irritation of the intestines.

Lumbar puncture
Removal of spinal fluid for examination. This simple procedure—also called a spinal tap—involves numbing the skin of the back with a local anesthetic and placing a needle into the numbed area to remove the spinal fluid.

LVN
Licensed vocational nurse. A nurse trained to do more limited tasks than a registered nurse (RN).

Lymph nodes
Oval-shaped organs, often the size of peas or beans, that are located throughout the body and contain clusters of cells called lymphocytes. They produce infection-fighting lymphocytes and also filter out and destroy bacteria, foreign substances and cancer cells. They are connected by small vessels called lymphatics. Lymph nodes act as our first line of defense against infections and the spread of cancer.

Lymphangiogram
An x-ray picture of the abdominal lymph nodes obtained by injecting a contrast substance under the skin on the feet. This test helps to determine if cancer has spread to the abdominal lymph nodes.

Lymphatic system
The system of lymph nodes and the lymphatic vessels that connect them.

Lymphedema

Swelling, usually of an arm or leg, caused by obstructed lymphatic vessels. It can develop because of a tumor or as an unusual late effect of surgery or radiotherapy.

Lymphocytes

A family of white blood cells responsible for the production of antibodies and for the direct destruction of invading organisms or cancer cells.

M

Macrophages

White blood cells that destroy invading organisms by ingesting them.

Malaise

Tiredness or lack of "drive."

Malignant

An adjective meaning cancerous. Two important qualities of malignancies are the tendency to sink roots into surrounding tissues and to break off and spread elsewhere ("metastasize").

Markers

Chemicals in the blood that are produced by certain cancers. Measuring the markers is useful for diagnosis, but especially useful for following the course of treatment. (See CEA)

Metastasis

The spread of cancer from one part of the body to another by way of the lymph system or bloodstream. Cells in the new cancer are like those in the original tumor.

Modality

A general class or method of treatment. The basic modalities of cancer therapy include surgery, radiation therapy, chemotherapy and immunotherapy.

Monilia

A common fungal infection often seen as white patches on the tongue or the inside of the mouth.

Monoclonal antibodies (MAbs)

Highly specific antibodies, usually manufactured in a laboratory, that react to a specific cancer antigen or are directed against a specific type of cancer. Current research is studying their role in therapy. One potential use is to deliver chemotherapy and radiotherapy directly to a tumor, thus killing the cancer cells and sparing healthy tissue. Studies are also trying to find out if monoclonal antibodies can be produced to detect and diagnose cancer cells at a very early and curable stage.

Mortality

Death as a result of disease.

MRI (magnetic resonance imaging)

A method of creating images of the body using a magnetic field and radio waves rather than xrays. Although the images are similar to those of CT scans, they can be taken in all three directions (planes) rather than just in cross-sections. There is no x-ray exposure.

Mucosa; mucous membrane

The inner lining of the gastrointestinal tract or other structures such as the vagina and nose.

Mucositis

Inflammation of the mucous membranes. Soreness—like "cold sores"—can develop in the mouth as a side effect of chemotherapy.

Multimodality

Using a combination of two or more types of therapy—for example, radiotherapy plus chemotherapy, radiation plus surgery, or chemotherapy plus surgery.

Mutation

A permanent change in a cell's DNA that alters its genetic potential. It may be a response to a chemical substance (mutagen) or result from a physical effect such as radiation. Sometimes the daughter cells may be cancerous.

N

Narcotics

Pain-relieving (analgesic) substances whose use is closely regulated by government. There are natural and synthetic types.

National Cancer Institute

A highly regarded research center in Bethesda, Maryland, that conducts basic and clinical research on new cancer treatments and supervises clinical trials of new treatments throughout the United States.

National Surgical Adjuvant Breast/Bowel Project (NSABP)

A group of dedicated research and clinical physicians who have formed a large cooperative group to study new treatments. Many major advances in treatment are attributed to this group.

Natural killer (NK) cells

Large, granular lymphocyte cells normally present in the body whose normal function is to kill virally infected cells. Some methods of cancer treatment take advantage of this ability of NK cells.

Necrosis

The disintegration of tissues caused by some physical or chemical agent or by lack of blood supply. Cancers treated effectively by chemotherapy, radiotherapy, heat or biological agents undergo necrosis.

Nerve block

Removing pain by numbing a nerve temporarily (with a local anesthetic) or permanently (with an alcohol injection).

Neuropathy

Malfunction of a nerve, often causing numbness (sensory nerve) or weakness (motor nerve). It is sometimes a side effect of anticancer drugs.

Neurotoxicity

Toxic effects (usually of drugs) on the nervous system.

Neutrophils

One of the white blood cells that fights infection. Also called granulocytes, polys or PMNs.

NK cell

See Natural killer cells

Nodes

See Lymph nodes

Non-cell-cycle specific

Chemotherapeutic drugs capable of destroying cells that are not actively dividing.

O

Oncologist

A physician who specializes in cancer therapy. There are surgical, radiation, pediatric, gynecologic and medical oncologists. The term oncologist alone generally refers to medical oncologists, who are internists with expertise in chemotherapy and handling the general medical problems that arise during the disease.

Oncology

The medical specialty that deals with the diagnosis, treatment and study of cancer.

Ostomy

A surgically created opening in the skin, leading to an internal organ, for purposes of drainage.

P

Palliative

Treatment that aims to improve well-being, relieve symptoms or control the growth of cancer, but not primarily intended or expected to produce a cure.

Parenteral nutrition

Artificial feeding by the intravenous administration of concentrated amino acid, sugar and fat solutions. (See TPN)

Pathologist

A physician skilled in the performance and interpretation of laboratory tests and in the examination of tissues to provide a diagnosis.

Persistent Vegetative State
The condition of a person who is in a coma and has no hope of regaining consciousness even with medical treatment.

Phlebitis
Inflammation of the veins, often causing pain and tenderness.

Placebo
An inactive substance, used in a research study or clinical trial, that looks like the medication. It is used to eliminate the improvement that may result from the belief that a medication is being given, rather than the actual effect of a medication.

Platelet
One of the three kinds of circulating blood cells. The normal platelet count is about 150,000 to 300,000. Platelets are responsible for creating the first part of a blood clot. Platelet transfusions are used in cancer patients to prevent or control bleeding when the number of platelets has significantly decreased.

Polyp
A growth that protrudes from mucous membranes, often looking like a tiny mushroom. Polyps may be found in the nose, ears, mouth, lungs, vocal cords, uterus, cervix, rectum, bladder and intestine. Some polyps occurring in the cervix, intestine, stomach or colon can eventually become malignant and should be removed.

Potassium
An important mineral in the body that is often lost during illness, especially with diarrhea. Low potassium levels can cause weakness.

Primary tumor
The place where a cancer first starts to grow. Even if it spreads elsewhere, it is still known by the place of origin. For example, breast cancer that has spread to the bone is still breast cancer, not bone cancer.

Progesterone
One of the female hormones (the other is estrogen). It causes the buildup of the uterine lining in preparation for conception and performs other functions before and during pregnancy. Certain synthetic forms of the hormone are used in cancer treatment.

Prognosis
A statement about the likely outcome of disease—the prospect of recovery—in a particular patient. In cancer, it is based on all available information about the type of tumor, staging, therapeutic possibilities, expected results and other personal or medical factors. For example, breast cancer patients who are diagnosed early usually have a good prognosis.

Progression
The growth or advancement of cancer, indicating a worsening of the disease.

Prophylactic
Treatment designed to prevent a disease or complication that is likely to develop but has not yet appeared. Also may be called adjuvant treatment.

Prostate-specific antigen (PSA)
A substance in the blood derived from the prostate gland. Its level may rise in prostatic cancer and is useful as a marker to monitor the effects of treatment.

Prosthesis
An artificial replacement or approximation of a body part—such as a leg, breast or eye—that is missing because of disease or treatment.

Protocol
A carefully designed and written description of a cancer treatment program. It includes dosages and formulas for any drugs to be administered.

R
Radiotherapist
A physician who specializes in the use of radiation to treat cancer.

Radiation therapy
See Radiotherapy

Radiosensitizer
A drug or biological agent that is given together with radiation therapy to increase its effect.

Radiotherapy
The use of high energy radiation from x-ray machines, cobalt, radium or other sources for control or cure of cancer. It may reduce the size of a cancer before surgery or be used to destroy any remaining cancer cells after surgery. Radiotherapy can be helpful in treating recurrent cancers or relieving symptoms.

Recurrence
The reappearance of a disease after treatment had caused it to apparently disappear.

Red blood cells
Cells in the blood that bring oxygen to tissues and take carbon dioxide from them.

Regression
The shrinkage of a cancer usually as the result of therapy. In a complete regression, all tumors disappear. In a partial regression, some tumor remains.

Rehabilitation
Programs that help patients adjust and return to a full productive life. Rehabilitation may involve physical measures such as physical therapy and prostheses, as well as counseling and emotional support.

Remission
The partial or complete shrinkage of cancer usually occurring as the result of therapy. Also the period when the disease is under control. A remission is not necessarily a cure.

Residual disease
Cancer left behind after surgery or other treatment.

Ribonucleic acid (RNA)
A nucleic acid present in all cells and similar to DNA. It is the biochemical blueprint for the formation of protein by the cells.

S
Scans (isotope)
Diagnostic procedures for assessing organs such as the liver, bone or brain. Radioactive tracers are introduced intravenously and if a malignant tumor or other foreign material is present pictures of the organ will show abnormalities that may indicate the presence of a tumor. There is no significant risk with this small, brief radiation exposure.

Screening
The search for cancer in apparently healthy people who have no cancer symptoms. Screening may also refer to coordinated programs in large populations.

Seizure
Shaking of a part or all of the body, often with loss of consciousness. This can be caused by an injury, a benign condition (such as idiopathic epilepsy) or a brain tumor.

Sigmoidoscopy
An examination of the rectum and lower colon with a hollow lighted tube called a sigmoidoscope. It is used to detect colon polyps and cancer, to find the cause of bleeding and to evaluate other bowel diseases. A newer instrument using fiberoptics—the flexible sigmoidoscope—permits easier, safer and more extensive examination. Also called proctoscopy.

Sodium
An important mineral in the body that helps maintain fluid balance. It is measured as part of an electrolyte panel.

Staging
An organized process of determining how far a cancer has spread. Staging involves

a physical exam, blood tests, x-rays, scans and sometimes surgery. Knowing the stage helps determine the most appropriate treatment and the prognosis.

Stem cells
Primitive or early cells found in bone marrow and blood vessels that give rise to all of our blood cells. To protect patients from low blood counts and the resulting complications after high-dose chemotherapy, a complex device is used to remove stem cells from a vein in the arm and give them back intravenously a few days later. They find their way back into the bone marrow and replace the marrow that was depressed by chemotherapy. The use of peripheral stem cell transplants has made the need to collect bone marrow itself much less important. This procedure should really be called peripheral stem cell protection rather than transplantation since patients get their own cells back.

Steroids
A class of fat-soluble chemicals—including cortisone and male and female sex hormones—that are vital to many functions within the body. Some steroid derivatives are used in cancer treatment.

Stool
Feces or bowel movement.

Suppository
A way to administer medications by absorbing the drug into a wax preparation, then inserting it into the rectum or vagina. Suppositories are used to treat local conditions such as vaginitis or hemorrhoids and are also used when pills cannot be swallowed or kept down because of nausea, sore mouth or narrowing of the esophagus. Antinausea suppositories such as Compazine and Tigan are often used to combat this side effect of chemotherapy.

Systemic disease
Disease that involves the entire body rather than just one area.

T

T cell
Lymphocytes are the cells in the body that are intimately involved in the immune response. They occur in the blood, in lymph nodes and in various organs. The two types of lymphocytes are T cells and B cells. Special techniques are needed to tell them apart because they look the same when viewed by ordinary methods under a microscope.

Terminal
This term has a number of definitions. Some people use it when cure is not possible, even if treatment can add years to the patient's life. Others say a patient is terminal when he or she has a specific short life expectancy, perhaps six months or one month. Still others mean that no other treatment can be given and "nature will take its course." If this term comes up, discuss with your doctor exactly what is meant by it.

Tissue
A collection of cells of the same type. There are four basic types of tissues in the body: epithelial, connective, muscle and nerve.

TPN (total parenteral nutrition)
The use of complex protein and fat solutions to supply enough calories and nutrients to sustain life. The solutions are delivered intravenously.

Tumor
A lump, mass or swelling. A tumor can be either benign or malignant.

Tumor necrosis factor
A natural protein substance produced by the body, which may make tumors shrink.

Tumor-suppressor gene
A class of genes that suppresses cell growth.

U
Ulcer
A sore resulting from corrosion of normal tissue by some irritating process or substance such as stomach acid, chemicals, infections, impaired circulation or cancerous involvement.

Ultrasound
The use of high-frequency sound waves to create an image of the inside of the body. Also called ultrasonography.

V
Virus
A tiny infectious agent that is smaller than bacteria. Many common infections such as colds and hepatitis are caused by viruses. Viruses invade cells, alter the cells' chemistry and cause them to produce more virus. Several viruses produce cancers in animals. Their role in the development of human cancers is now being studied.

W
White blood cells
Cells in the blood that fight infection. These are composed of monocytes, lymphocytes, neutrophils, eosinophils and basophils. The normal count is 5,000 to 10,000. It may be elevated or depressed in a wide variety of diseases. Chemotherapy and radiotherapy usually cause low white counts.

INDEX